Adolescent Medicine:

A Handbook for

D1457443

Victor C. Strasburger, MD

Division of Adolescent Medicine
Department of Pediatrics
University of New Mexico School
    of Medicine
Albuquerque, New Mexico

Robert T. Brown, MD

Section of Adolescent Health
Children's Hospital
Department of Pediatrics
The Ohio State University College
    of Medicine
Columbus, Ohio

Paula K. Braverman, MD

Division of Adolescent Medicine
Cincinnati Children's Hospital
    Medical Center
Cincinnati, Ohio

Peter D. Rogers, MD, MPH

Section of Adolescent Health
Children's Hospital
Department of Pediatrics
The Ohio State University College
    of Medicine
Columbus, Ohio

Cynthia Holland-Hall, MD,
    MPH

Section of Adolescent Health
Children's Hospital
Department of Pediatrics
The Ohio State University College
    of Medicine
Columbus, Ohio

Susan M. Coupey, MD

Department of Pediatrics
Albert Einstein College of Medicine
Section of Adolescent Medicine
Children's Hospital at Montefiore
Bronx, New York

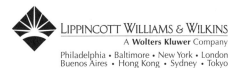

LIPPINCOTT WILLIAMS & WILKINS
A **Wolters Kluwer** Company
Philadelphia • Baltimore • New York • London
Buenos Aires • Hong Kong • Sydney • Tokyo

Acquisitions Editor: Anne M. Sydor
Developmental Editor: Louise Bierig
Managing Editor: Nicole Dernoski
Project Manager: Nicole Walz
Senior Manufacturing Manager: Ben Rivera
Senior Marketing Manager: Kathy Neely
Design Coordinator: Holly McLaughlin
Cover Designer: Christine Jenny
Production Services: Laserwords Private Limited
Printer: Edwards Brothers

© 2006 by **Lippincott Williams & Wilkins**
530 Walnut Street
Philadelphia, PA 19106

Printed in the United States

Library of Congress Cataloging-in-Publication Data
Adolescent medicine: a handbook for primary care / Victor Strasburger ... [et al.].
    p. ; cm.
Includes bibliographical references.
ISBN 0-7817-5315-5
1. Adolescent medicine--Handbooks, manuals, etc. 2. Teenagers--Diseases--Handbooks, manuals, etc. 3. Teenagers--Health and hygiene--Handbooks, manuals, etc. I. Strasburger, Victor C., 1949-
[DNLM: 1. Adolescent Medicine--methods. 2. Adolescent Health Services. 3. Mental Disorders--Adolescent. WS 460 M294 2005]
RJ550.M366 2005
616'.00835--dc22

                                                      2005005661

Care has been taken to confirm the accuracy of the information presented and to describe generally accepted practices. However, the authors, editors, and publisher are not responsible for errors or omissions or for any consequences from application of the information in this book and make no warranty, expressed or implied, with respect to the currency, completeness, or accuracy of the contents of the publication. Application of this information in a particular situation remains the professional responsibility of the practitioner.

The authors, editors, and publisher have exerted every effort to ensure that drug selection and dosage set forth in this text are in accordance with current recommendations and practice at the time of publication. However, in view of ongoing research, changes in government regulations, and the constant flow of information relating to drug therapy and drug reactions, the reader is urged to check the package insert for each drug for any change in indications and dosage and for added warnings and precautions. This is particularly important when the recommended agent is a new or infrequently employed drug.

Some drugs and medical devices presented in this publication have Food and Drug Administration (FDA) clearance for limited use in restricted research settings. It is the responsibility of health care providers to ascertain the FDA status of each drug or device planned for use in their clinical practice.

The publishers have made every effort to trace copyright holders for borrowed material. If they have inadvertently overlooked any, they will be pleased to make the necessary arrangements at the first opportunity.

To purchase additional copies of this book, call our customer service department at (800) 638-3030 or fax orders to (301) 824-7390. International customers should call (301) 714-2324. Lippincott Williams & Wilkins customer service representatives are available from 8:30 am to 6:30 pm, EST, Monday through Friday, for telephone access. Visit Lippincott Williams & Wilkins on the Internet: http://www.lww.com.

Dedication

To my two teenagers, Max & Katya, who continue to teach me more than I want to know about Adolescent Medicine, and to Alya with love.
—Victor C. Strasburger

To William A. Daniel, Jr., who remains a guiding light for me.
—Robert T. Brown

To my father, Irwin, who has been a source of support and encouragement as well as a role model throughout my career in medicine.
—Paula K. Braverman

To my best friend and beautiful wife, Emilie, the woman I love.
—Peter D. Rogers

To my husband Mark for his unwavering support.
—Cynthia Holland-Hall

To all of my former and current adolescent medicine fellows from whom I have learned so much.
—Susan M. Coupey

Contents

Contributing Authors

Paula K. Braverman, MD

Professor of Clinical Pediatrics, Pediatrics, University of Cincinnati College of Medicine; Director of Community Programs, Division of Adolescent Medicine, Cincinnati Children's Hospital Medical Center, Cincinnati, Ohio

Robert T. Brown, MD

Professor of Clinical Pediatrics and Obstetrics/Gynecology, The Ohio State University College of Medicine; Chief, Section of Adolescent Health, Children's Hospital, Columbus, Ohio

Jane Chang, MD
Syncope
Eating Disorders

Post-Doctoral Fellow, Department of Pediatrics, Section of Adolescent Medicine, Albert Einstein College of Medicine of Yeshiva University, Children's Hospital at Montefiore, Bronx, New York

Susan M. Coupey, MD

Professor of Pediatrics, Director, ICM Program, Albert Einstein College of Medicine, Chief, Adolescent Medicine, Children's Hospital at Montefiore, Bronx, New York

Cynthia Holland-Hall, MD, MPH

Assistant Professor of Clinical Pediatrics, The Ohio State University College of Medicine; Section of Adolescent Health, Children's Hospital, Columbus, Ohio

Unab Khan, MD
Adolescent Growth and Development
Hypertension

Post-Doctoral Fellow, Section of Adolescent Medicine, Department of Pediatrics, Albert Einstein College of Medicine of Yeshiva University, Children's Hospital at Montefiore, Bronx, New York

Peter D. Rogers, MD, MPH, FAAP, FSAM, FASAM

Clinical Associate Professor of Pediatrics, The Ohio State University College of Medicine; Section of Adolescent Health, Children's Hospital, Columbus, Ohio

Victor C. Strasburger, MD

Professor of Pediatrics and Family and Community Medicine, Division of Adolescent Medicine, Department of Pediatrics, University of New Mexico School of Medicine, Albuquerque, New Mexico

Foreword

It is frequently said that adolescence is the neglected age group; perhaps it is more sound to say that that it is physicians' training in the care of adolescents which has been given relatively little attention. This astute observation was made by Dr. J. Roswell Gallagher in 1957 and remains credible today, despite the intervening half century of developments in the field of adolescent medicine. Pioneers such as Gallagher realized that adolescents are special and have different medical needs; they realized too that young people are better served, as they always will be, when their health care providers are appropriately informed.

Many health care professionals feel ill-equipped to deal with adolescents in their practices, particularly in relation to sexuality and substance use. Adolescents want to discuss health behaviors but often feel too embarrassed to initiate discussion in these sensitive areas. And while parents also want clinicians to discuss health issues with their adolescents, many fail to do so. How can clinicians feel more comfortable talking with teens and better able to facilitate the conversation?

This excellent manual of adolescent health has the answers to this and many other crucial questions. It has been designed as a handy, pertinent and useful book for primary care clinicians. Content has been selected for its clinical relevance and does not purport to cover all known facts within the diverse range of topics covered. But little of importance has been excluded—from obesity and ADHD to sports medicine, hypertension and eating disorders. In a clear and accessible format, key issues are highlighted and well explained; suggested treatments reflect best current knowledge and practice. And each chapter concludes with a "pearls and pitfalls" section followed by a brief bibliography and helpful Web sites for both parents and clinicians.

At adolescence, perhaps more powerfully than at any other period in the lifespan, organic and psychosocial issues are complexly intertwined. Psychosomatic illness is "a diagnosis of inclusion as well as exclusion," not what the person has "when no organic illness can be discovered." With chronic abdominal pain, we are reminded to "do the minimal necessary laboratory/imaging workup" and not "...forget about gynecologic causes of pain in female adolescents." Likewise, "Syncope can be a presenting symptom of early pregnancy in an adolescent girl."

It is useful to know that parents may report periorbital oedema in a teenager with infectious mononucleosis and that "petechiae of the soft palate are also frequently overlooked" in this common condition. The almost universal affliction of acne in adolescents is rife with myths and common management mistakes, and yet "treating it (properly) can establish an immediate and long-lasting rapport with adolescent patients."

In working with adolescents, the challenge is to engage their trust, make a meaningful assessment of the presenting problem or issue, and intervene in a helpful and supportive way. Confidentiality is extremely important and, in regard to legal concerns generally, common sense must prevail—"no physician has ever been successfully sued for prescribing birth control to a minor" (also true in Australia). Whether an experienced adolescent health physician, a family physician or fellow in training, all will benefit from having this concise, comprehensive and highly accessible resource close at hand.

David Bennett, AO, MBBS, FRACP, FSAM
Clinical Associate Professor and Senior Staff Specialist
Department of Adolescent Medicine and Head,
NSW Centre for the Advancement of Adolescent Health
The Children's Hospital at Westmead
Sydney, Australia

Preface

"I see no hope for the future of our people if they are dependent on the frivolous youth of today, for certainly all youth are reckless beyond words....When I was a boy, we were taught to be discreet and respectful of elders, but the present youth are exceedingly wise and impatient of restraint."

Hesiod, 8th century Egyptian historian

Adolescents have always been a challenge. From Hesiod's complaint that they disrespect their elders to Aristotle's observation that they lack "sexual restraint" to Shakespeare's suggestion that they be put into suspended animation until age 23, the history of Western civilization is replete with a litany of complaints about teenagers. Yet we sometimes forget how adolescents have changed the world. Many of the signers of the Declaration of Independence were still in their teens. In the 1960s, student unrest on college campuses catalyzed public opinion against the Vietnam War. Many of today's most gifted athletes whom adults spend hours watching on TV are, in fact, adolescents.

Adolescents sometimes make challenging patients as well. Not just "sex, drugs, rock 'n' roll," but acne, eating disorders, and depression may complicate adolescence. In the movie "One-Eyed Jacks," Brando's character is asked, "What are you rebelling against?" He answers: "What've you got?" But while the image of a motorcycle-jacketed Marlon Brando or a James Dean rebel-without-a-cause may represent parents' (or clinicians') worst fears, most teenagers get through adolescence with little or no difficulty (80%, according to the psychiatric literature).

Physicians, nurse practitioners, and others who treat teenagers need to be vigilant about the pitfalls encountered during adolescence but also need to be nonjudgmental and tolerant as well. Clinicians also need to enjoy seeing teenagers. Adolescents are unique creatures and deserve special care. This small handbook is designed to be a practical and quick guide to diagnosing and treating common adolescent problems. It is not intended to be a comprehensive academic tome but rather, since "brevity is the soul of wit" according to Polonius in "Hamlet," this book is meant to be useful above all else. Take it to clinic with you, keep it at your desk in your consulting room, refer to it often. We hope that you will find it indispensable in treating your adolescent patients.

Acknowledgments

We would like to thank Carole Clark for her technical assistance, as well as Lisa S. Blackwell, Serials/Reference Librarian at the Children's Hospital Library of Columbus, Ohio.

Many thanks also to the Department Chair of the School of Medicine at the University of New Mexico, Dr. Robert Katz, who allowed Dr. Strasburger time to write, and to his colleague, Dr. Karen Campbell, who allowed him time to think.

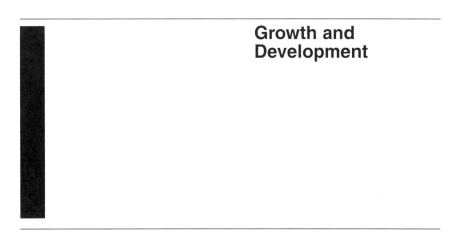

Growth and Development

Adolescent Growth and Development

I. **Description of normal growth:** Adolescence is a dynamic period of development, with rapid changes in body size, shape, and composition. Along with physical changes, cognitive, psychological, and social development occur, making this a very important period in a person's life. *Puberty* is described as the transitional period between childhood and the reproductive maturity of adulthood. However, adolescence is a biopsychosocial process, and cognitive changes may start before the appearance of secondary sexual characteristics and may go well beyond attainment of reproductive maturity and cessation of physical growth.

A. Endocrine changes at puberty:
- The hormonal regulation of puberty depends on the release and interaction of various hormones, including gonadotropins, growth hormone (GH), thyroid hormones, and leptin. The signal for onset of puberty originates in the hypothalamus.
- An increase in the frequency and amplitude of the pulsatile release of gonadotropin-releasing hormone (GnRH) causes the release of follicle-stimulating hormone (FSH) and luteinizing hormone (LH). The rising level of these hormones, in turn, causes the production of sex steroids (estrogen and testosterone), which promotes the development of secondary sex characteristics and changes in body composition.
- In females, the development of a positive feedback of estrogen causes further release of GnRH, which leads to LH stimulation to initiate ovulation.
- In males, LH causes the Leydig cells to release testosterone. Testosterone is then converted to dihydrotestosterone. Both lead to development of secondary sexual characteristics.
- In both males and females, secretion of sex steroids from the adrenal gland occurs independently of the hypothalamic-pituitary-gonadal axis. At adrenarche, an increase in dehydroepiandrosterone (DHA) and dehydroepiandrosterone sulfate (DHEA-S) levels leads to pubic hair development, body odor, and changes in the pilosebaceous gland apparatus.
- Adrenal androgens are not necessary for pubertal development or the adolescent growth spurt.
- Activation of GH and insulin like growth factor-1 (IGF-1) axis occurs. GH levels increase, causing an increase in growth velocity.
- There is relative insulin resistance secondary to increased GH levels, and this results in increased insulin secretion. Insulin, in turn, increases somatic growth along with GH.
- Nutritional and metabolic factors also influence the onset of puberty. Leptin, a hormone that regulates body fat, increases LH release.
- Insulin and glucocorticoids also increase the release of leptin, whereas androgens decrease it.
- Other hormones that play a vital role in the adolescent growth are thyroid hormones and cortisol, and adequate levels of both are prerequisites for normal growth.

B. Physical growth:
- The physical growth seen at puberty involves an interaction between the body's endocrine and skeletal systems. The key hormone is GH, which affects bone growth through IGF-1.

- Bone maturation is under the control of thyroid hormones, adrenal androgens, and estrogen. Increased secretion of these hormones can cause advanced bone maturation, and deficiency causes delayed bone maturation.
- It is important to remember that puberty begins nearly 2 years later in males. Hence, females may appear more physically mature than their male counterparts.
- *Growth spurt* accounts for 20% of the final adult height. This period of rapid height increase can last 24 to 36 months.
- The growth spurt occurs at different times in the two sexes. It occurs earlier in females, and the peak height velocity (PHV) is less. This accounts for females appearing taller at the beginning of puberty, but their adult height is shorter compared to males.
- PHV in females is reached just before menarche, between Tanner stages 2 and 3, and is approximately 9 cm per year, whereas PHV in males is approximately 10 cm per yr and is reached between Tanner stages 3 and 4.
- The end of the growth spurt is secondary to epiphyseal closure due to the action of sex steroids, mainly estrogen. Epiphyseal closure is approximately 2 years later in males, adding to their adult height.
- *Weight growth* during puberty accounts for 50% of adult body weight. Peak weight velocity (PWV) in males coincides with the PHV. In females, the maximum weight gain occurs approximately 6 months after the PHV. This is an important time in development of body image, and hence questions about the body should be addressed openly and nonjudgmentally.
- Changes in *body composition* are also noted during puberty. In females, the lean body mass decreases to 75% to 80% because of an increase in the adipose tissue, whereas in males, the lean body mass increases to about 90% secondary to the effect of androgens.
- Bone mineral density (BMD) increases in both sexes and depends on heredity, nutrition, weight, exercise, and endocrine function, especially estrogen levels.

C. **Development of secondary sexual characteristics:** Sexual Maturity Ratings (SMRs), as described by Marshall and Tanner, are based on pubic hair and breast development in females and pubic hair and genital development in males.

The development of breasts and genitalia is through the hypothalamic-pituitary-gonadal axis, and pubic hair development represents the activation of the hypothalamic-pituitary-adrenal axis. Hence it is common to see a variation between the stages of breast/genital and pubic hair development in the same individual.

It is important to remember that there are vast individual variations, not only in the time of initiation of puberty but also in the time between the different stages. However, the progression is consistent, as will be described.

1. **Female sexual development:**
   - Breast budding (thelarche) is usually the first physical sign of puberty, although approximately 15% of females may start with adrenarche.
   - Thelarche can start between the ages of 8 and 14 and is seen earlier in non-Hispanic blacks than in non-Hispanic whites.
   - Adrenarche leads to pubic and axillary hair development.
   - The typical sequence is breast budding, adrenarche, PHV, continued breast and pubic hair development, menarche, and completion of puberty.
   - Accelerated growth begins about 1 year before breast development and is followed in an average of 1.1 years by peak height velocity. Menarche occurs approximately 1 year after the female has reached PHV.
   - Menarche is one of the major developmental landmarks of female puberty. It occurs fairly consistently in pubertal development (by pubic hair stage 3 in 19% of females and by pubic hair stage 4 in 56%).
   - It should be remembered that maturation of the hypothalamic–pituitary–ovarian axis is not complete at menarche and ovulatory cycles might not be established for 2 to 3 years.
   - Full fertility is usually reached within 2 years of menarche, between 14 and 15 years of age on average.

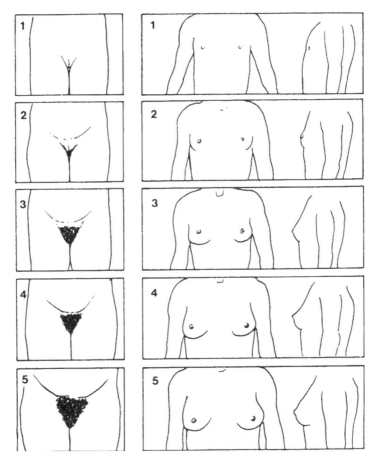

Figure 1-1. Sexual maturity rating in females by breast and pubic hair development.

Figure 1-2. Sequence of female physical and sexual development. (From the standards established by Tanner JM, Davies PW. Clinical longitudinal standards for height and weight velocity for North American children. *J Pediatrics* 1985;107:317, with permission.)

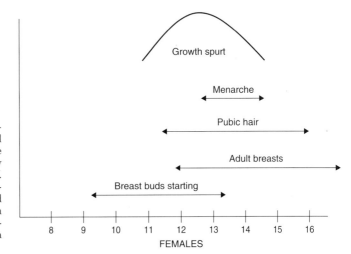

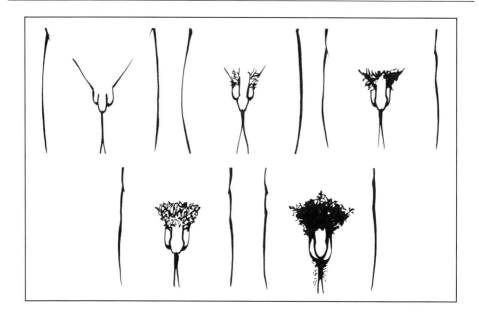

Figure 1-3. Sexual maturity ratings in males by pubic hair and genital development. From Neinstein L, ed. *Adolescent health care: A practical guide*, 4th ed. Philadelphia, PA: Lippincott Williams & Wilkins, 2002, with permission.

2. **Male sexual development:**
   - The first physical sign of puberty is testicular enlargement.
   - The typical sequence is testicular enlargement, adrenarche, continued testicular and penile enlargement, and then PHV.
   - Spermarche, an early pubertal event, precedes PHV in most adolescents and usually occurs 1 year after testicular enlargement begins. Ejaculation first occurs at SMR3.
   - The average length of time for completion of puberty is 2 to 5 years, with an average of 3 years.
   - Complete sexual maturity is usually reached by 17 or 18 years of age.

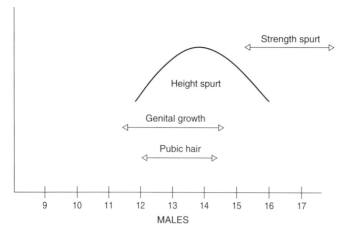

Figure 1-4. Sequence of male physical and sexual development. (From the standards established by Tanner JM, Davies PW. Clinical longitudinal standards for height and weight velocity for North American children. *J Pediatrics* 1985; 107:317, with permission.)

D. Psychosocial development: No outline of psychosocial development can adequately describe each and every adolescent. The transition from childhood to adulthood is not a continuous, uniform, synchronous process. Although adolescence is a stressful period, 80% of adolescents cope well with this developmental process and do not have any lasting problems.

    As most of adolescent morbidity and mortality is preventable, it is important to understand the patient's developmental level to appropriately teach the patient about health-promoting behaviors. Understanding psychosocial development helps the clinician to communicate with the teenager and to tailor questions, explanations, and instructions to the level of the teenager.

1. **Early adolescence:** Early adolescents are defined as 10 to13 year olds. They attend middle school.

   Family
   - The hallmark of this stage is the quest for autonomy. Adolescents show less interest in activities with family. They are able to recognize parental flaws and may be reluctant to accept parental advice.
   - As the adolescent attempts to better define his or her self by testing authority, increased tension between the adolescent and authority figures is noted.
   - Emotional lability, leading to wide mood swings, is seen.

   Friends
   - An emotional void is created due to separation from parents, leading to a search for new people to love.
   - Solitary friendships with members of the same sex are more common. These strong emotional and tender feelings toward peers may lead to homosexual exploration.
   - The adolescent becomes aware of feelings of sexual attraction. However, there is usually little or no action on these feelings.

   Physical Development
   - There is an uncertainty about appearance, and frequent comparisons are made of one's own body to those of peers. Body image issues can develop at this stage.
   - An increased interest in sexual anatomy and physiology is seen, and anxieties about menstruation or nocturnal ejaculations and masturbation and breast or penis size are common.

   Cognitive Development
   - Early adolescents have concrete thinking and have little understanding of consequences.
   - There is lack of impulse control, and the need for instant gratification results in experimentation and high risk-taking behaviors.
   - There is a tendency to set unrealistic vocational goals.

2. **Middle adolescence:** This group comprises 14 to 17 year olds who are attending high school.

   Family
   - Conflicts with parents become more prevalent as the adolescent exhibits less interest in parents and devotes more time to peers.

   Friends
   - Peer groups now include both sexes, and conformity with peer values and codes is of utmost importance.
   - Relationships tend to be experimental and exploitative as teens explore their own boundaries and the boundaries of others.

   Physical Development
   - Linear growth peaks, decelerates, and then ceases.
   - Middle adolescents are focused on making themselves attractive to peers.

   Cognitive Development
   - Formal operational thinking is noted, with the beginning of abstract reasoning. However, there is reversion to concrete thinking in times of stress.
   - The feeling of omnipotence and immortality persists and increases, leading to risk-taking behaviors.
   - There is increased intellectual ability and creativity and more realistic vocational aspirations.

3. **Late adolescence:** The 17 to 21 year olds fall into this category. They are going to college or to vocational schools, are in the military, or are already working and may be starting families.

Family
- The adolescent renegotiates relationships with parents, and the relationships become more positive.
- Moral, religious, and sexual values start to mirror the family's value system.

Friends
- Peer group values become less important, and late adolescents become more comfortable with their own values and identity.
- Relationships become less exploitative, and mutual understandings with a selected partner are reached.

Physical Development
- There is a realistic body image.

Cognitive Development
- Abstract reasoning is established. The sense of perspective improves, with the ability to compromise and set limits. A rational and realistic conscience develops.
- Interests are more stable, and there is greater ability to delay gratification.
- Financial independence may be attained. However, some adolescents may decide to continue with higher education, thus delaying this step.

For many reasons, it is important to understand and remember the normal physical and psychosocial development of adolescents. First, with the many variations of normal, it is the physician's job to reassure both the patient and the parent of normal physical development. At the same time, it is imperative to understand the patient's level of psychosocial development in order to offer relevant preventive and anticipatory guidance. In addition, health promotion and disease prevention during these years can help establish habits that carry into adulthood. Our job, therefore, is to deliver age-appropriate care that is accessible and attractive to teenagers.

II. **Clinical pearls and pitfalls:**
- Adolescent development is a biopsychosocial process with physical, psychological, cognitive, and social changes taking place simultaneously but at different rates. When one of these developmental processes is very far ahead of or behind the others, the individual adolescent often has difficulties adjusting, for example, the 10-year-old female whose body is developed like that of a 16-year-old or the 16-year-old male with a 10-year-old body.
- It is important for clinicians to be aware not only of normal pubertal development but also of its variations, in order to avoid overdiagnosing pathological development.
- The neuroendocrine signal for the onset of puberty originates in the hypothalamus.
- Adrenal androgens are not necessary for pubertal development or the adolescent growth spurt.
- Puberty begins nearly 2 years later in males than in females. Hence females appear more physically mature than their male counterparts.
- The *growth spurt* occurs earlier in females and PHV is less than in males. Hence females appear taller at the beginning of puberty, but their adult height is shorter compared to males.
- Weight growth also occurs at different times in the two sexes. In males PWV coincides with the PHV. In females the maximum weight gain occurs approximately 6 months after the PHV.
- Pubertal changes in *body composition* include a decrease in lean body mass in females and an increase in lean body (muscle) mass in males, as well as an increase in fat mass in females and a decrease in males.
- It is common to see a variation between the stages of breast/genital and pubic hair development in the same individual.
- Early adolescents think concretely and have little understanding of the consequences of their actions. Abstract reasoning begins in middle adolescence, but feelings of omnipotence and immortality persist, leading to risk-taking behaviors. In late adolescence the sense of perspective improves, along with the ability to compromise and set limits.
- Understanding an individual adolescent's psychosocial developmental level helps the clinician to tailor questions, explanations, and instructions appropriately.

BIBLIOGRAPHY

For the clinician

Frankowski BL, and the Committee on Adolescence. Sexual orientation and adolescents. *Pediatr* 2004;113:1827–1832.

Ginsburg KR, Slap GB. Unique needs of the teen in the health care setting. *Curr Opin Pediatr* 1996;8:333–337.

Goldenring JM, Rosen DS. Getting into adolescent heads: an essential update. *Contemp Pediatr* 2004;21:64–90.

Neinstein L, Kaufman FR. Normal physical growth and development. In: Neinstein L, ed. *Adolescent health care: A practical guide*, 4th ed. Philadelphia, PA: Lippincott Williams & Wilkins, 2002:3–49.

Ozer EM, Adams SH, Lustig JL, Gee S, et al. Increasing the screening and counseling of adolescents for risky health behaviors: a primary care intervention. *Pediatrics* 2005;115:960–968.

Plant TM. Neurophysiology of puberty. *J Adolesc Health* 2002;31:185–191.

Preece M. Assessment of physical growth and pubertal development. *Adolesc Med State Art Rev* 1994;5(1):1–17.

Rosen DS. Physiologic growth and development during adolescence. *Pediatr Rev* 2004;25(6): 194–200.

Sun S, Schubert CM, Chumlea WC, et al. National estimates of timing of sexual maturation and racial differences among US Children. *Pediatrics* 2002;110(5):911–919.

Tanner JM. *Growth at adolescence*, 2nd. ed. London: Blackwell Scientific Publications, 1962.

For patients and parents

Walsh D, Bennett N. *WHY do they act that way?: A survival guide to the adolescent brain for you and your teen*. New York: Free Press, 2004.

WEB SITES

www.youngwomenshealth.com   Teen-friendly website from the Children's Hospital, Boston

www.connectforkids.org   For parents and guardians and people who want to be more actively involved with adolescents

www.teenshealth.org   Good site for parents and patients about coping with adolescent issues

www.brightfutures.org   Affiliated with the American Academy of Child and Adolescent Psychiatry

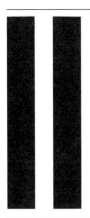

Office Problems

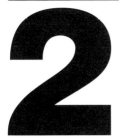

The Office Visit

I. **Background:**
   A. **Overall health status of adolescents:** Adolescence is a time of profound change in several areas including physical, psychosocial, and cognitive development. The majority of adolescents are healthy and come to a medical office setting for preventive health maintenance examinations or for an acute illness or injury. Many of the diseases that present in adolescents are a result of lifestyle choices that cause morbidity and mortality. The negative consequences of these choices are preventable and include complications of substance use and sexual activity; future heart disease related to smoking, exercise behaviors, and nutrition; and accidental injuries such as those related to motor vehicle accidents.

   Data from the National Survey of Children with Special Health Care Needs Chartbook 2001 show that 15.8% of 12 to 17 year olds have special health care needs that include chronic physical, developmental, and behavioral problems. Males have higher rates of special health care needs than do females, possibly related to a higher number of behavioral diagnoses. These adolescents present special challenges because they individually make more office visits than do their healthy peers while still presenting with issues similar to those of other adolescents.
   B. **Use of services by adolescents:**
   - Overall, adolescents are less likely to utilize health care services than are younger children or adults.
   - National data from the Commonwealth Fund Survey of the Health of Adolescent Girls in 1997 show that approximately 90% of adolescents identify a primary care source [physician's office (62%), health care center (24%), hospital-based clinic (7%)]. Five percent report the emergency room as their only source of care. Females are more likely to report a regular source of care than are males.
   - Data from the 2000 National Ambulatory Medical Care Survey indicate that for 11 to 17 year olds, 37.4% of nonsurgical physicians' office visits are with pediatricians while 40.4% are with family physicians (family practice, general medicine). In the past 20 years, the proportion of visits to pediatricians has increased by 11.1%, with a parallel decline in visits to family physicians. Overall, family physicians see more adolescents than younger children.
   - National data show that 68% to 85% of adolescents have received a "checkup" or physical exam in the past year and 77% to 94% have received one in the past 2 years. Older adolescents are more likely than younger ones to miss recommended preventive care visits, and females are more likely than males to have had a regular checkup in the previous year. Analysis of national data sets has also shown that the gender discrepancy appears to be related to the differential use of services by older males (16–20 years) compared to females in the same age group. Some of these gender differences may be due to differences in health beliefs, more use of reproductive health services by females, and insurance status.
   - In the Commonwealth Fund Study, almost one-third of adolescents reported missing needed care. National studies have found that factors related to missing care include lack of insurance, low family income, not wanting to tell parents, lack of time, lack of transportation, race/ethnicity (nonwhite), and low parental education. Missing care is also more common for youth who cannot identify a regular source of primary care. In this study, females were more likely than males to report concerns about confidentiality and embarrassment.

II. **The health encounter:**
   A. **Adolescents *do* want to discuss health issues with their health care provider:** Adolescents want to discuss health behaviors including sexuality and substance use with their clinician. An analysis from the 1997 Commonwealth Fund Survey of the Health of Adolescent Girls found that among fifth to twelfth graders of both sexes, a doctor

Table 2-1. Comparison of health topics of interest adolescents want to discuss with physicians vs. actual discussions

Topic	Discussion desired %	Topic discussed %
Exercise	86	42
Growth	80	47
STD	70	18
Contraception	66	22
Depression	59	16
Alcohol	52	23
Drugs	50	23
School	48	37
Smoking	47	30

STD, sexually transmitted disease.
Adapted from Malus M, LaChance PA, Lamy L, et al: Priorities in adolescent health care: the teenager's viewpoint. *J Fam Practice* 1987;25:159–162.

or nurse was the second most common source of health information after their mother.

Discrepancies between what adolescents wish to discuss and actual discussions continue to be shown in studies conducted over the past decade. A 1987 study found that discussions about reproductive health and substance use occurred much less frequently than other topics such as school, exercise, and growth (see Table 2-1). This difference remained in the recent analysis of the 1997 Commonwealth Fund Survey of the Health of Adolescent Girls in which the topics adolescents were most interested in discussing were not the same ones as those actually discussed (see Table 2-2) The top three topics desired were drugs, sexually transmitted diseases (STDs), and smoking while the top three subjects actually addressed were good eating habits, weight, and exercise. There was clearly a need for discussion about substance use and sexuality in this group; however, conversations with youth engaged in these risk-taking behaviors occurred less than one-half of the time (see Table 2-3). **Multiple studies have indicated that many adolescents feel embarrassed or are not able to initiate these discussions themselves. It is crucial that clinicians feel comfortable talking with teens and that they facilitate the conversation.**

Clinicians must also remember that adolescents with chronic illness engage in risk behaviors and need to have similar discussions. This point was illustrated in a recent study among 11 to 19 year olds attending subspecialty clinics in a tertiary care children's hospital. The patients had a minimum 2-year history of juvenile rheumatoid arthritis, sickle cell disease, inflammatory bowel disease, or cystic fibrosis. A

Table 2-2. Differences between health topics adolescents would like to discuss and actual discussions, 1997 Commonwealth Fund Survey

Topic	Discussion desired		Topics discussed	
	Males %	Females %	Males %	Females %
Drugs	64.9	65.1	34.2	27.7
STD	57.5	65.4	24.3	27.6
Smoking	57.9	59.1	31.8	27.1
Alcohol	56.3	56.0	27.2	23.1
Eating habits	50.8	62.9	43.8	53.1
Weight	48.0	65.3	37.7	47.7
Exercise	47.2	55.6	40.5	41.1

STD, sexually transmitted disease.
Adapted from Ackard DM, Neumark-Sztainer D. Health care information sources for adolescents: age and gender differences on use, concerns, and needs. *J Adolesc Health* 2001;29(3)170–176.

Table 2-3. Discussions with adolescents engaged in specific risk-taking behaviors

Risk behavior	% Reporting behavior	Of those reporting behavior, % discussed
High stress	37.3	32.7
Alcohol use	34	28.2
Smoking	27.2	40.2
Exercise less than 2 times per week	20.9	34.2
Willing to have sex without contraception	17.5	30.5
Drug use past month	15.6	37.3
Binging and purging	12.3	32.3

Adapted from Klein JD, Wilson KM. Delivering quality care: adolescents' discussion of health risks with their providers. *J Adolesc Health* 2002;30:190–195.

substantial proportion of these adolescents had engaged in sexual activity and substance use (see Table 2-4).

B. **Parents *do* want clinicians to discuss health issues with their adolescents:** A study conducted in the early 1990s among parents from ten pediatric practices in central New York indicated that parents want clinicians to discuss health topics with adolescents. More than 90% of parents indicated that discussions on nutrition, substance abuse, breast or testicular self exam, smoking, exercise and sports, STDs, and skin care were very to somewhat important, while 85% to 88% placed suicide, pregnancy, contraception, safe sex, depression, and menstruation in these categories. Very few parents reported that any of these topics should not be discussed. There were slightly higher rates for the no discussion category for safe sex (8%), contraception (7%), and pregnancy (6%).

C. **Qualities adolescents value in their health care provider:** Studies have indicated that adolescents value certain qualities in their health care provider. These include being:
- Friendly, caring
- Not rushed
- Trustworthy, honest, open
- Nonjudgmental
- Knowledgeable, experienced
- Careful
- Respectful
- Willing to assure confidentiality

A study of high school students, utilizing ideas generated by adolescents in focus groups, provided particularly powerful information on the opinions of adolescents. This study confirmed that characteristics of health care providers such as honesty, cleanliness in preventing disease transmission, respect, and experience were more important than the physical or operational characteristics of clinical sites. Although confidentiality was important and highly rated by 63% of the subjects, it was surpassed by knowledge, respect, honesty, and cleanliness. In another study, adolescents with chronic illnesses reported similar preferences. Honesty, knowledge, caring, and listening to their concerns and opinions were most important while communication

Table 2-4. Risk behaviors among youth with chronic illness

Risk behavior	% Reporting behavior
Ever smoking	28
Ever marijuana use	16
Ever alcohol use	42
Ever sexual intercourse (≥age 13)	27
Inconsistent seatbelt use	42

Adapted from Britto MT, DeVellis RF, Hornung RW, et al. Health care preferences and priorities of adolescents with chronic illness. *Pediatrics* 2004;114:1272–1280.

about outside activities or hobbies, convenience of the office, and a physical environment tailored to adolescents were less important.

D. Reasons why desired discussions on health topics do not occur: Several factors that may hinder ideal delivery of health services to adolescents include:
- Lack of knowledge and poor self-efficacy regarding competence to address certain issues

  Historically this has been the case for reproductive health issues but also is applicable to mental health and substance abuse
- Discomfort in addressing certain issues

  Belief that providing contraception condones sexual activity

  Belief that it is morally wrong to discuss abortion during options counseling

  Belief that homosexuality is abnormal
- Dislike of working with adolescents
- Time constraints
- Problems ensuring confidentiality

  Interventions that provide training to help clinicians implement preventive health services have successfully increased office-based services to adolescents. Examples cited in the literature include training on implementation clinical preventive services including the Guidelines for Adolescent Preventive Services (GAPS) from the American Medical Association (AMA) and delivery of smoking prevention and cessation services.

E. Confidentiality: Confidentiality is crucial in providing health care to adolescents. Discussions between health care providers and adolescents are more likely to occur when the adolescents have private time alone without parents. The need for privacy is in part related to the specific medical issue. In general, adolescents are not concerned about parental knowledge about a routine physical, an acute febrile illness, or a weight problem. However, adolescents are much less likely to want to disclose information and are more likely to express concern about parental knowledge regarding sensitive topics such as sexuality, substance use, and mental health. A study of females under the age of 18 attending the 33 Planned Parenthood family planning sites in Wisconsin indicated that 59% would stop all reproductive health services including STD and human immunodeficiency virus (HIV) testing if there was mandatory parental reporting of those who were prescribed contraception. Lack of confidentiality in just one area has the potential to spill over to other services where adolescents legally have a right to access confidential services.

Among 14 to 19 year olds in Monroe County, New York, one study found that only 5% of adolescents identified their primary care physician as a source of confidential health services, and 46% did not know where to access these services. The problem of access is further compounded by the fact that many clinicians do not consistently discuss confidentiality with adolescents and in some cases inappropriately guarantee unconditional confidentiality. Confusion also can occur when the front desk staff does not deliver the same confidentiality messages as do the clinicians. In a telephone survey of 615 physicians in 372 practices, office staff and physicians disagreed about provision of confidential services. In general, the office staff were less likely to report that confidential services were available even though the physician did affirm their availability. Written policies on adolescent confidentiality improved consistency in the responses. Providing confidential services including reproductive health and substance abuse counseling can serve to increase patient satisfaction by expanding the capability of the primary care office. However, it is important to recognize that some adolescents may choose to seek confidential services elsewhere because they feel safer in an environment where they can remain more anonymous.

As a general approach, **the concept of confidentiality should be discussed with both the parent and adolescent at the first visit,** making it clear that there are certain specific situations such as harm to oneself (suicide) or harm to others that cannot be kept confidential. There are also specific state laws about mandatory reporting of sexual or physical abuse and certain infectious diseases including STDs (see Chapter 29, "Legal Issues"). When the clinician feels that a particular issue falls into the disclosure category, it is important that the adolescent is told about the need for disclosure before informing the parent. Under the Health Insurance Portability and Accountability Act (HIPAA) Privacy Rule, if the particular state permits adolescents to consent to health care on their own or the parent has assented to confidential services, the parent does not necessarily have a right to the health information in the medical record regarding that particular medical problem. Some states may specifically permit or prohibit parental access to the minor's health information, and state law takes precedence. If the law is silent, the provider can use his or her own professional judgment to decide whether to disclose the information.

Physicians caring for adolescents constantly juggle the best interests of adolescents and their families. Open, honest communication between adolescents and their families is usually the best way to resolve conflict on these difficult issues. Parents can be invited to a three-way conversation with the clinician and adolescent with the understanding that information cannot be revealed without the consent of the adolescent unless the potential for significant harm has been determined.

F. Interviewing adolescents: There are many different formats for the office visit, and each clinician must tailor the approach to his or her own personality and style. Some clinicians meet with both the adolescent and parent together and then with each separately, while others meet with the adolescent first and then bring in the parent. There are several principles that can help guide the structure of the visit:
- The adolescent should always have an opportunity to meet with the clinician alone
- In order to avoid lack of full disclosure, risk-taking behaviors should not be discussed in front of the parent
- It is frequently helpful to meet with the adolescent and parent together to:
  Observe the parent–adolescent interaction
  Facilitate communication between the parent and adolescent
  Enable the adolescent to learn about his or her own personal and family medical history and promote future independence in seeking health care
  Define the roles and responsibilities of both the parent and adolescent (e.g., making appointments, calling the clinician when there is acute illness)

  The interview should include review of past and present medical problems as well as a detailed psychosocial history. The American Academy of Pediatrics' Bright Futures has sample questions that clinicians can utilize in addressing these issues. The acronym HEADSSS is helpful to remind clinicians about the content of the psychosocial history, which includes:

  H: Home: family relationships and living arrangements
  E: Education: academic performance and future goals
  A: Activities: recreational activities, information on peers, vocational activities
  D: Drugs: substance use and evaluation for potential abuse
  S: Sexuality: sexual activity, contraception, STDs, dating, sexual preference
  S: Suicide: suicide and other mental health issues including eating disorders
  S: Safety: use of seatbelts, bike helmets, etc.

  The following is a framework that utilizes a developmental approach to the adolescent interview:
- **Parent–adolescent collaborative model.** This model is appropriate for early adolescents, prior to the emergence of emancipation issues, where the parent and adolescent are addressed as a pair in terms of obtaining the history and developing the treatment plan. Both are present in the room at the same time and share in the decision-making process.
- **Adolescent primary/parent secondary model.** This model is appropriate for middle and late adolescents with the emergence of emancipation. The adolescent is primarily addressed by the clinician, has private time with the clinician to discuss confidential issues, and engages in initial discussions about the treatment plan with the clinician. The parent is then brought into the room at the end of the visit to review the visit. In many cases, it is useful for the adolescent to relate the details to the parent because this contributes to self-esteem and self-sufficiency. It is particularly important to permit adolescents with chronic illness to have a voice in their treatment decisions.
- **Adolescent primary/parent-optional model.** This model is appropriate for teens who are ready to assume responsibility for their own health care. In this case, the clinician does not communicate directly with the parent unless there is concern about harm (e.g., suicide). It is the responsibility of the patient to relay information to the parent.

  Specific interviewing techniques to elicit information include the use of:
- A **time frame** such as number of days, weeks, or relationship to a particular event
- A **numerical rating scale** (e.g., pain rating)
- **Empathy:** For example saying, "If I were in the situation, I would feel…"
- **Advance notice of understanding:** For example saying, "Many young people your age smoke…Do you?"
- **Indirection and projection:** For example saying, "Do any of your friends smoke?" or "What do people in your school think about…?"

III. The office setting:

A. Office hours: A new comprehensive office visit takes 30 to 45 minutes; however, in reality many visits last 15 minutes or less. Having the patient and parent fill out health surveys that include physical health and psychosocial issues prior to talking with the clinician can help focus the content of the encounter and facilitate the clinician's ability to address crucial issues when there are time constraints. The adolescent should complete this survey in private to maintain confidentiality. As an example, GAPS has adolescent and parent/guardian surveys that clinicians can administer in the office. In addition, support staff can help with patient education and provide anticipatory guidance. It is helpful to consider office hours that take into account the busy schedule of adolescents and include late afternoon or evening hours as well as weekends.

B. Office space: The office space should include a waiting area and exam rooms with appropriately sized furniture for adolescents and with literature and decorations that are age appropriate. Examination tables with stirrups permit inclusion of gynecologic services

C. Support personnel: Support personnel who answer the phones and provide initial screenings provide the first impression for adolescents and their parents. It is important for these personnel to be sensitive to the needs of adolescents and to demonstrate enjoyment in working with this age group.

D. Office fees: Reimbursement issues are a challenge. Issues of inadequate coverage, particularly for older adolescents, continue to limit access to care. Providing confidential services can be another challenge since itemized bills may automatically go home to the parents. Clinicians should be aware of this possibility. Adolescents may be willing to pay for confidential services on their own to maintain care with their clinicians. A sliding scale or reduced payment options have been successfully instituted to facilitate access to care. Clinicians also should be aware of services in their community that adolescents can access for free, such as health departments or federally funded family planning clinics.

IV. The physical examination:

A. The physical examination should include an assessment of pubertal maturation and attention to particular disease entities that are common during adolescence.

The AMA (GAPS) recommends a complete physical exam three times during adolescence between the ages of 11 to 13, 15 to 17, and 18 to 21. GAPS also recommends annual screening for health risk behaviors and health guidance. The American Academy of Pediatrics (AAP) has recommended annual examinations.

B. All adolescents should have height, weight, and blood pressure checked. Essential hypertension can present in adolescence, and clinicians should refer to published norms for age in determining abnormal values. The body mass index should be calculated and plotted to determine if the adolescent meets criteria for being underweight or obese.

C. Several screening areas remain controversial among the different recommending organizations:

1. **Hearing:** Bright Futures (AAP) recommends screening those with risk of hearing loss. Examples include family history of delayed onset hearing loss, exposure to excessive noise or ototoxic medications, or concerns by parents or educators. The AMA (GAPS) and US Preventive Services Task Force (USPSTF) do not have specific recommendations.

2. **Vision:** Myopia develops in adolescence. Bright Futures does recommend screening. However, AMA (GAPS) and USPSTF do not have specific recommendations.

D. Specific attention to the following areas on the physical examination include:

1. **Skin:** acne, warts, fungal infections, dermatitis, piercings, and tattoos. Skin complications of piercings and tattoos can include allergic dermatitis to metals or dyes and pigments, keloids, and local skin infections.

2. **Mouth/Teeth:** caries, gingivitis, enamel erosion from self-induced vomiting, mucosal/gum changes from smokeless tobacco use, and tongue piercings. Complications of tongue piercings can include swelling and edema, gingival injury, increased salivation, and tooth fractures and chipping.

3. **Neck:** thyromegaly, lymphadenopathy

4. **Cardiovascular:** murmurs

5. **Musculoskeletal:** joint instability, injury, Osgood-Schlatter Disease, scoliosis (especially in premenarchal females)

6. **Breast:** asymmetry, masses, gynecomastia in males

7. **Genitourinary (GU) male:** sexual maturity rating (SMR) of pubic hair, testicular volume, assess for masses, hernia, varicocele, penile discharge, tenderness

8. **GU female:** SMR of pubic hair, assess for normal external anatomy and any lesions. A pelvic exam is not necessary for a female who has not been sexually active and has no GU complaints. Even for those who are sexually active, STD testing can be performed with urine-based nucleic acid amplification testing, and a vaginal swab without a speculum can be done to perform a wet mount to look for trichomonas, yeast, or bacterial vaginosis. Unless the adolescent is having pelvic pain or an undiagnosed menstrual disorder, a speculum or bimanual examination may not be needed.

V. **Laboratory/screening tests:**

A. **Anemia:** Hemoglobin screening is not recommended by GAPS or USPSTF. The AAP has recommended screening at least once during adolescence and in those at risk including those with a history of iron deficiency anemia, menorrhagia, or poor dietary intake of iron. Menstruating females are at increased risk for anemia because of the blood loss during menses that further compounds the poor dietary intake of iron commonly found during adolescence.

B. **Lipids:**

1. **For adolescents (up to age 18):**
   AAP guidelines
   Adolescents up to age 18 should be screened for hyperlipidemia when there are certain risk factors.
   Screen with total cholesterol
   • Parent with cholesterol ≥240
   • Unknown family history
   Screen with fasting lipoprotein analysis
   • Parent or grandparent 55 years old or younger with documented myocardial infarction (MI), angina, peripheral vascular disease, cerebrovascular disease, sudden cardiac death, coronary atherosclerosis
   GAPS guidelines
   Same as AAP but GAPS also adds screening with a nonfasting total cholesterol if there is a personal history of hypertension, obesity, diabetes mellitus, or smoking

2. **For young adults (19 and older):** Screen everyone with nonfasting total cholesterol at least once

C. **Tuberculosis:**
   Immediate screening should be done when there is:
   • Contact with a person with known or suspected tuberculosis (TB)
   • Radiologic or clinical evidence of TB
   • Emigration from endemic countries
   • Travel from an endemic area
   • Significant contact with an individual from endemic country
   Annual screening should be done for
   • HIV-infected individuals
   • Incarcerated youth
   Some experts recommend screening every 2 to 3 years for individuals exposed to
   • HIV-positive individuals
   • Homeless people
   • Residents of nursing homes
   • Users of illicit drugs
   • Migrant workers
   See Table 2-5.

D. **STD screening:**
   • USPTF recommends screening all sexually active females up to age 25 for *Chlamydia Trachomatis* annually. GAPs and AAP also include males in this recommendation.
   • Additional recommendations from USPTF, AAP, and GAPS include adding annual screening for *Neisseria Gonorrhoeae* in high-risk individuals, particularly those with two or more partners
     Screening for chlamydia and gonorrhea is facilitated by the current availability of urine-based nucleic acid amplification testing, which permits noninvasive screening without a urethral swab or pelvic examination
   • HIV screening should be offered to individuals at risk

E. **Pap smears:**
   • Initial Papanicolaou (Pap) smears should be performed within 3 years of the onset of sexual activity or by age 21 if the patient is not sexually active. Reasons for the 3-year grace period include:
     Human papillomavius (HPV) infection is common and usually transient in sexually active adolescents

Table 2-5. Definitions of positive TB tests

Induration ≥5 mm
- Close contact with known or suspected case of TB
- Radiologic or clinical findings of TB
- Immunosuppression

Induration ≥10 mm
- Patients with other chronic medical conditions such as lymphoma, diabetes, chronic renal failure
- Those with increased exposure to TB, e.g., lived in endemic part of world, exposure to HIV-positive individuals

Induration ≥15 mm
- Everyone

TB, tuberculosis; HIV, human immunodeficiency virus.
Adapted from Red Book, 26th edition 2003 Report of the Committee on Infectious Diseases. American Academy of Pediatrics.

Many low grade lesions spontaneously resolve without intervention
Cervical cancer is rare in adolescents
- After the initial smear, repeat Pap smears should be done annually with conventional Pap and every 2 years with liquid-based cervical cytology
- Patients with HIV infection should get two Pap smears 6 months apart in the first year, and annually thereafter
- There are several options for follow up of an abnormal smear:
     Option 1: All ASC-H, LSIL, and HSIL are referred for colposcopy. ASC-US Pap are followed up with reflex HPV-DNA testing. If the DNA indicates high risk HPV then the patient should be referred for colposcopy.
     Option 2 for LSIL: If LSIL, repeat Pap in 6 and 12 months. If any Pap is ASC-US or higher, the patient should be referred for colpscopy.
     Option 3 for LSIL: If LSIL, perform HPV-DNA testing in 12 months and if positive for high risk HPV, the patient should be referred for colposcopy (see Table 2-6).
- VI. **Immunizations:**
     - **dT boosters** should be given between 11 and 12 years of age if at least 5 years have passed since the last dose, and then a booster should be given every 10 years after the initial series is completed. In May 2005, a combination vaccine containing Tetanus toxoid, Diptheria toxoid, and Acellular pertussis was approved by the FDA for use in adolescents. It will be indicated as a single dose booster in 10 to 18 year olds.
     - **Varicella** should be given to those without a history of clinical varicella disease. For patients age 13 and older, two doses should be given 1 month apart.
     - **Hepatitis B** series should be given to complete a three-dose regimen. There must be a minimum of 1 month between the first and second, and 4 months between the first and third, as well as 2 months between the second and third doses.
     - **Measles, Mumps, and Rubella (MMR)** should be given if there have not been two doses. Both doses must have been given after 12 months of age.
     - **Hepatitis A** should be given in parts of the country at high risk for hepatitis A and for certain high-risk groups such as homosexual males. Two doses are given 6 months apart.
     - **Meningococcal vaccine:** In May of 2005, recommendations for the use of the meningococcal vaccine were revised following the release of the quadravalent conjugate vaccine named Menactra. The new recommendations, which are endorsed by the American Academy of Pediatrics, Society for Adolescent Medicine, and the CDC's Advisory Committee on Immunization Practices, recommend routine vaccination of 11 to 12 year olds, vaccination of previously unvaccinated 15 year olds, and routine

Table 2-6. Definitions of Pap smear results

ASC-US	Atypical cells of undetermined significance
ASC-H	Atypical cells cannot exclude high grade lesion
LSIL	Low grade squamous intraepithelial lesion
HSIL	High grade squamous intraepithelial lesion

vaccination of college freshmen living in dormitories as well as other populations at increased risk, such as military recruits.

Catch up immunizations for primary series in individuals older than age 7
- **dT:** There should be three dT immunizations, with 4 weeks between dose 1 and 2 and 6 months between dose 2 and 3. The booster should be given in 10 years.
- **Inactivated Polio vaccine (IPV):** There should be three IPV immunizations, with 4 weeks between dose 1 and 2 and 4 weeks between doses 2 and 3.

VII. **Clinical pearls and pitfalls:**
- Adolescents *do* want to discuss health topics with their health care providers but may be unable to initiate the discussions.
- Parents *do* want health care providers to discuss health topics with their adolescents.
- Ensuring confidentiality is important in facilitating open communication with adolescents, particularly about sensitive topics such as sexuality and substance use.

BIBLIOGRAPHY

Akinbami LJ, Ganhi H, Cheng TL. Availability of adolescent health services and confidentiality in primary care practices. *Pediatrics* 2003;111:394–401.
Cavanaugh RM, Hastings-Tolsma M, Keenan D, et al. Anticipatory guidance for the adolescent. Parents' concerns. *Clin Pediatr* 1993;32:542–545.
Ford CA, Millstein SG. Delivery of confidentiality assurances to adolescents by primary care physicians. *Arch Pediatr Adolesc Med* 1997;151:505–509.
Freed GL, Nahra TA, Wheeler JRC. Which physicians are providing health care to America's children. Trends and changes in the past 20 years. *Arch Pediatr Adolesc Med* 2004;158:22–16.
Ginsburg KR, Slap GB, Cnaan A, et al. Adolescents' perceptions of factors affecting their decisions to seek health care. *JAMA* 1995;273:1913–1918.
Greydanus DE, Strasburger VC, eds. Office practice of adolescent medicine, primary care clinics. 2006 (in press).
Hofmann AD, Greydanus DE. *Adolescent medicine*, 3rd ed. Stamford, CT: Appleton & Lange, 1997.
Kahn JA, Hillard PA. Human papillomavirus and cervical cytology in adolescents. *Adol Med Clin N Am* 2004;15:301–321.
Klein JD, McNulty M, Flatau CN. Adolescents' access to care. Teenagers' self-reported use of services and perceived access to confidential care. *Arch Pediatr Adolesc Med* 1998;152:676–682.
Marcell AK, Klein JD, Fischer I, et al. Male adolescent use of health care services: where are the boys? *J Adolesc Health* 2002;30:35–43.
Rainey DY. Office-based care of adolescents: part 1. Creating a teen-friendly office. *Adolescent Health Update* 2003;16:1–9.
Rainey DY, Brandon DP, Krowchuk DP. Confidential billing accounts for adolescents in private practice. *J Adolesc Health* 2000;26:389–391.
Rappo PD. Office-based care of adolescents: part 2. Practice strategies and coding procedures for proper payment. *Adolescent Health Update* 2004;16:1–9.
Reddy DM, Fleming R, Swain C. Effect of mandatory parental notification on adolescent girls' use of sexual health care services. *JAMA* 2002;288:710–714.

WEB SITES

www.cmwf.org   The Commonwealth Fund: Quality of Health Care for Children and Adolescents: A Chartbook, and Health of Adolescent Girls, 1997
www.aap.org   The American Academy of Pediatrics: Bright Futures and Patient Education Information
www.ama.org   The American Medical Association: GAPS
www.mchb.hrsa.gov   Health Resources and Services Administration—The National Survey of Children with Special Health Care Needs
www.adolescenthealth.org   Society for Adolescent Medicine. Position paper on confidential health care
www.arhq.gov   US Preventive Services Task Force

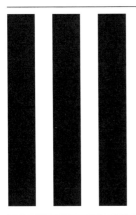

Common Medical Problems

Headache

I. **Description of the condition:**
   A. **Epidemiology:**
   - The vast majority of adolescents have experienced headache at least once, and 16% of persons over 14 years of age report experiencing headaches at least monthly.
   - About 1% of adolescents experience chronic daily headache.
   - By mid-to-late adolescence up to 20% of adolescents have experienced a migraine headache.
   - Female adolescents and adults are more likely to report frequent headaches than are male adolescents and adults.
   - Up to 25% of female migraineurs experience their first migraine headache shortly after menarche.
   - Most frequent headache sufferers do not seek medical care explicitly for their headaches, but the complaint often comes up during routine office visits.
   B. **Classification:** Clarifying the headache pattern is a critical step in headache evaluation (see Figure 3-1). Headaches may be acute or chronic. *Acute* headaches may last hours to days. A patient's acute headache may be an isolated event, such as the headache accompanying a viral infection, or it may be one of a series of *acute recurrent* headaches, such as migraines. No specific criteria exist to define *chronic* headache; some suggest that this nomenclature be used when headaches occur at least 15 times a month for over 4 months. The *chronic progressive* headache, a headache that increases in frequency and/or severity over time, is the least common but most worrisome headache pattern. Prompt and aggressive evaluation is required to rule out serious intracranial pathology. *Chronic nonprogressive* headaches are most frequently encountered by primary care providers; while they rarely represent serious pathology, they are challenging to treat and often are associated with significant morbidity. Some patients present with a *mixed* headache pattern, such as chronic daily tension-type headaches with intermittent migraines. This pattern may evolve from the acute recurrent headache pattern, possibly as the result of analgesic overuse.

II. **Making the diagnosis:**
   A. **History:** A careful history is the most important step in headache diagnosis and management. An entire office visit dedicated to the management of this complaint is recommended, particularly for patients with chronic headaches that cause significant functional impairment. Important elements of the history include:
   - Establishing the headache pattern: timing, frequency, and progression of headaches
   - Headache quality (throbbing, dull aching, "squeezing," etc.) and severity
   - Precise location of pain in the head
   - Associated pain (eyes, neck, shoulders, tooth, jaw, or facial pain)
   - Are all headaches the same, or do they vary in quality and/or severity?
   - Are headaches preceded by an aura or prodrome?
   - Is pain aggravated by physical activity (e.g., climbing stairs, walking)?
   - Are associated symptoms present: nausea/vomiting, photophobia or other visual disturbance, phonophobia, neurologic symptoms?
   - Are symptoms present that suggest elevated intracranial pressure (ICP): nausea/vomiting, early morning wakening with pain, ataxia, mental status change, other neurologic deficits?
   - Are symptoms present that suggest systemic illness and/or infection: fever, neck stiffness, malaise, myalgia, weight loss?
   - Does anything "trigger" headaches: stress, fatigue, caffeine use and/or withdrawal, alcohol, chocolate, other foods, menstruation?
   - History of head trauma, seizure, hydrocephalus, presence of ventriculo-peritoneal shunt, other neurologic problems

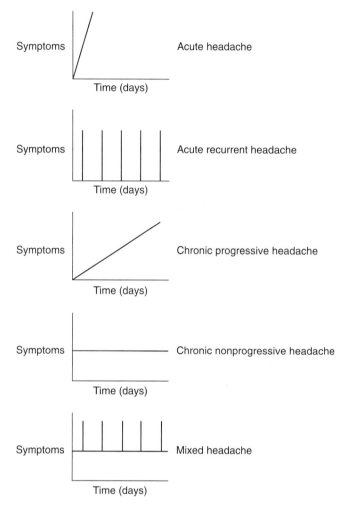

Figure 3-1. Temporal patterns of headache. (Adapted from Rothner AD. The evaluation of headaches in children and adolescents. *Semin Pediatr Neurol* 1995;2:109, with permission.)

- Family history of migraine
- Mental health history/symptoms, psychosocial stressors
- Detailed medication use history: medications that have been tried, doses, frequency of use, efficacy
- Other measures taken to alleviate symptoms (sleep, avoidance of noise or light)
- Drug use (prescription, nonprescription, and illicit substances).

For patients with chronic nonprogressive headaches, a *headache diary* can be a valuable evaluation tool, revealing triggers, patterns, and associations that the patient was not previously aware of. A diary also provides documentation of medication use/overuse.

Lastly, to determine the *headache burden*, that is, the impact of the headache on the patient's life, the following questions should be answered:

- How debilitating are the headaches?
- Do they impair normal functioning and quality of life?
- Are school attendance and performance, peer activities, or work affected?
- How do the headaches affect the patient's family?
- What is the family's response to the patient's pain?

B. Differential diagnosis:
1. **Acute headache:** Most acute, nonrecurrent headaches in adolescents are caused by upper respiratory infections, viral syndromes, and acute sinusitis. Migraine and tension-type headaches certainly may present as acute headache, but often are part of a chronic or recurrent headache pattern and should be diagnoses of exclusion in the patient with acute, severe headache. The large differential diagnosis of acute headache includes:
    *   Trauma, concussion, or postconcussive state
    *   Infection, such as meningitis, encephalitis, or intracranial abscess
    *   Toxins, including environmental toxins (e.g., carbon monoxide), medications (e.g., stimulants), or illicit substances
    *   Cerebrovascular accident, aneurysm, or other vascular insult
    *   Intracranial or subarachnoid hemorrhage
    *   Hypertension
    *   Dental pathology.

    Most of these conditions can be ruled out with a careful history and physical examination. More extensive discussion of the approach to the patient with severe acute headache may be found in the emergency medicine and neurology literature.

2. **Chronic progressive headache:** This is the most likely headache pattern to be associated with severe pathology, such as a brain tumor, abscess, or other intracranial mass lesion. Hydrocephalus, vascular malformations, aneurysms, vasculitis, and chronic or intermittent subarachnoid hemorrhage can cause this headache pattern as well. Chiari malformations and other congenital malformations may cause intermittent increases in intracranial pressure; the associated pain is often occipital and is worsened with the Valsalva maneuver. Although these conditions are relatively uncommon, they must be considered and ruled out, either clinically or with the appropriate use of laboratory and neuroimaging studies.

    Idiopathic intracranial hypertension (pseudotumor cerebri) is characterized by elevated cerebrospinal fluid (CSF) pressure in the absence of a mass lesion or obstruction to CSF flow. Patients present with generalized headache; sixth and third cranial nerve palsies and loss of vision are common. Neuroimaging is normal. Adolescents at greatest risk are obese, post-pubertal females. Certain medications including tetracycline and nitrofurantoin, excessive intake of vitamin A derivatives, and cessation of corticosteroid use have been associated with this condition. The association of oral contraceptive pill use with idiopathic intracranial hypertension has been suggested but remains unclear. Formerly known as "benign intracranial hypertension," this condition is far from benign; permanent vision loss may result, especially if untreated. Treatment may include weight loss, the use of acetazolamide, and repeated lumbar punctures to reduce ICP and relieve the pain.

    Posttraumatic and postconcussive headaches are common and may follow even mild head injuries. They may be progressive or nonprogressive, persisting up to 3 to 6 months following the injury and resolving gradually. The headache may have migrainous and/or tension-type features.

3. **Chronic nonprogressive headache:** This is the most common headache pattern encountered by primary care providers. Most adolescents with chronic nonprogressive headache experience migraine, tension-type, or analgesic withdrawal headaches.

    Migraine headaches are characterized by a specific constellation of symptoms, described by the International Headache Society, that distinguish them from tension-type headaches (see Table 3-1). Special considerations must be made when diagnosing migraine in a child or younger adolescent. The duration of the attack may be shorter, lasting as little as 1 hour. The pain is usually frontotemporal, but it is often bilateral in younger people, whereas adults typically experience unilateral pain. The pain may be associated with photophobia *or* phonophobia; both are not necessary to meet diagnostic criteria in an adolescent. Migraine pain can be severe and debilitating; many migraine sufferers report that they are unable to function and must lie down in a dark, quiet room and sleep to relieve their symptoms. A recurrent pattern is critical for the diagnosis of migraine; a patient who appears to be experiencing his or her first migraine headache should be approached with the broad differential diagnosis of acute headache. Although the pathophysiology remains somewhat uncertain, migraine headache appears to be a primarily neuronal event that causes vascular inflammation and dilatation and subsequent pain. Migraine-specific therapies target these vascular changes.

Table 3-1. Diagnostic criteria for migraine

Migraine without aura ("common" migraine)
A. At least five attacks fulfilling B–D
B. Headache lasts 4 to 72 h (untreated/unsuccessfully treated)
C. Headache has at least two of the following characteristics:
  • Unilateral location
  • Pulsating quality
  • Moderate or severe intensity
  • Aggravation by physical activity (e.g., climbing stairs, walking)
D. During headaches at least one of the following:
  • Nausea, vomiting, or both
  • Photophobia and phonophobia
E. Not attributed to another disorder

Migraine with aura ("classic" migraine)
A. At least two attacks fulfilling B
B. Migraine aura fulfills criteria for typical aura, hemiplegic aura, or basilar-type aura
C. Not attributed to another disorder

Typical aura
• Fully reversible visual, sensory, or speech symptoms without motor weakness
• Homonymous or bilateral visual symptoms including positive features (e.g., flickering lights, spots, lines) or negative features (e.g., loss of vision), or unilateral sensory symptoms including positive features (e.g., visual loss, pins and needles) or negative features (e.g., numbness) or any combination
• At least one of:
  i. At least one symptom develops gradually over at least 5 minutes
  ii. Each symptom lasts 5–60 min
• Headache meeting criteria for migraine without aura begins during aura or following aura within 60 minutes

Adolescents with *menstrual migraine* experience migraine during at least two-thirds of their menstrual cycles. The pain occurs between days -2 to $+3$ of the cycle and may occur with or without exogenous hormonal cycle control. *Prospective* documentation of cycles and headache pattern is important when making this diagnosis. The etiology is uncertain. Several other migraine variants exist, including basilar-type migraine and familial or sporadic hemiplegic migraine. These migraine variants are distinguished by the discrete neurological symptoms that accompany them. Full discussion of these entities is beyond the scope of this chapter.

Tension-type headaches are the most common type of chronic nonprogressive headache in adolescents. They may occur daily or several times a week in many adolescents. The pain of tension-type headache is typically mild-to-moderate, and patients often are able to continue functioning during the headache. The pain may be dull or squeezing in character and may be located anywhere in the head or neck. Sleep typically does not provide relief. Psychosocial stress may contribute to the patient's experience of the pain and the functional impairment caused by the headache. Adolescents may have headaches with features of both vascular and tension-type headache symptoms, clouding the diagnosis.

Analgesic withdrawal headache commonly follows analgesic overuse in the treatment of chronic daily headache. It may occur following the withdrawal of any analgesic [including acetaminophen and nonsteroidal anti-inflammatory drugs (NSAIDs)] that has been used three times a week or more for several weeks or months for the treatment of headache. It may be particularly common following the overuse of combination medications that contain multiple drugs, such as aspirin, acetaminophen, caffeine, and sedative medications.

Less common causes of chronic nonprogressive headache include:
• Cluster headache. This is a rare diagnosis in adolescents.
• Temporomandibular joint disorder. Jaw pain and tenderness typically are present with this disorder.
• Posttraumatic headache.

- Obstructive sleep apnea (OSA). Patients with OSA may experience morning headaches secondary to chronic hypoxemia and hypercapnia overnight.
- Mental health disturbance, such as depression or excessive psychosocial stress.
- Refractive error. Although headaches are often attributed to this, it actually is a *rare* cause of chronic headache in a patient who reports no eye pain.

   C. Physical examination: A complete physical examination should be performed, with special attention paid to the following areas:
- General appearance: Is the patient clearly in pain? Ill in appearance? Has he or she turned out the lights in the exam room?
- Vital signs: Fever? Hypertension? Elevated heart rate or blood pressure indicating acute pain?
- Growth and development: Recent weight loss? Obesity? Normal pubertal progression?
- HEENT: Tenderness with palpation of head, sinuses, temporomandibular joint? Sharp disc margins on fundoscopic exam? Photophobia? Evidence of otitis media or externa? Restricted jaw opening? Dental caries or tenderness of teeth with palpation?
- Neck: Nuchal rigidity? Tenderness or spasm of neck muscles?
- Complete neurologic examination: Mental status changes or altered level of consciousness? Papilledema? Abnormal eye movements or cranial nerve exam? Ataxia or other coordination disturbance? Asymmetric or abnormal findings on assessment of strength, sensation, or deep tendon reflexes?

   D. Laboratory evaluation and neuroimaging: Often no ancillary testing is necessary, particularly in the evaluation of chronic, nonprogressive headache. A complete blood count, differential, and erythrocyte sedimentation rate may be useful if infection, vasculitis, or malignancy is suspected. A toxin screen may be performed if acute intoxication is suspected. A lumbar puncture may be indicated for evaluation for meningitis/encephalitis, subarachnoid hemorrhage, or idiopathic intracranial hypertension. Opening pressures greater than 200 to 250 mm H_2O suggest the latter diagnosis. Electroencephalography (EEG) is rarely useful in the absence of other evidence of seizure activity.

   Neuroimaging is rarely useful in the evaluation of headache in patients without objective neurologic findings on physical exam; over 95% of adolescents with brain tumors have such findings. It should be considered, however, particularly in a patient with chronic progressive headache. Several indications for neuroimaging are listed in Table 3-2. Computed axial tomography (CT) should be used for evaluation for hemorrhage, hydrocephalus, subdural fluid, sinus disease, or abscess. Magnetic resonance imaging (MRI) is best for visualizing the posterior fossa and evaluating for congenital malformations, vasculitis, and venous sinus thrombosis. It may be used in conjunction with angiography for evaluation of vascular abnormalities. MRI is significantly more expensive than CT, takes longer to perform, and is less readily available in the acute setting. CT can subject the patient to significant radiation exposure.

III. Management:

   A. Goals of treatment: For patients whose headaches are a symptom of a systemic infection or other illness, treatment of the underlying illness should be the focus of therapy. A variety of analgesics may be used to treat concurrent headache pain. The remainder of this chapter is dedicated to the treatment of chronic and/or recurrent headache.

   Treatment of patients with chronic nonprogressive headache can be extremely challenging and may require several visits. Although complete pain relief is the ultimate goal of headache treatment, this may not be a realistic goal in patients with

Table 3-2. Indications for neuroimaging in an adolescent with headache

Acute mental status changes
Focal neurologic symptoms and/or abnormal neurologic exam
Visual disturbance (other than photophobia)
Progressively worsening symptoms
Evidence or suspicion of increased intracranial pressure
Growth/pubertal arrest
"Worst headache in life"
Posttraumatic headache

chronic headache. Focus should be placed on increasing functionality and decreasing (rather than eliminating) pain. Consistent school attendance may be an appropriate specific goal for many adolescents.

B. **Treatment:** Once serious systemic and/or intracranial pathology has been ruled out, either clinically or with appropriate laboratory and/or imaging studies, patients and their parents must be reassured that the provider knows the diagnosis and is prepared to treat it. Specific mention that brain tumor is not the cause of the headache may be particularly reassuring. The importance of lifestyle changes must not be underestimated. Patients should eat meals regularly, not skip breakfast, and consider reducing or eliminating caffeine intake. Any foods or food additives that are *known* to trigger migraines should be eliminated as well, although broad "elimination" diets are not recommended. Good hydration should be maintained; 64 oz of water a day (approximately the equivalent of two large sports bottles) should be the goal. Sleep hygiene and exercise habits should be optimized. Mental health counseling may be useful to address underlying mood or anxiety symptoms, assist with stress management, and help the patient identify appropriate coping strategies.

Nonpharmacologic techniques may be used to treat acute headache as well. Self-hypnosis, biofeedback, and relaxation techniques may all be useful. Patients with migraines that respond well to sleep should be encouraged to think of sleep as an alternative to abortive medication. Other complementary therapies such as acupuncture may be considered.

C. **Medications:** Pharmacologic treatment options for acute headache (i.e., abortive therapies) are listed in Table 3-3. Nonspecific analgesics such as NSAIDs often are effective and should be used in appropriately high doses. Triptans are the mainstay of migraine treatment when nonspecific treatments are ineffective. Although they are not approved by the FDA for migraine treatment in adolescents, there is good evidence for their safety and efficacy in this age group. The response to different triptans may be idiosyncratic; failure to respond to one medication in this family should not lead to the assumption that others will be ineffective. Greatest efficacy has been demonstrated for subcutaneous sumatriptan, but side effects (hypertension, flushing, dizziness) are also greatest for this formulation. Concomitant use of an antiemetic can enhance the absorption of oral triptans. Dihydroergotamine may be used in adolescents 18 years of age and older; hypertension and vasospasm may be significant side effects, and it should not be used within 24 hours of triptan use. Opioids should be avoided in the treatment of adolescent headache. Abortive therapies should be readily available so that treatment may be initiated as soon as possible with the onset of headache. This includes making them available at school as well as at home. In order to avoid analgesic withdrawal headache, they should not be used more than two to three times a week.

Patients who experience migraine headache two or more times a week, have severe and debilitating headaches, or have a poor response to abortive treatments may be candidates for daily prophylactic therapy. Medications used for prophylactic

Table 3-3. Acute (abortive) therapies for adolescent headache[a]

Nonspecific analgesics
- Acetaminophen
- Ibuprofen
- Naproxen sodium
- Ketorolac

Combination products
- Midrin® (isometheptene, dichloralphenazone, acetaminophen)
- Fioricet® (butalbital, acetaminophen, caffeine)
- Excedrin® (acetaminophen, aspirin, caffeine)

Migraine-specific therapies
- Sumatriptan (oral, intranasal, or subcutaneous)
- Rizatriptan
- Zolmitriptan
- Naratriptan
- Dihydroergotamine mesylate (with caffeine) (intranasal)

[a]Many used "off-label" in adolescents. All oral formulations, unless otherwise indicated.

Table 3-4. Prophylactic therapies for adolescent migraine^a

- Amitriptyline
- Cyproheptadine
- Propranolol (and other beta-blockers)
- Verapamil
- Carbamazepine
- Valproic acid
- Topiramate
- Gabapentin
- Lamotrigine
- Riboflavin (vitamin B$_{12}$)

^{a}Many used "off-label" in adolescents.

therapy are listed in Table 3-4. Prophylactic medications may require trials of 2 to 6 months to show effectiveness. When used, they should be discontinued after several months, and the patient's need for ongoing treatment should be reassessed. Good evidence is accumulating for the use of topiramate, valproate, and other antiepileptic drugs for this indication. Calcium channel blockers and beta blockers may have significant side effects and have not been shown to be effective in adolescents. Daily low-dose amitriptyline is widely used for treatment of migraine, tension-type headache, and analgesic rebound headache, although evidence of its efficacy is limited. Many of the medications listed in Tables 3-3 and 3-4 are used "off label" in adolescents, because safety and efficacy in headache treatment have not been definitively demonstrated in this age group.

Treatment of rebound headaches associated with analgesic overuse can be quite difficult. All analgesics should be discontinued for at least 1 month. Patients and their parents often are skeptical of the diagnosis and resistant to this treatment. Use of a prophylactic medication such as amitriptyline may be considered, as well as non-pharmacologic treatments.

Evidence-based recommendations for the treatment of menstrual migraine are lacking. Abortive therapies may be used, as previously described. Combination oral contraceptive pills (COCs) often are used and may be effective. Continuous cycling (i.e., continuous use of hormonally active pills and elimination or reduction of the frequency of the placebo pills) to reduce the frequency of menses is a reasonable treatment option. COCs are contraindicated in the treatment of migraine with focal neurologic symptoms. Naproxen sodium may be used from days −7 to +6 of the menstrual cycle as menstrual migraine prophylaxis.

D. **Criteria for referral:** Patients with focal neurologic findings or headaches refractory to treatment should be referred to a neurologist. Referral to a mental health provider may be warranted for evaluation and treatment of an underlying mood or anxiety disorder, for stress management, and to assist with nonpharmacologic treatment strategies. Family counseling may be useful to assist family members in responding appropriately to a patient with chronic pain. Comprehensive headache treatment centers often employ multidisciplinary teams to address all of these needs.

IV. **Clinical pearls and pitfalls:**
- The vast majority of acute headaches in adolescents are associated with viral and/or upper respiratory infections.
- The vast majority of chronic headaches in adolescents are migraine or tension-type headaches.
- A chronic, progressive headache pattern is the most likely to represent serious underlying pathology, such as a brain tumor or other cause of increased intracranial pressure.
- Neuroimaging is rarely indicated in the presence of a completely normal neurologic exam, particularly in evaluation of chronic, nonprogressive headache.
- The development of analgesic rebound headache can be avoided by limiting the use of abortive therapies to an absolute maximum of three times per week.
- Lifestyle changes, including optimizing diet, hydration, exercise, and sleep patterns, may play a critical role in headache management.
- Migraine headache should be treated early and aggressively, including having abortive medications available at school, in order to achieve the most rapid relief.
- A multidisciplinary team approach may be appropriate for treatment of chronic headaches.

BIBLIOGRAPHY

For the clinician

Gladstein J, Mack KJ. Chronic daily headache in adolescents. *Pediatr Ann* 2005;34:472–479.
Goadsby PJ, Lipton RB, Ferrari MD. Migraine—current understanding and treatment. *New Engl J Med* 2002;346(4):257.
Headache Classification Committee. The international classification of headache disorders, 2nd ed. *Cephalalgia* 2004;24(S1):1–160.
Lewis D, Ashwal S, Hershey A, Hirtz D, et al. Pharmacological treatment of migraine headache in children and adolescents. *Neurology* 2004;63:2215–2224.
Lewis DW. Migraine headaches in the adolescent. *Adolesc Med State Art Rev* 2002;13(3):413.
Pakalnis A. New avenues in treatment of paediatric migraine: a review of the literature. *Fam Pract* 2001;18:101.
Pakalnis A. Nonmigraine headaches in adolescents. *Adolesc Med State Rev* 2002;13(3):433.
Silberstein SD. Migraine. *Lancet* 2004;363:381.
Winner P, Rothner AD, Saper J, et al. A randomized, double-blind, placebo-controlled study of sumatriptan nasal spray in the treatment of acute migraine in adolescents. *Pediatrics* 2000; 106:989.

WEB SITES

www.headaches.org (1-888-NHF-5552)   The Web site of the National Headache Foundation has useful information and tools for both headache sufferers and health care providers, including a headache diary and several assessment tools that may be downloaded. Several pages are designed specifically for teens
www.achenet.org   The Web site of the American Council for Headache Education contains several resources for child and adult headache sufferers, including a list of books that may be ordered

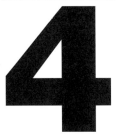

Seizures

Seizures are one of the more common chronic neurological problems of adolescents. As might be expected, they bridge the gap between those typical of childhood and those more associated with maturity. Seizures in adolescents can be idiopathic or they can be due to a primary condition such as a mass lesion in the brain or misuse of drugs.

I. **Description of the condition:**
   A. **Definitions and causes: Seizures can be defined as stereotypical, paroxysmal occurrences due to abnormal electrical activity in the brain.** This abnormal activity can either be from over-excitation of or insufficient inhibition of electrical impulses. The presentation of this abnormal electrical activity depends on where in the brain it occurs. Disturbances can be motor, sensory, autonomic, or psychic. Numerous conditions that impair brain function can provoke seizures. These include infections of the central nervous system (CNS), trauma, or stroke.

   Generalized seizures begin in both hemispheres whereas **partial seizures** emanate from one hemisphere. Generalized seizures involve immediate loss of consciousness. **Partial seizures are either simple or complex. Simple ones** involve no loss of consciousness while **complex seizures** do involve loss of consciousness.

   Epilepsy is a condition in which there are recurrent, unprovoked seizures. There are several syndromes, as listed in Table 4-1. These syndromes are either primary, i.e., with no discernible cause, or secondary, that is, due to a CNS injury or problem.

   Status epilepticus is a condition in which a seizure lasts for longer than 5 minutes. Patients in this situation should be transported to an emergency department as soon as possible. Benzodiazepines are the preferred drugs to treat status epilepticus. Newer treatments include fosphenytoin, rectal diazepam, and parenteral valproate. Rectal diazepam also can be used by lay people or primary care clinicians to treat status in situations where expeditious transport to an emergency room may be difficult.

   B. **Syndromes:** Epilepsy syndromes change from childhood to adulthood. Some benign syndromes of childhood, for example, typical absence epilepsy and benign epilepsy with centrotemporal spikes (BECT; "rolandic epilepsy") stop needing treatment with medications some time in adolescence. Treatment of partial and generalized seizures

Table 4-1. International League Against Epilepsy (ILAE) seizure classification

1. Partial
   A. Simple
   B. Complex
      With secondary generalization

2. Generalized
   A. Nonconvulsive
      Absence
      Atypical absence

   B. Convulsive
      Tonic
      Clonic
      Tonic-Clonic
      Myoclonic
      Atonic (drop attacks)

Adapted from Commission on Classification and Terminology of the ILAE. Proposal for revised clinical and electroencephalographic classification of epileptic seizures. *Epilepsia* 1981;22:498–501.

Table 4-2. Epilepsy syndromes and adolescence

Change	Syndrome affected
Remit	Typical absence epilepsy
	Benign epilepsy with centrotemporal spikes
	Benign occipital epilepsy
Persist	Lennox-Gastaut syndrome
	Symptomatic partial epilepsy
	Symptomatic generalized epilepsy
Begin	Juvenile myoclonic epilepsy
	Juvenile absence epilepsy
	Epilepsy with grand mal on awakening
	Progressive myoclonic epilepsy
	Temporal lobe epilepsy with mesial temporal
	Sclerosis

can also stop at this stage. Table 4-2 lists syndromes and states whether they start, continue, or end in adolescence.

1. **Juvenile myoclonic epilepsy (JME):** This is the **most common form of idiopathic generalized seizures (GTC, i.e., generalized tonic-clonic seizures).** It has an incidence of 5% to 10% in the general population, with more than 75% of patients presenting between 12 and 18 years of age. Its **features** include:
   * morning myoclonic jerks,
   * generalized tonic-clonic seizures in 90%, and
   * absence seizures in 10%.

   Seizures begin with myoclonic jerks that can be subtle at the start. These then progress to GTC. They are **precipitated frequently by adolescent behaviors,** e.g., lack of sleep, abuse of alcohol/drugs, and by stress. Patients have normal intelligence, normal neurological examination, and positive family history for similar seizures. This is a lifelong syndrome.

2. **Juvenile absence epilepsy (JAE) and grand mal on awakening (GMA):** These types of epilepsy **share common features, and they may overlap.** They may share a common genetic focus with childhood absence epilepsy. JAE presents in adolescents who are neurologically normal. Ninety percent also have GTC.

3. **Mesial temporal lobe epilepsy (MTLE):** MTLE, which starts in adolescence, is due to mesiotemporal lobe sclerosis and is the most common epileptic syndrome of adults. Frequently these patients have partial complex seizures in childhood that become more difficult to control in adolescence. A seizure begins with an aura 90% of the time. Automatisms are common. The seizures last 1 to 2 minutes and are followed by postictal confusion or lethargy.

4. **Lennox-Gastaut syndrome (LGS):** LGS consists of mental retardation and a generalized seizure disorder. There is significant disability by the time a child reaches adolescence.

5. **Nonepileptic events (NEE):** When an adolescent has a paroxysmal event, one must first ask if this is a true epileptic seizure or if it is a **nonepileptic event (NEE).**

   NEEs are common in adolescents, with one series reporting them in 20% to 25% of children referred for evaluation. As listed in Table 4-3, the **causes of NEE in adolescents are usually discernible by history.**

II. **Making the diagnosis:**
   A. **History:** Diagnosis of seizures begins, as always, with **a thorough history.** The history should emphasize past head trauma; illnesses that might have caused brain impairment; metabolic problems; history of seizures with fever as a small child;

Table 4-3. Nonepileptic events

Vasovagal syncope
Migraine and variants
Narcolepsy
Pseudoseizures

exposure to toxins both voluntary (e.g., drugs of abuse) and unintended; travel history; and family history of epilepsy.

B. **Physical examination:** A **thorough physical examination,** including a meticulous neurologic examination, is mandatory. If there are positive CNS findings, especially signs of increased intracranial pressure, immediate neuroimaging is mandatory. Any visual loss or focal weakness, even though it could be a postictal finding, demands immediate imaging as well.

C. **Imaging and laboratory evaluation:**
   1. **Nonacute evaluation:** In the nonacute situation, an adolescent should have an electroencephalogram (EEG). **The American Academy of Neurology, Child Neurology Society, and the American Epilepsy Society all recommend a routine EEG in all children with a first, afebrile seizure.** Twice as many children with abnormal EEGs after a paroxysmal event have recurrent seizures compared to those with a normal EEG.
   2. **Acute evaluation:** When there is an **acute seizure episode,** one first should rule out metabolic, traumatic, and toxic causes. A complete blood count, electrolyte and blood glucose evaluations, a pregnancy test where appropriate, and a screen for drugs of abuse should be done. **Head imaging** in the acute situation should be done immediately. Either a CT or an MRI should be done, with MRI more sensitive for more subtle abnormalities, for example, medial temporal sclerosis (MTS), or scar tissue in the hippocampal region of the temporal lobe, the most common cause of symptomatic temporal lobe epilepsy in adolescents. Other MRI findings might include atrophy, stroke, signs of past trauma, cerebral dysgenesis, and cortical dysplasia.
   3. **Evaluation for specific syndromes:** For JME, **the EEG is characteristic and diagnostic,** that is, 4 to 6 Hz polyspike and wave complexes. They are activated by sleep and sometimes by photic stimulation. These are usually responsive to anti-epileptic drugs (AED). **For JAE/GMA,** the EEG shows a 3.5 to 4 Hz spike and wave pattern. GMA peaks in its initiation at puberty. **For MTLE,** the EEG shows temporal slowing and epileptiform discharges that may be bilateral. The MRI is characteristic with findings including hippocampal atrophy. **For LGS,** the disability that begins in childhood and the somewhat uncontrollable seizures ensure that the diagnosis is made by the time the child reaches adolescence.

   For possible NEE, if there is still a question as to cause, a patient can be observed with a video EEG to make the diagnosis. One of the problems with NEE is that **almost three fourths of patients with NEE also suffer from epilepsy.** Video EEG, then, is most effective in differentiating what is causing a particular type of spasm. This is also helpful in showing parents and the affected teens "proof" that a paroxysmal event may not be a manifestation of true epilepsy.

III. **Management:** The cornerstone of management is the proper use of AEDs. In JME, the seizures are usually responsive to AEDs. Phenytoin and carbamazepine can exacerbate this type of epilepsy; therefore, they should be avoided. Valproic acid causes weight gain, so **the drugs of choice** are lamotrigine or topiramate, as well as possibly a newer AED. JAE and GMA require lifelong treatment with AED. In MTLE, carbamazepine, oxcarbazepine, and gabapentin all can be effective AEDs. One third of patients with MTLE become resistant to AED therapy and require surgical intervention. Surgery works in 80% to 90% of cases refractory to AED; therefore, clinicians should refer patients who have undergone two failed trials of AED. Most adolescents with this syndrome are already supervised by neurologists, and they should be the ones to refer to neurosurgeons. LGS needs broad spectrum AEDs. Potentially it can be helped with an implantable vagus nerve stimulator. Finally, clinicians should remember that the blood levels of some AEDs can be affected by combined hormonal contraceptives, and there can be a converse effect as well.

IV. **Clinical pearls and pitfalls:**
   • **Puberty:** Obviously, puberty is the major physical milestone of adolescence, with its attendant changes in body size and configuration and with the onset of reproductive capability. With the change in body mass and surface area, there is increased opportunity for underdosing of AEDs. Therefore it is necessary to monitor treatment more frequently via clinical reassessments and via plasma levels of the drugs. With the progression of pubertal processes, types of seizures can change and syndromes can vary in their impact or occurrence.
   • **Compliance:** Adolescents are notorious for supposed noncompliance with treatment regimens for chronic illnesses, but in reality they are no less compliant than are adults. During adolescence, compliance becomes an issue because it can become entangled with issues of developing independence from parents and authority figures, with psychological defense mechanisms that allow denial and similar mechanisms to interfere with optimum treatment, and with changing schedules and life activities.

- **Driving:** A frequent issue that arises during adolescence is the risk of allowing the adolescent who has a seizure disorder to drive. Each state has statutes that say how long adolescents have to be seizure free before they can drive. Many states require, for example, that the adolescent be seizure free for at least 1 year. If an adolescent is being considered for AED cessation, this process should take place before driving becomes an issue.
- **Sexuality:** The issues in this area include sexual function/enjoyment, pregnancy, and menstrual disorders. Adolescents on AEDs report an increased rate of deficits in libido and arousal. Adolescent women on AED also are at increased risk of endocrine malfunctions such as polycystic ovary syndrome, particularly with valproic acid and its attendant weight gain. Also, efficacy of combined hormonal contraceptive pills can be compromised to some degree with certain AEDs.

  Adolescents should seriously consider the *negative impact of their disease and of AED on a pregnancy.* Overall, women taking an AED in pregnancy have a two to three fold increased risk of having abnormal infants. The more AEDs a woman is taking, the greater are her chances of having an infant with a birth defect such as cleft palate, neural tube defect, or cardiac abnormality.

  For all these reasons, *contraceptive counseling* is most important for this group of adolescents, and these young women need to be on the right form of contraception. If they take oral contraceptive pills, the brand should contain 50 μg. of ethinyl estradiol if their AED is carbamazepine, phenobarbital, phenytoin, or topiramate. A barrier method also should be used, and a progestin-only method should be considered.
- **Peers:** Adolescence is a time of intense involvement with peers, particularly with those of the same sex early in adolescence and with both genders in middle adolescence. Intimate relationships with single partners begin during this time as well. Adolescents with epilepsy have a condition that may make them feel so different from other teens that they don't socialize properly, with consequent social isolation and possibly depression. These effects should be anticipated, and prophylactic counseling should be considered for all children who enter adolescence with epilepsy or for those who acquire it during this stage of life.
- **Transition to adulthood:** Adolescents with any chronic illness, including epilepsy, may have increased difficulty in negotiating the transitions necessary to become an adult.
  - They may have difficulty finding appropriate medical care in the adult medical arena.
  - They may have difficulty finding insurance that not only covers their needs but also allows them to work.
  - They may have difficulty pursuing higher education.
  - They may have difficulty entering into intimate relationships.
  - They may have difficulty getting jobs.

For all these reasons, adolescents with epilepsy should be cared for by clinicians who are cognizant of these transition issues and who can help their patients negotiate them.

BIBLIOGRAPHY

For the clinician

French JA. Efficacy and tolerability of the new antiepileptic drugs I: treatment of new onset epilepsy. Report of the Therapeutics and Technology Assessment Subcommittee and Quality Standards Subcommittee of the American Academy of Neurology and the American Epilepsy Society. *Neurology* 2004;62(8):1252–1260.

Paolicchi JM. Epilepsy in adolescents: diagnosis and treatment. *Adolesc Med State Art Rev* 2002;13:443–459.

Sirven JI. Management of status epilepticus. *Am Fam Physician* 2003;68:469–476.

Stores G. Practitioner review: recognition of pseudoseizures in children and adolescents. *J Child Psychol Psychiatry* 1999;40:851–857.

Wheless JW, Kim HL. Adolescent seizures and epilepsy syndromes. *Epilepsia* 2002;43 (suppl. 3):33–52.

For patients and parents

Freeman JM, Vining EPG, Pillas DJ. *Seizures and epilepsy in childhood: A guide*, 3rd ed. Baltimore, MD: Johns Hopkins University Press, 2002.

WEB SITES

www.epilepsy.com.au

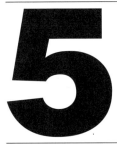

Syncope

I. **Description of the condition:**
   A. **Epidemiology:** Syncope is defined as a sudden and transient loss of consciousness and postural muscle tone resulting from decreased cerebral perfusion, followed by spontaneous recovery without resuscitation. Presyncope is the term used to describe the premonitory symptoms of syncope, such as dizziness and nausea, without actual loss of consciousness. Approximately 30% of healthy teenagers experience a syncopal episode during their adolescence. The peak ages are between 15 and 19 years, and females are more likely to present to a clinician for evaluation than are males.
   B. **Etiology:** Though the vast majority of episodes are neurocardiogenic (vasovagal), any condition that decreases cerebral perfusion, cardiac or noncardiac, as well as metabolic disturbances and psychiatric conditions, may cause syncope. The causes of syncope can be categorized as **neurocardiac, cardiac,** and **noncardiac.**
      1. **Neurocardiac** (vasovagal) syncope is the most common type of syncope in adolescents. Approximately a quarter of cases are precipitated by acute illness, anemia, or noxious stimuli such as pain, fear, anxiety, exhaustion, hunger, prolonged standing, overcrowding, or the sight of blood. The pathophysiology of neurocardiac syncope involves peripheral venous pooling from an upright posture, which leads to decreased ventricular filling and increased circulating catecholamines. The ventricle then contracts vigorously, which stimulates mechanoreceptors and produces a paradoxic withdrawal of sympathetic activity and parasympathetic activation that causes vasodilation, hypotension, and bradycardia, resulting in the syncopal episode.
      2. **Cardiac** causes of syncope should be considered in the adolescent with a history of syncope of sudden onset, syncope during vigorous exercise, or syncope occurring while lying down in a recumbent position (see Table 5-1).
      3. **Noncardiac causes** (see Table 5-2).
II. **Making the diagnosis:**
   A. **History:** The history of the event is critical for the diagnosis and should be obtained from both the adolescent patient and, if possible, from an eyewitness. The history should include:
      • Time of day
      • Time of last meal
      • Situation and antecedents of the event, including position of patient
      • Associated prodromal symptoms such as palpitations, chest pain, headache, shortness of breath, nausea, diaphoresis, and visual changes
      • Duration of episode
      • Loss of consciousness
      • Family history of sudden death, arrhythmia, congenital heart disease, seizures, or metabolic disorders
      • Medications, including illicit drugs
   B. **Differential diagnosis:**
      • Seizure
      • Atypical migraine headache
      • Narcolepsy
      • Vertigo
   C. **Physical examination:** Any adolescent who has a syncopal episode should undergo a complete physical examination with particular attention to the cardiac and neurologic examination. Vital signs should be obtained with the patient supine and after he or she has stood for 5 to 10 minutes. The results of most physical examinations for adolescents with syncope are entirely normal.

Table 5-1. Cardiac causes of syncope

Obstruction to flow	Myocardial dysfunction	Arrhythmias
Aortic stenosis	Cardiomyopathy	Ventricular tachycardia
Hypertrophic cardiomyopathy	Myocarditis	Prolonged QTc syndrome
Primary pulmonary hypertension	Ischemia	Wolff-Parkinson-White Syndrome

    D. Laboratory evaluation and tests: The history and physical examination should guide clinicians in choosing the diagnostic tests that apply to a given adolescent with syncope. Patients often present several hours or even days after the event occurred.
- All patients should have a 12-lead electrocardiogram
- Postmenarchal females should be tested for pregnancy
- A complete blood count, serum glucose, electrolytes, urinalysis (to assess dehydration), and/or toxicology screen should be considered
- If episodes are associated with palpitations, a 24-hour Holter monitor or an event recorder may help to capture the cardiac rhythm when these patients are symptomatic
- Further outpatient studies may include echocardiography, electroencephalography, and *tilt-table testing.*

    Tilt-table testing may be helpful in confirming the diagnosis of neurocardiac syncope if the episodes are recurrent and the history, physical examination, and electrocardiogram (ECG) are all normal. Tilt-table testing is based on the theory that orthostatic stress is often the precipitating factor for syncopal events. After lying flat for a period of time, the patient is tilted upright for a time sufficient to reproduce symptoms and changes in cardiovascular function (hypotension or bradycardia). Positive responses include dizziness, lightheadedness, nausea, visual changes, and frank syncope.

III. **Management:** The etiology of the syncopal event determines the appropriate therapy. Cardiac disease may require antiarrhythmics or surgery. For situational syncope, the precipitating stimulus should be avoided. For patients with typical features of neurocardiac syncope, reassurance and instructions regarding avoidance of both dehydration and postural hypotension should be provided. Specific therapy is seldom necessary.

    A. Behavioral management of neurocardiac syncope: Avoid the noxious stimuli that precipitate syncope. Wear elastic hose to prevent venous pooling in the legs. Eat regularly and increase salt and water intake. Contract leg muscles intermittently to increase venous return when standing.

    B. Pharmacologic management of neurocardiac syncope: If episodes are frequent and do not respond to simple measures, beta-blockers may inhibit the initial tachycardia and inotropic response to catecholamines. Other pharmacologic treatment of neurocardiac syncope includes alpha-adrenergic agonists, which cause arteriolar vasoconstriction and venoconstriction, and mineralocorticoids, which cause volume expansion and alpha-receptor sensitization.

    C. Criteria for referral: Referral to a pediatric cardiologist for specialized testing or management should be made if the adolescent is in a high-risk group such as:
- Episodes that are exercise-induced or recurrent
- Associated chest pain, palpitations, or dyspnea
- Cardiac disease
- Positive family history for conditions associated with sudden death
- If history obtained is suggestive of alternate diagnoses, the appropriate referral may be to a pediatric neurologist, endocrinologist, or psychiatrist

Table 5-2. Noncardiac causes of syncope

- Migraine
- Orthostatic hypotension
- Metabolic disease (hypoglycemia, electrolyte imbalance)
- Situational (cough, neck stretching, micturition, hair grooming)
- Toxins/drugs
- Hyperventilation
- Hysteria

IV.   **Clinical pearls and pitfalls:**
- A thorough and detailed history and physical examination is critical in the evaluation of adolescents with syncope.
- All adolescents with syncope should undergo an ECG, but other laboratory tests should be selected based on specific information obtained from the history and physical examination.
- The most common type of syncope in otherwise healthy adolescents is neurocardiac (vasovagal) syncope, which is generally a benign and transient condition.
- Syncope can be a presenting symptom of early pregnancy in an adolescent female.
- All syncope associated with exertion or exercise should be considered dangerous, as it can be a predictor of sudden cardiac death. Appropriate screening must be performed on these patients.

BIBLIOGRAPHY

For the clinician

Kapoor WN. Syncope. *N Engl J Med* 2000;343:1856–1862.

Lewis DA, Dhala A. Syncope in the pediatric patient: the cardiologist's perspective. *Pediatr Clin North Am* 1999;46:205–219.

Prodinger RJ, Reisdorff EJ. Syncope in children. *Emerg Med Clin North Am* 1998;16:617–626.

Walsh CA. Syncope and sudden death in the adolescent. *Adolesc Med* 2001;12:105–132.

Weimer LH. Syncope and orthostatic intolerance for the primary care physician. *Prim Care* 2004;31(1):175–199.

Willis J. Syncope. *Pediatr Rev* 2000;21:201–204.

WEB SITES

www.americanheart.org

cpmcnet.columbia.edu/dept/syncope/

Common Respiratory Infections

BACTERIAL RHINOSINUSITIS

I. **Description of the condition:**
   A. **Definition:** Rhinosinusitis is the more correct term for sinusitis in children and adolescents because most sinus infections begin with or have a concomitant rhinitis. Rhinosinusitis denotes an array of acute and chronic neutrophilic and eosinophilic allergic and nonallergic inflammatory processes in the nasal and sinus mucosa. Acute bacterial rhinosinusitis is defined by the American Academy of Pediatrics (AAP) as a "bacterial infection of the paranasal sinuses lasting less than 30 days in which symptoms resolve completely."

   In the United States, bacterial rhinosinusitis is the fifth most common diagnosis requiring an antimicrobial prescription. Rhinosinusitis is a common disorder in the United States and affects more than 30 million individuals each year. Between 5% and 10% of upper respiratory infections are complicated by acute bacterial infections of the paranasal sinuses.

   B. **Etiology:** The sinus *ostia* (1–3 mm in diameter) provide a conduit for drainage of the maxillary, frontal, ethmoid, and sphenoid sinuses into the nasal cavity. Persistent obstruction of the sinus ostia by inflammatory edema may provide a favorable environment for secondary bacterial colonization.

   Bacteria or virus-induced mucosal inflammation inhibits mucociliary transport, which in turn promotes stagnation of secretions, decreased pH, and lowered oxygen tension; this results in the optimal environment for bacterial multiplication. The absence of normal mucociliary clearance and reduced mechanical drainage allow bacteria present on the surface of the respiratory mucosa to increase in density, leading to a bacterial superinfection. The drainage tract of the maxillary sinus resists gravitational drainage and allows fluid to accumulate, predisposing the maxillary sinus to bacterial infection as a complication of an upper respiratory viral infection. In the ethmoid sinuses, the slightest mucosal inflammation may block the narrow caliber drainage openings. This may result in infection of the orbit, especially in younger children because of the thin partition between their ethmoid sinuses and the orbit.

   Viral upper respiratory tract infections and, less frequently, allergic inflammation, are by far the most common causes of mucosal swelling and lead to ostial obstruction. In general the pathophysiology of bacterial sinusitis is related to poor drainage of secretions in the paranasal sinuses as a result of obstruction of the sinus ostia, reduction in the number or impaired function of the cilia, or increase in the viscosity of secretions.

II. **Making the diagnosis:**
   A. **Clinical manifestations:** Two characteristic clinical syndromes suggest **bacterial rhinosinusitis.**
      1. The most common clinical syndrome consists of persistent signs and symptoms of an upper respiratory tract (URI) infection beyond 10 days without significant improvement. Although patients with an uncomplicated URI may still be symptomatic by the tenth day, their condition has improved. The respiratory symptoms include nasal discharge and cough. The nasal discharge usually is purulent but may be clear or mucoid. The cough is present during the daytime although it often worsens at night because of the irritation of the pharyngeal wall by the postnasal drip while the patient is in a recumbent position.
      2. The second and less common syndrome is a URI that is more severe than usual. The severe features are a temperature higher than 39°C (102.2°F) and purulent nasal discharge lasting for at least 3 days.

      Table 6-1 lists the most common signs and symptoms of acute bacterial sinusitis.

Table 6-1. Common clinical findings in acute rhinosinusitis in older children and adolescents

- Rhinorrhea
- Cough
- Fever
- Halitosis
- Poor appetite
- Headache
- Erythematous nasal mucosa
- Tenderness over the sinuses
- Postnasal drip
- Pain in the upper teeth

The above table is not inclusive and not all signs and symptoms listed need to be present in order for this diagnosis to apply.

If the signs and symptoms of bacterial rhinosinusitis last longer than 30 days, **chronic rhinosinusitis** must be considered as the diagnosis.

B. **Diagnostic imaging:** The diagnostic imaging available to help in the diagnosis of sinusitis includes plain sinus radiographs, computed tomography (CT), magnetic resonance imaging (MRI), and ultrasound. The American Academy of Pediatrics has stated that "imaging modalities have no clear role in the diagnosis of **uncomplicated acute bacterial sinusitis.**" There are no data to suggest any imaging modality, which is recommended over the others. The American College of Radiology believes that the diagnosis of acute, uncomplicated bacterial rhinosinusitis should be made on clinical grounds.

III. **Treatment:**
A. **Antimicrobials:** Once acute or chronic sinusitis has been diagnosed, the choice of the appropriate antimicrobial is based on the most common causative organism. See Table 6-2.

In the adolescent, most of the organisms responsible for acute bacterial rhinosinusitis are:

1. H. influenza
2. Strep pneumonia
3. *Moraxella catarrhalis*
4. Penicillin sensitive anaerobes

The American Academy of Pediatrics recommends the antimicrobials listed in Table 6-3.

Adolescents with acute rhinosinusitis should be treated for 10 to 14 days. For chronic sinusitis, the adolescents should be treated for 3 to 4 weeks. Symptoms should dramatically improve in the teen who has been treated for 48 hours. If the adolescent has not improved in 48 hours, he or she should be reevaluated and consideration may be given to changing antibiotics.

B. **Ancillary measures:** The American Academy of Pediatrics, in a statement published in 2001 on the treatment of acute bacterial sinusitis, states that there are no data to suggest that antihistamine-decongestants, steroid nasal sprays, or over-the-counter nasal sprays have a place in the treatment of acute bacterial sinusitis.

C. **Indications for referral and admission:** Complications of sinus disease can cause substantial morbidity and, occasionally, mortality. The most common complication of sinusitis is preseptal cellulitis or, more properly, inflammatory edema. Inflammatory edema is actually not an infection but rather soft tissue swelling of the periorbital area caused by impedance of the local venous draining. Preseptal cellulitis (inflammatory edema) is almost always associated with an ipsilateral ethmoidal sinusitis. The management of these patients must be individualized, and referral to an ophthalmologist or an ear, nose, and throat (ENT) specialist should be considered.

The adolescent with acute bacterial sinusitis that includes the frontal sinus must be observed closely because infection of this sinus cavity may lead to intracranial, intraorbital, or osseous complications. If the patient has high fever (>39°C, 102.2°F) or the periorbital swelling that has resulted in greater than 40% closure of the eye, hospital admission and parenteral antimicrobials are a reasonable treatment.

Table 6-2. Etiologic agents in sinusitis analyzed by patient age and type of illness

	Frequency			Age group (y)
	Overall	Acute	Chronic	>12
Aerobic Bacteria				
Haemophilus influenzae	++++	++++	++++	++++
Streptococcus pneumoniae	++++	++++	++++	++++
Moraxella catarrhalis	+++	+++	+	++
Staphylococcus aureus	++	+	++	++
Streptococcus pyogenes		++	++++	++
Alpha- and nonhemolytic				
Streptococci		+	+	++
Staphylococcus epidermis	+		+	++
Alcaligenas species	+		+	++
Escherichia coli	+		+	++
Pseudomonas aeruginosa	+		+	++
Other[a]	+		+	++
Anaerobic Bacteria				
Peptococcus species	++	+	++	++
Peptostreptococcus species	++	+	++	++
Bacteroides species	++	+	++	++
Veillonella	++	+	++	++
Other[b]	+	+	++	
Mycoplasma				
Mycoplasma pneumoniae	+	+		+
Other				
L-forms	+		+	+
Mixed: aerobes and anaerobes	++	+	++	++
Mixed *Haemophilus influenzae*				
with other organisms	++	+	++	++
Other[c]	+	+	+	+

[a]*Serratia*, diphtheroids, *Enterococcus* species, *Neisseria* species, *Haemophilus* species, *Proteus* species, *Acinetobacter*, *Citrobacter* species, Elkenella corrodens.
[b]*Fusobacterium* species, *Bifidobacterium, Propionibacterium.*
[c]Rhinovirus, adenovirus, *Aspergillus* species, other fungi.
From Feigin RD, Cherry JD, Demmler GJ, et al. *Textbook of pediatric infectious disease.* Philadelphia, PA: Elsevier, 2004:204, with permission.

Table 6-3. Antimicrobials and dosage schedules for the treatment of rhinosinusitis in adolescents

Antimicrobial	Dosage (adolescent[a])
Amoxicillin Standard dose	250 mg 3 times daily
Amoxicillin-potassium clavulanate Standard dose	250 mg 3 times daily
Cefuroxime axetil	250 mg 2 times daily
Cefpodoxime proxetil	200 mg 2 times daily
Cefdinir	300 mg once daily or 600 mg once daily
Clindamycin	150–450 mg 3–4 times daily
Clarithromycin	500 mg 2 times daily or 1,000 mg once daily
Azithromycin	500 mg once daily on day 1,250 mg once daily thereafter
Trimethoprim-sulfamethoxazole	160/800 mg 2 times daily
Erythromycin-sulfisoxazole	Not indicated

[a]Generally defined as a patient 13 years or older.
From Burg FS, Ingelfinger JR, Polin RA, et al. *Gellis and Kagan's current pediatric therapy.* Philadelphia, PA: W.B. Saunders, 2002:17:926, with permission.

IV. Clinical pearls and pitfalls:
- Bacterial sinusitis often occurs simultaneously with rhinitis.
- The signs and symptoms of bacterial sinusitis often persist after the rhinitis has resolved.
- By the time the child is 12 years old the nasal cavity and the paranasal sinuses are usually completely developed.
- There is poor correlation between nasopharyngeal cultures and the organism causing sinusitis.
- Systemic and/or local decongestants and steroid nasal sprays have not been shown to help in the treatment of rhinosinusitis.
- Less than 5% of upper respiratory infections are complicated by acute sinusitis.
- Imaging studies of the sinuses should probably be reserved for the adolescent who has signs and symptoms of sinusitis that do not respond to medical therapy. Which imaging study should be ordered remains controversial. Some authors suggest that a CT scan of the sinuses is optimal.
- The length of antibiotic treatment for rhinosinusitis is controversial and has not been studied adequately. One author (Dr. Ellen Wald) suggests that for acute sinusitis, the antibiotic should be continued for 7 days after symptoms have resolved. In chronic sinusitis, the same author recommends that antibiotic treatment be for 3 weeks and for 7 days after the patient has resolution of symptoms.

PHARYNGITIS

I. Description of the condition:
  A. Epidemiology and classification: Pharyngitis encompasses infection or irritation of the pharynx and tonsils. It is rarely found in infants younger than 2 years. **Pharyngitis peaks between the ages of 5 to 10 years, but recurs throughout life.**
  B. Etiology:
   1. Although **group A beta-hemolytic streptococcus (GABHS)** causes only 15% to 30% of all pharyngitis, it is the usual bacterial cause and may cause significant non-suppurative sequelae in the form of acute rheumatic fever (ARF) or acute glomerularnephritis (AGN). All types of pharyngitis can lead to suppurative complications including cervical lymphadenitis, peritonsillar abscess, retropharyngeal abscess, sinusitis, and otitis media. Rhinitis and cough are rare in GABHS pharyngitis.
   2. **Viral causes of pharyngitis:** Most cases of acute pharyngitis are the result of **viral infection.**
     a. Rhinoviruses (100 types) cause 20% of all pharyngitis.
     b. Coronavirus (at least three types) causes 5% of all pharyngitis infections.
     c. Adenovirus (types 17, 9, 1416, and 21) and parainfluenza virus (type 14) each cause 5% of cases of pharyngitis.
     d. Other common viral causes include influenza virus (A and B), herpes simplex virus (1 and 2), and coxsackievirus A and B.
     e. Epstein-Barr virus (EBV) and cytomegalovirus (CMV) can produce pharyngitis that is difficult to distinguish clinically from GABHS.
     f. With few exceptions, such as **infectious mononucleosis**, viral pharyngitis tends to develop after rhinitis.
       - About 50% of people with rhinovirus or coronavirus colds have a scratchy, sore throat.
       - Similarly, 50% to 80% of those with influenza A, parainfluenza, or adenovirus have significant pharyngeal discomfort.
       - In adults with viral pharyngitis, fever and cough tend to be absent. Edema and redness of the pharynx are usual, but the degree of exudate is less effusive than in GABHS. (For more information, see Chapter 9, "Infectious Mononucleosis.")
   3. **Bacterial causes of pharyngitis:** GABHS is the most important agent in acute pharyngitis because of its ability to produce local suppurative disease such as peritonsillar abscess, overwhelming systemic illness such as toxic shock, and the non-suppurative sequelae of ARF and AGN. The throat and skin are favorite targets for infection with GABHS because of host-dependent receptor sites. The streptococcal M protein is the key to the communality of this organism and its link to ARF. The structure of all M proteins is strikingly similar to myocardial muscle protein. Antibodies to M proteins therefore cross-react with myocardial cells, resulting in carditis.
     a. **Epidemiology of GABHS:** In the first 2 years of life, pharyngitis is rare. ARF does not occur in infants younger than 2 years. As many as 30% of school

Table 6-4. Microbial causes of acute pharyngitis

Agent	Syndrome or disease	Estimated occurrence
Bacterial		
Group A B-hemolytic *Streptococcus* (*S. pyogenes*)		
Pharyngitis/tonsillitis		15–30
Group C B-hemolytic *Streptococcus*	Pharyngitis/tonsillitis	1–5
Neisseria gonorrhoeae	Pharyngitis	<1
Arcanobacterium haemolyticum	Pharyngitis, rash	<1
Corynebacterium diphtheriae	Diphtheria	<1
Mixed anaerobic infection	Pharyngitis, gingivitis (Vincent's angina)	<1
Francisella tularensis	Oropharyngeal tularemia	<1
Viral		
Rhinovirus (100 types)	Common cold	20
Coronavirus (4 or more types)	Common cold	≥5
Adenovirus (types 3, 4, 7, 14, 21)	Pharyngoconjunctival fever, acute respiratory disease	5
Herpes simplex viruses (types 1 and 2)	Gingivitis, stomatitis, pharyngitis	4
Parainfluenza viruses (types 1–4)	Common cold, croup	2
Influenza viruses (types A and B)	Influenza	2
Coxsackieviruses (types 2, 4–6, 8, 10)	Herpangina	<1
Epstein-Barr virus	Infectious mononucleosis	<1
Cytomegalovirus	Infectious mononucleosis	<1
Other		
Mycoplasma pneumoniae	Pneumonia, bronchitis, pharyngitis	
Chlamydia pneumoniae	Pneumonia, bronchitis, pharyngitis	<1
Unknown		40

From Jensen HB, Baltimore RS, *Pediatric infectious disease: Principle and practice*, 2nd ed. Philadelphia, PA: W.B. Saunders; 2002:712, with permission.

children carry streptococci in their throats each winter, yet a bout of significant GABHS occurs, on the average, only about every 4 years for each child. The peak occurrence of GABHS is late winter and early spring.
  b. **Clinical presentation of GABHS:** After an incubation period of 2 to 5 days, patients develop the sudden onset of sore throat, painful swallowing, chills, and fever up to 40.5°C (104.9°F).
      Headache, nausea, vomiting, and abdominal pain are common. There is marked erythema of the throat and tonsils, accompanied by patchy, discrete tonsillar exudate. There are usually enlarged, tender, anterior cervical lymph nodes, uvular edema, and sometimes a typical scarlet fever rash or palatal petechiae. An initial white strawberry tongue denudes to become a classic red strawberry tongue.
      Untreated GABHS pharyngitis is short-lived, rarely lasting longer than 5 to 6 days. The appropriate antibiotic speeds recovery to 1 to 3 days.
  c. **Diagnosis of GABHS:** Throat culture on a sheep blood agar plate remains the most effective method for diagnosis of GABHS. The plate can be read in 24 hours. A positive culture shows beta hemolysis, a ring of inhibition around a bacterium disc placed on the agar. Rapid streptococcal antigen detection kits are approximately 90% specific (true negatives) and 60% to 80% sensitive (true positives). Rapid streptococcal kits cost between $2 and $4 each and take about 20 minutes to read.
  d. **Treatment of GABHS:** Definitive treatment for adolescents is penicillin V 500 mg two to three times daily for 10 days. GABHS is most often sensitive to penicillin. Clinical improvement is seen in 24 to 72 hours. A 10-day regimen of penicillin V is strongly recommended because recovery of the organism from

the throat may last as long as 7 days of treatment. The 10-day course is recommended to prevent ARF. Intramuscular benzathine penicillin G, 1.2 million units for those over 60 pounds, is also a recommended therapy.

Amoxicillin, 500 mg twice per day for 10 days, is an acceptable alternative to penicillin. For those allergic to penicillin, erythromycin up to 1 gram per day in two to four divided doses for 10 days is recommended. Clarithromycin and azithromycin are alternative macrolide antibiotics acceptable for the treatment of GABHS, although these antibiotics are considerably more expensive than erythromycin.

Up to 50% of children and adolescents with sore throats and culture positive GABHS do not have serologic evidence of streptococcal infection and may be "carriers" of GABHS. The failure rate of penicillin treatment for carriers is quite high. Carriers of GABHS are thought to be at low risk for developing ARF. The treatment for carriers of GABHS includes oral clindamycin or a mixture of amoxicillin and clavulanic acid plus rifampin, along with a 10 day course of penicillin V.

IV.   **Clinical pearls and pitfalls:**
- Acute nasopharyngitis (pharyngitis with nasal symptoms) is almost always of viral etiology. Pharyngitis without nasal symptoms is more likely to be bacterial.
- Small, ulcerative lesions of the soft palate, uvula and pharyngeal wall are most often caused by an enterovirus.
- A reasonable approach to diagnosing streptococcal pharyngitis is to perform a rapid test. If the rapid test is positive, specific therapy should be instituted. If the rapid test is negative, a routine culture is performed and therapy is withheld pending the culture results.
- In all instances of acute pharyngitis, ruling out streptococcal disease is mandatory.
- The ampicillin (or amoxicillin) "rash" associated with oral use or intramuscular injection (IM) is not a hypersensitivity reaction.

ACUTE UNCOMPLICATED PNEUMONIA

I.   **Description of the condition:** Acute, uncomplicated pneumonia, also known as community acquired pneumonia (CAP), is defined as pneumonia acquired outside the hospital setting.

    A. **Epidemiology:** Although the incidence of pneumonia with specific pathogens is not well-defined for the adolescent population with CAP, the estimated annual incidence of CAP in older children and adolescents is six to twelve cases per 1,000.

    B. **Etiology:** The specific pathogens thought to be the most common cause of pneumonia in the adolescent population are:
- *Streptococcus pneumonia*
- *Mycoplasma pneumonia*
- *Chlamydia pneumonia*
- *Influenza viruses.*

Table 6-5 lists the common etiologic agents of pneumonia in adolescents and the most common presenting signs and symptoms.

II.   **Making the diagnosis:**

    A. **Clinical manifestations:** The signs and symptoms of pneumonia are variable and depend on the causative organism and when in the course of illness the patient is seen. If the adolescent has a fever, cough, and increased respiratory rate, the diagnosis of pneumonia must be considered. Abdominal pain may be a presenting symptom. It is often difficult to distinguish viral and bacterial pneumonia in adolescents on the basis of clinical and radiographic findings.

Table 6-5. Microbial causes of CAP in adolescents

Etiologic agent	Clinical features
1. *Mycoplasma pneumoniae*	1. The major cause of pneumonia in adolescents. Radiographic appearance variable.
2. *Chlamydia pneumonia*	2. An important cause of pneumonia in older children and adolescents.
3. *Streptococcus pneumoniae*	3. Most often the cause of lobar pneumonia.
4. Viruses – Influenza A & B adenovirus	4. Often indistinguishable from early stages of other causes of pneumonia.

Table 6-6. Outpatient antimicrobial therapy for common pneumonias in adolescents

Drug	Suspected etiologic agent
1. Oral azithromycin 500 mg p in 1 dose followed by 250 mg on days 2–5 *or* oral clarithromycin XL 1,000 mg/d in 1 dose for 10 days	1. *Mycoplasma pneumonia* 2. *Chlamydia pneumonia* 3. *Streptococcal pneumonia*

III. **Treatment of pneumonia:** Table 6-6 lists the antibiotics of choice for the common etiologic agents causing pneumonia in adolescents.

IV. **Clinical pearls and pitfalls:**
- *Streptococcus pneumoniae, Mycoplasma pneumonia,* and *Chlamydia pneumoniae* are the major treatable causes of pneumonia in children 10 or older.
- *M. pneumoniae* account for 50% or more of pneumonias during adolescence.
- *M. pneumoniae* are among the smallest free-living organisms, have no cell walls, and are thus resistant to β-lactam antibiotics.
- The three most common causes of CAP in adolescents are sensitive to the macrolide antibiotics.

BIBLIOGRAPHY

American Academy of Pediatrics. Clinical practice guideline: management of sinusitis. *Pediatrics* 2001;108(3):798–808.
Bisno AL, Gerber MA, Gwaltney JM, et al. Diagnosis and management of group a streptococcal pharyngitis: a practice guideline. *Clin Infect Dis* 1997;25:574–583.
Burg FS, Ingelfinger JR, Polin RA, et al. *Gellis and Kagan's current pediatric therapy.* Philadelphia, PA: W.B. Saunders, 2002:17.
Chernick V, Boat TF, Kendig EL. *Disorders of the respiratory tract in children,* 6th ed., Philadelphia, PA: W.B. Saunders, 1998.
Feigin RD, Cherry JD, Demmler GJ, et al. *Textbook of pediatric infectious disease.* Philadelphia, PA: Elsevier, 2004.
Gordon RC. Community-acquired pneumonia in adolescents. *Adolesc Med State Art Rev* 2000;11(3): 681–695.
Hammerschlag MR. Chlamydia trachomatis and Chlamydia pneumoniae in children and adolescents. *Pediatr Rev* 2004;25:43–51.
Neinstein LS, *Adolescent health care: A practical guide,* 3rd ed., Baltimore, MD: Williams & Wilkins, 1996.
Strasburger VS, Brown RT. *Adolescent medicine: A practical guide,* 2nd ed., Philadelphia, PA: Lippincott Williams & Wilkins, 1998.
Taussig LM, Landau LT. *Pediatric respiratory medicine,* St. Louis: Mosby, 1998.
Wald ER. Sinusitis. In *Ambulatory pediatric care,* 3rd ed. Dershewitz, RA, ed. Philadelphia, PA: Lippincott Williams & Wilkins, 1999.

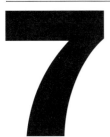

Asthma

I. **Description of the condition:**
   A. **Epidemiology:** Asthma, the most common chronic disease among children and adolescents, is a chronic inflammatory disease of the airways that has become a significant public health problem in terms of morbidity and mortality. Children and adolescents (ages 5–17) have the highest prevalence rates of asthma. In 2001, more than 6% of all children younger than 18 reported having an asthma attack.

   In 1999 asthma was responsible for 2 million emergency room visits and 478,000 hospitalizations with asthma as the primary diagnosis. In 2001 there were 4,269 deaths due to asthma. The highest death rate was among African-American females. The rates of hospitalization have remained the same or lower since 1980 for all age groups except children younger than 15 years. Death rates due to asthma have declined overall since 1995. Asthma mortality is nearly 3 times higher in African-American males than in white males and 2.5 times higher in African-American females than in white females.

   B. **Pathogenesis:** Asthma is a chronic inflammatory disorder of the airways in which many cells and cellular elements play a role, in particular, mast cells, eosinophils, T lymphocytes, neutrophils, and epithelial cells. In susceptible individuals, this inflammation causes recurrent episodes of wheezing, breathlessness, chest tightness and cough, particularly at night and in the early morning.

   Nocturnal awakening is a symptom of uncontrolled asthma. There is increased excretion of inflammatory mediators in conjunction with a decreased airway caliber at night in patients with nocturnal symptoms. These episodes are usually associated with widespread but variable airflow obstruction that is often reversible either spontaneously or with treatment. The inflammation also causes an associated increase in the existing bronchial hyper-responsiveness to a variety of stimuli. Treatment with anti-inflammatory drugs can, to a large extent, reverse some of these processes; however, the successful response to therapy often requires weeks to achieve and, in some situations, may be incomplete.

II. **Diagnosis of asthma:** Although adolescents with asthma may present in a variety of ways, most have certain common historical features and often asthma can be diagnosed on the basis of history alone.
   A. **Physical exam–auscultation during asthma exacerbation:** Expiratory airway obstruction usually is manifested by wheezing produced by airflow turbulence in the large airways below the thoracic inlet. Asthma can occur without wheezing if the obstruction involves small airways predominantly. Wheezing also occurs with inspiration when asthma worsens and may disappear altogether as obstruction becomes more severe and airflow is limited. Examination of the lungs frequently reveals coarse crackles or uneven breath sounds.

   Vocal cord dysfunction (VCD) syndrome should be considered in the differential diagnosis of the adolescent with wheezing who is apparently refractory to all therapy. In this condition, wheezing may occur on inspiration and expiration and is loudest over the central, anterior chest. VCD responds poorly to bronchodilator therapy, unless the patient has coexisting asthma.

   B. **Lung function tests:** Pulmonary function tests (PFTs) are objective, noninvasive, and extremely helpful in the diagnosis of asthma. Documentation of reversibility of airflow obstruction following inhalation of a bronchodilator is central to the definition of asthma. Spirometry, particularly the forced expiratory volume in 1 second (FEV_1), is considered the standard for assessing asthma severity and response to therapy. If airway obstruction is demonstrated on spirometry, a bronchodilating aerosol such as albuterol should be administered and spirometry should be repeated in 10 to 20 minutes. An improvement of at least 15% in the FEV_1 is indicative of asthma. Peak expiratory flow rates (PEF) can be measured in the office or clinic, emergency department, or the patient's home. PEF measure maximal expiratory flow generated at total lung capacity. PEF is an effort-dependent maneuver so the patient must be well instructed on the proper technique in order to obtain accurate results.

After optimal control of the patient's asthma, the adolescent's PEF "personal best" is established. A "zone" system, which is determined by the percentage of the patient's personal best, can be used to guide therapy. The "green" zone is usually 80% of the patient's personal best, the "yellow" zone is between 50% and 80%, and the "red" zone less than 50% and requires immediate emergency care.

III.   **Management of the patient with asthma:**
   A. **Medications:** The medications required to maintain long-term control of asthma are determined by the clinical features of the asthmatic patient before treatment or

Table 7-1. Stepwise approach to managing asthma in adults and children older than 5 years

Classify severity: clinical features before treatment or adequate control	Symptoms/day Symptoms/night	PEF or FEV$_1$ PEF Variability	Daily medications required to maintain long-term control
Step 4 (severe persistent)	Continual Frequent	<60% >30%	*Preferred treatment:* High-dose inhaled corticosteroids *and* long-acting inhaled β$_2$-agonists *and, if needed* corticosteroid tablets or syrup long term (2 mg/kg/d, generally do not exceed 60 mg/d). Make repeat attempts to reduce systemic corticosteroids and maintain control with high-dose inhaled corticosteroids.
Step 3 (moderate persistent)	Daily >1 night/wk	>60%–<80% >30%	*Preferred treatment:* Low-to-medium dose inhaled corticosteroid and long-acting inhaled β$_2$-agonists. *Alternative treatment (listed alphabetically):* Increase inhaled corticosteroids within medium-dose range *or* low-to-medium dose inhaled corticosteroids and either leukotriene modifier or theophylline if needed (particularly in patients with recurring severe exacerbations). *Preferred treatment:* Increase inhaled corticosteroids within medium-dose range and add long-acting inhaled β$_2$-agonists *Alternative treatment:* Increase inhaled corticosteroids within medium-dose range and add either leukotriene modifier or theophylline.
Step 2 (mild persistent)	>2/wk but <1X/d >2 nights/mo	>80% 20%–30%	*Preferred treatment:* Low-dose inhaled corticosteroids *Alternative treatment (listed alphabetically):* cromolyn, leukotriene modifier, nedocromil, *or* sustained release theophylline to serum concentration of 5–15 μg/mL

(continued)

Table 7-1. *(Continued)*

Classify severity: clinical features before treatment or adequate control	Symptoms/day Symptoms/night	PEF or FEV$_1$ PEF Variability	Daily medications required to maintain long-term control
Step 1 (mild Intermittent)	≤2 d/wk ≤nights/mo	≥80% <20%	No daily medications needed. Severe exacerbations may occur, separated by long periods of normal lung function and no symptoms. A course of systemic corticosteroids is recommended.
Quick relief			Short acting bronchodilator: 2–4 puffs
For all patients			Short-acting inhaled β$_2$ agonists as needed for symptoms. Intensity of treatment will depend on severity of exacerbation; up to three treatments at 20-min intervals or a single nebulizer treatment as needed. Course of systemic corticosteroids may be needed. Use of short-acting β$_2$ agonists >2 times

PEF, peak expiratory flow rates.

The stepwise approach is meant to assist, not replace, the clinical decision making required to meet individual patient needs.

To classify severity, assign patient to most severe step in which any feature occurs. PEF is % of personal best; FEV$_1$ is % predicted.

Gain control as quickly as possible (consider a short course of systemic corticosteroids). Then step down to the least medication necessary to maintain control.

Provide education on self-management and controlling environmental factors that make asthma worse (e.g., allergens and irritants).

Refer to an asthma specialist if there are difficulties controlling asthma or if step 4 care is required. Referral may be considered if step 3 care is required.

Step down: Review treatment every 1 to 6 months. A gradual stepwise reduction in treatment may be possible.

Step up: If control is not maintained, consider step up. First, review patient medication technique, adherence, and environmental control.

Adapted from NAEPP Expert Panel Report. Guidelines for the diagnosis and management of asthma: Update on selected topics 2002. Report available at http://www.nhlbi.nih.gov/guidelines/asthma (accessed 10/12/02).

adequate control (see Tables 7-1 and 7-2). Table 7-3 gives the estimated comparative daily dosages for **inhaled** corticosteroids.

B. **Environmental modification:** One of the most important nonpharmacologic interventions in asthma control measures is the identification of environmental triggers.

Indoor hazards include possible allergens such as dust mites, cat or dog dander, molds, and cockroach antigens. Measures such as dust covers over bedding, adequate and clean room air filters, removal of carpets or drapes, and low humidity may reduce allergen exposure. Outdoor allergens may include a wide variety of grasses, pollens, trees, or molds. Irritants in the environment that can contribute to increased asthma symptoms include cigarette smoke, strong chemical odors, perfumes, and the

Table 7-2. Usual dosages for long-term-control medications

Medication	Dosage form	Adult dose	Child dose[a]
Inhaled corticosteroids (see estimated comparative daily dosages for inhaled corticosteroids)			
Systemic corticosteroids			
Methylprednisolone	2,4,8,16, 32 mg tablets	7.5–60 mg daily in a single dose	0.25–2.0 mg/kg daily in a single dose in a.m. or q.i.d as needed for control

(continued)

Table 7-2. *(Continued)*

Medication	Dosage form	Adult dose	Child dose[a]
		Short-course "burst" to achieve control 40–60 mg/d as single or two divided doses for 3–10 d	Short course "burst": 1–2 mg/kg/d, maximum 60 mg/d for 3–10 d
Prednisolone	5 mg.tablets, 5 mg/5 mL, 15 mg/5 mL	See above	See above
Prednisone	1,2.5,5,10,20, 50 mg	See above	See above

Long-acting Inhaled β₂ agonists (should not be used for symptom relief or for exacerbations; use with inhaled corticosteroids)

Salmeterol	MDI 21 μg/puff	2 puffs q 12 h	1-2 puffs q 12 h
	DPI 50 μg/blister	1 blister q 12 h	1 blister q 12 h
Formoterol	DPI 12 μg/single-use capsule	1 capsule q 12 h	1 capsule q 12 h

Combined medication

Fluticasone-salmeterol	DPI 100, 250, or 500 μg/ 50 μg	1 inhalation b.i.d.; dose depends on severity of asthma.	1 inhalation b.i.d.; dose depends on severity of asthma.

Cromolyn and Nedocromil

Cromolyn	MDI 1 mg/puff	204 puffs t.i.d.-q.i.d.	1-2 puffs t.i.d.-q.i.d.
	Nebulizer 20 mg/ampule	1 ampule t.i.d.-q.i.d.	1 ampule t.i.d.-q.i.d.
Nedocromil	MDI 1.75 mg/puff	2-4 puffs b.i.d.-q.i.d.	1-2 puffs b.i.d.-q.i.d.

Leukotriene modifiers

Montelukast	4 or 5 mg chewable 10 mg tablet	10 mg q.h.s.	4 mg q.h.s. (2–5 yr); 5 mg q.h.s. (6–14 yr) 10 mg. q.h.s. (>14 yr)
Zafirlukast	10 or 20 mg tablet	40 mg daily (20 mg tablet b.i.d.)	20 mg daily (7–11 yr)
Zileuton	300 or 600 mg tablet	2,400 mg daily (give tablets q.i.d.)	

Methylxanthines (serum monitoring is important [serum concentration of 5–15 μg/mL at steady state])

Theophylline	Liquids, sustained release tablets, and capsules	Starting dose 10 mg/kg/d up to 300 mg. max; usual max 800 mg/d	Starting dose 10 mg/kg/d; usual max: 16 mg/kg/d

DPI, dry powder inhaler; MDI, metered dose inhaler.
[a]Children younger than 12 years of age.
Adapted from NAEPP Expert Panel Report. Guidelines for the diagnosis and management of asthma: Update on selected topics 2002. Report available at http://www.nhlbi.nih.gov/guidelines/asthma (accessed 10/12/02).

Table 7-3. Estimated comparative daily dosages for inhaled corticosteroids

Drug	Low daily dose		Medium daily dose		High daily dose	
	Adult	Child[a]	Adult	Child[a]	Adult	Child[a]
Beclomethasone CFC 42 or 84 μg/puff	168–504 μg	84–336 μg	504–840 μg	336–672 μg	>840 μg	>672 μg
Beclomethasone HFA 40 or 80 μg/puff	80–240 μg	80–160 μg	240–480 μg	160–320 μg	>480 μg	>320 μg
Budesonide DPI 200 μg/inhalation	200–600 μg	200–400 μg	600–1200 μg	400–800 μg	>1200 μg	>800 μg
Inhalation suspension for nebulization (child dose)		0.5 mg		1.0 mg		2.0 mg
Flunisolide 250 μg/puff	500–1000 μg	500–750 μg	1000–2000 μg	1000–1250 μg	>2000 μg	>1250 μg
Fluticasone MDI: 44,110,or 220 μg/puff	88–264 μg	88–176 μg	264–660 μg	176–440 μg	>660 μg	>440 μg
DPI: 50,100, or 250 μg/ inhalation	100–300 μg	100–200 μg	300–600 μg	200–400 μg	>600 μg	>400 μg
Triamcinolone acetonide 100 μg/puff	400–1000 μg	400–800 μg	1000–2000 μg	800–1200 μg	>2000 μg	>1200 μg

MDI, metered dose inhaler; DPI, dry powder inhaler.
[a]Children younger than 12 years of age.
Adapted from NAEPP Expert Panel Report. Guidelines for the diagnosis and management of asthma: Update on selected topics 2002. Report available at http://www.nhlbi.nih.gov/guidelines/asthma (accessed 10/12/02).

use of wood-burning stoves. Evaluation by an allergist to determine specific allergen avoidance may be helpful in establishing a trigger-free environment. Allergen immunotherapy is beneficial in a selected group of patients with allergy-based asthma.

C. **Exercise-induced asthma:** Exercise-induced asthma (EIA) is defined as transient narrowing of the airway that follows vigorous exercise. In healthy individuals the fall in FEV_1 is less than 5%. In patients with EIA the fall in FEV_1 with exercise is 10% to 15%. In patients with EIA, the drop in lung function may be manifested as cough, shortness of breath, wheezing, or inability to perform physical activities and exercise. EIA occurs in 70% to 90% of patients with persistent asthma and 10% of the general population.

See Table 7-4 for controlling EIA.

D. **Goals of therapy for asthma:**
- Minimal or no chronic symptoms day or night.
- Minimal or no exacerbations.
- No limitations on activities and no school or work missed.
- Maintain (near) normal pulmonary function.
- Minimal use of short acting inhaled β_2 agonist (<1 per day, <1 canister per month).
- Minimal or no adverse effects from medication.

IV. **Clinical pearls and pitfalls:**
- Asthma is the most common chronic disease among adolescents and has the highest prevalence rate among children and adolescents ages 5 to 17.
- Asthma is a chronic inflammatory disorder of the airways.
- Nocturnal awakening is a symptom of uncontrolled asthma.
- Vocal cord dysfunction should be considered in the differential of the adolescent who does not respond to therapy.

Table 7-4. Controlling exercise-induced asthma

Step	Measure
1	Control environmental conditions (use mask in cold weather; indoor exercise)
	Breathe through nose
	If not controlled, go to step 2 measures.
2	Use inhaled β-agonists or mast-cell stabilizers
	Short acting: albuterol 2–4 puffs 15–20 min before exercise
	Long acting: salmeterol 2 puffs MDI (or 1 puff DPI) 60 minutes before exercise; formoterol DPI 1 puff 15–30 minutes before exercise
	Cromolyn sodium or nedocromil sodium 2 puffs 15–20 min before exercise (mild EIA)
	If not controlled, go to step 3 measures.
3	Cromolyn or nedocromil 21 puffs in conjunction with β-agonist *or*
	Leukotriene inhibitor or antagonist (zileuton, montelukast, zafirlukast) 1 hour before exercise *or*
	Sustained release theophylline or inhaled corticosteroid on a regular basis if not already part of daily asthma management program
	If not controlled by step 3 measures, refer for evaluation.

DPI, dry powder inhaler; MDI, metered dose inhaler.
Adapted from Randolph CD. Exercise-induced asthma, part 2: Treatment options. *J Respire Dis* 2002;23:423–432; and Marks JH, Homnick DN. Opening the door to exercise for teens with chronic pulmonary disease. *Contemp Pediatr* 2002;19:71.

- Pulmonary function testing or eucapnic hyperventilation is needed to confirm the diagnosis of asthma by documenting reversibility of airflow obstruction following inhalation of a bronchodilator.
- Environmental modifications are often needed to be made to help control asthma.
- If adequate control of the patient is not maintained, first review patient mediation technique, adherence, and environmental control.

BIBLIOGRAPHY

Cabana MD, Slish KK, Lewis TC, et al. Parental management of asthma triggers within a child's environment. *J Allergy Clin Immunol* 2004;114:352–357.

Flores G, Abrew M, Chausson CE, et al. Keeping children out of hospitals: parent's and physicians' perspectives on how pediatric hospitalizations for ambulatory care-sensitive conditions can be avoided. *Pediatrics* 2003;112:1201–1230.

Guill MF. Asthma update: Epidemiology and pathophysiology. *Pediatr Rev* 2004;25:299–305.

Asthma update: Clinical aspects and management. *Pediatr Rev* 2004;25:335–344.

Rosenstreich DL, Eggleston P, Kahan M, et al. The role of cockroach allergy and exposure to cockroach allergen in causing morbidity among inner-city children with asthma. *N Engl J Med.* 1997;336:1356.

US Department of Health and Human Services. *Expert Panel Report Guidelines for the Diagnosis and Management of Asthma Education and Prevention Program.* NIH Publication. No. 02-5074, 2003.

Weiss ST, Horner A, Shapiro G, et al. The prevalence of environmental exposure to perceived asthma triggers in children with mild-to-moderate asthma: data from the Childhood Asthma Management Program. (CAMP). *J Allergy Clin Immunol* 2001;107:634–640.

Williams SG, Schmidt DK, Redd SC. Key clinical activities for quality asthma care. Recommendations of the national asthma education and prevention program. *MMWR Recomm Rep.* 51RR-6:2003.

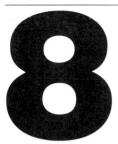

Acne

I. **Description of the condition:**

  A. Epidemiology: Acne is a nearly universal affliction of adolescents, with an incidence approaching 80% to 90% (Table 8-1). To the average teenager, however, acne has a tremendous impact on his or her sense of well-being. Given adolescents' normal self-consciousness about themselves and their appearance, it is extremely important to help them deal with this disorder. In one study, 58% of adolescents with acne were upset with their appearance, 75% felt embarrassed, and more than half were socially inhibited. Teens with acne are more likely to be depressed, suffer from lower self-esteem, or withdraw socially compared with their clear-complexioned peers.

  Clinicians need to realize how crucial this disorder is and also how treating it can establish an immediate and long-lasting rapport with adolescent patients.

  Few teens will actually go to see a clinician for treatment for their acne. Instead, they spend more than $100 million per year on less than effective over-the-counter preparations. Primary care providers can treat approximately 90% of teenagers with acne, leaving only those with severe nodular or cystic acne for referral. Early treatment can prevent permanent **scarring** (Figure 8-1). Males tend to have worse acne than do females due to their higher levels of androgen.

  B. Clinical features: Acne is a skin disorder characterized by a variety of different lesions—comedones, papules, pustules, nodules, cysts, and scars—that can appear on the face, chest, and back, typically during adolescence. Not all forms of acne are necessarily associated with adolescence.

  C. Etiology: Acne typically occurs in adolescents because of androgenic stimulation of the sebaceous glands that are most numerous on the face, upper chest, and upper back. The exact pathogenesis of acne is unclear. Nevertheless, a multifactorial theory helps to explain the disorder and how different medications work (Figure 8-2).

  The disease originates in the **pilosebaceous apparatus,** which is a rudimentary hair follicle better explained to patients as a "pore." Each pilosebaceous duct is lined with epidermal cells, which, in acne patients, are abnormally sticky because of faulty keratinization. This makes the follicle more likely to plug. Under androgenic stimulation, sebaceous glands empty more sebum into the follicle as well. **Sebum** is a viscous, complex mixture of triglycerides, waxy esters, and other lipids. The sebum excretion rate is influenced by both heredity and androgens and is elevated in patients with acne, but it is not completely predictive of acne severity.

  Androgens also cause enlargement of the sebaceous glands and an increase in the density of *Proprionibacterium acnes,* a gram-positive anaerobe normally found in the skin. A rise in androgenic hormones may be the first endocrinologic sign of puberty; therefore, females as young as 8 or 9 years can develop acne. Earlier development

Table 8-1. Acne myths

1. Acne is caused or exacerbated by
   - Chocolate
   - Fried foods
   - Too much or too little sex
2. Only dermatologists can treat acne.
3. Blackheads are caused by dirt.
4. Scrubbing blackheads will get rid of them.
5. Long-term treatment with tetracycline is dangerous.
6. Acne is part of adolescence and will go away on its own.
7. All teenagers with acne need to take Accutane.

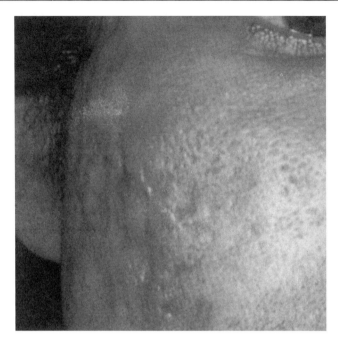

Figure 8-1. Keloidal and atrophic "ice-pick" scarring in a male teenager. Once they develop, such scars are difficult to eradicate, even with newer techniques. (From Hurwitz S. *Clinical pediatric dermatology*, 2nd ed. Philadelphia, PA: W.B. Saunders, 1993:140. Used with permission from Elsevier Science.)

of comedonal acne is predictive of later, more severe acne and seems to correlate with higher levels of dehydroepiandrosterone sulfate (DHEAS) and testosterone. A girl who develops acne at a relatively young age needs to be screened for disorders with androgen excess (e.g., a free testosterone level, a DHEAS level, and a determination of the LH/FSH ratio).

This initial lesion—the **microcomedone**—consists of keratin, sebum, and bacteria, particularly *P. acnes*. This is a blocked follicle (normally, sebum and other products of bacterial metabolism flow out of the follicle, giving the surface of the skin its oily feel). If the follicle's opening to the skin is tight, then the lesion is a closed comedone or

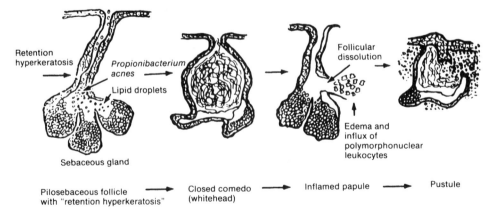

Figure 8-2. One comprehensive theory of the pathogenesis of acne. (From Hurwitz S. Acne vulgaris: Current concepts of pathogenesis and treatment. *Am J Dis Child* 1979;133:536–544. Copyright © 1979, American Medical Association. Reprinted with permission.)

"whitehead." If the pore opening is wide, then it is an open comedone or "**black-head**." "Blackheads" are relatively inert, with no back-pressure phenomenon and can be extruded simply by use of an eyedropper. Their blackness probably derives from melanin, not from dirt or surface oxidation. Although "whiteheads" look less objectionable than "blackheads," they potentially cause more trouble because they might rupture at the slightest provocation: if there is a slight increase in sebaceous material or if the skin is traumatized in any way (e.g., picking).

When this occurs, a cascade of events leads to inflammation and, occasionally, scarring as well. Once the thin follicular wall has ruptured, sebum escapes into the surrounding dermis. *P. acnes* breaks the triglycerides down into free fatty acids, which are extremely irritating to the skin. The inflammatory pathway is activated, complete with an influx of polymorphonuclear cells (PMNs) and activation of the complement pathway. Inflammation does not depend on follicular rupture, however. Proinflammatory substances can be released through the intact follicular wall, producing **papulopustules**. PMNs can then release hydrolytic enzymes, which increase duct permeability and lead to rupture and formation of pustules. Unfortunately, once inflammation occurs in the dermis, scarring may occur.

D. **Contributing factors:** Severe acne tends to have a genetic predisposition. Just as endogenous androgenic disorders may present with severe acne, exogenous androgens such as more androgenic oral contraceptive pills might make acne worse. Even the normal progesterone produced in the secretory phase of the menstrual cycle can result in premenstrual flares because the size of individual follicles actually decreases.

Other important factors may include:

- **Immunologic factors.** Tetracycline decreases neutrophil chemotaxis, which helps to explain its usefulness in treatment.
- **Mechanical factors.** Oil-based cosmetics will help to increase the blockage of follicles, thus worsening acne.
- **Climatic factors.** Sunny dry climates aid acne patients. Whether this is an effect of ultraviolet light or diminished stress is not known.
- **Genetic factors.** Patients with XYY genotypes often suffer from severe acne.
- **Stress and emotional factors.** Stress is a well-known cause of acne exacerbations, although the mechanism for this is not clear. Conversely, acne can cause stress, depression, anxiety, and social withdrawal.
- **Diet.** Excellent, controlled, double-blinded trials have demonstrated that large doses of chocolate, or other suspect foods, will not cause or exacerbate acne. However, if a teenager is convinced that a certain food makes her "break out," then certainly that food should be avoided.

E. **Presentation:** Acne can present as early as age 8 to 9 in girls or 10 to 11 in boys. It is broadly classified as being either noninflammatory or inflammatory but, in fact, the first category can shade into the second (see Table 8-2).

II. **Management:**

A. **Primary goals:** Early treatment of acne is essential to prevent scarring. Clinicians need to recognize that teenagers usually will *not ask* for anything to treat their acne, since they usually will be using over-the-counter medicines. However, an offer to prescribe superior medicines is often welcomed. Another underlying message for the teenager is that the doctor really cares. A coordinated plan is required, including prescribing the correct medications, counseling, and guidance about contributory factors. As one acne expert states, "Treatment failure is doctor failure." Experience with only a few drugs is all that is required (Table 8-3). The physician's arsenal is

---

Table 8-2. Classification of acne

Noninflammatory acne:
Comedonal
Papular

Transitional acne:
Papulopustular

Inflammatory acne:
Pustular
Nodulocystic

Table 8-3. Treatment of acne

Noninflammatory acne (comedonal or papular)	Benzoyl peroxide 2.5%–5% aqueous gel at bedtime *or* Retin-A 0.025%–0.05% cream at bedtime
Inflammatory papules (papulopustular)	Add: T-stat or Cleocin-T once or twice a day, begin tetracycline 500–1,000 mg twice a day if >4 pustules
Inflammatory acne (pustular)	Benzoyl peroxide 2.5%–5% aqueous gel in the morning *plus* Retin-A 0.025–0.05% cream or 0.025% gel at bedtime T-stat or Cleocin-T twice a day Tetracycline, 500–1,000 mg twice a day (Consider Azelex 20% cream twice a day instead of benzoyl peroxide and Retin-A if pustules or scars are hyperpigmented.)
Inflammatory acne with scarring (nodulocystic)	Candidate for Accutane. Begin treatment for pustular acne and immediately refer to a dermatologist.

far more powerful than what is available over-the-counter. Unfortunately, *there is no predicting when pustular lesions will scar.* Early treatment, especially of noninflammatory acne, is essential and is one of the most important preventative measures for adolescents.

B. Medications (Table 8-3): Many mainstays of acne treatment have been around for decades (e.g., benzoyl peroxide, tetracycline). Newer products tend to be more expensive and may not be included in a given formulary (e.g., BenzaClin, Differin, Azelex). Also the vehicle is nearly as important as the drug. It is important to minimize the drying effects of many agents. Therefore, medications in a water base may be preferable to those in an alcohol or acetone base. In addition, gels have greater penetrating power than creams or lotions, but they are more drying.

1. Mainstays: Benzoyl peroxide. Benzoyl peroxide is one of the foundations of acne treatment. It is an irritant that inhibits triglyceride hydrolysis, reduces free fatty acids, and functions as a topical antiseptic, eliminating as much as 95% of *P. acnes* within 5 days of twice-daily use. It comes in the form of a cream, lotion, wash, or gel, in concentrations of 2.5%, 5%, or 10%. Often, patients have been using an over-the-counter lotion, cream, or wash. Even a 10% lotion will not be as effective as a 2.5% prescription gel—an important point to emphasize to patients. The 2.5% gel is as effective against *P. acnes* as the 10% gel but is considerably less irritating and drying. Commonly used preparations can be seen in Table 8-4.

Benzoyl peroxide is synergistic with tretinoin (Retin-A): one can be used in the evening, the other in the morning. Benzoyl peroxide also can be combined with topical antibiotics (with 1% clindamycin, to make BenzaClin and Duac; with 3% erythromycin, to make Benzamycin). Patients who are likely to be less compliant, or those with dry skin, may benefit from these combination preparations.

Counseling should accompany the first prescription of benzoyl peroxide. Since it is a bleaching agent, benzoyl peroxide also can discolor T-shirts, blouses, and sheets. Patients with oily skin can better tolerate the alcohol or acetone-based products. An initial test application on the forearm for a few hours will detect those rare patients who will have an allergic contact dermatitis to the drug. Initially, a

Table 8-4. Some benzoyl peroxide preparations

Alcohol or Acetone base	Water base
Benzagel	—
Benzac	Benzac-W
Desquam-X	Desquam-E
PanOxyl	PanOxyl Aq
Persa-Gel	Persa-Gel W
	Xerac

low concentration (2.5%–5%) is applied as a thin film to all acne-prone areas, beginning every other day or even every third day and building up within 2 to 3 weeks to once or twice daily usage. Because absorption is increased by moisture, preparations should never be applied immediately after washing one's face, nor should benzoyl peroxide be used simultaneously with any other preparation (only the combination products have been specifically formulated to be used together). Patients should always be told to expect some dryness and tingling, especially initially, and to decrease the frequency of application if this occurs.

Acne on the chest or back is usually easier to treat since there are more layers of stratum corneum and therefore less irritation or dryness. Hence, a 5% to 10% aqueous gel is a reasonable start.

Because of the risk of bacterial resistance, some dermatologists prefer to start treatment with benzoyl peroxide, switch to tretinoin after several weeks, then return to "pulsing" the benzoyl peroxide on weekends only.

Tretinoin or Vitamin A acid (Retin-A) is a powerful drug that is superior to benzoyl peroxide at times but requires careful instruction. It works via several mechanisms: increased cell turnover in the follicles, decreased stickiness of the epidermal cells lining the follicles, expulsion of existing comedones, and prevention of new lesions.

Retin-A works to clean out follicles that have been plugged, especially microcomedones. For this reason, patients may feel that they are "breaking out" more in the first week or two of using this product. Its full effect may take 2 to 3 months to occur. Also, because it increases cell turnover, Retin-A should be used cautiously in patients who have dry skin or who are poorly compliant.

Retin-A is available in many different preparations (Table 8-5) but most clinicians will need to prescribe only the 0.025% or 0.05% cream. The most recent reformulation is 0.04% Retin-A-Micro, which uses microsphere technology in an effort to achieve faster onset and milder impact. If it is available on formulary, Retin-A Micro may be preferable to the older preparations. Although it is expensive compared with benzoyl peroxide, a 20-g tube of Retin-A or Retin-A Micro should last at least a month or two, when used sparingly (Figure 8-3). Because of its potential to produce erythema, peeling, and dryness, small amounts should be used.

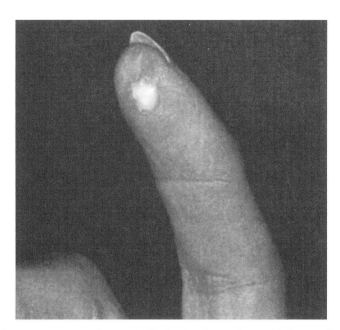

Figure 8-3. The proper amount of tretinoin (Retin-A) or benzoyl peroxide is a small, pea-sized dot. A dot can be used to cover an entire treatment area such as one cheek. (From Hurwitz S: *Clinical pediatric dermatology*, 2nd ed. Philadelphia, PA: W.B. Saunders, 1993:142. Copyright © 1993. Used with permission from Elsevier Science.)

Table 8-5. Potency of Retin-A preparations

Degree of irritation	Vehicle	Concentration
Lowest	Cream	0.025%
Cream		0.05%
Cream		0.1%
Gel		0.025%
Highest	Solution	0.05%

In most patients with comedonal acne, Retin-A is the drug of choice. For patients with inflammatory acne, it is an excellent drug used in combination with benzoyl peroxide and a topical or systemic antibiotic. Patients should be instructed never to apply Retin-A to wet skin and to wait at least 20 to 30 minutes after washing their faces before using it. In addition, they will need to use sunscreen with a sun protective factor (SPF) of 15 or greater during the summer or in sunny climates. Patients should begin using the lowest-strength preparation (0.025% cream) two or three times weekly, gradually increasing to every other night, then nightly, then twice daily if tolerated.

As with benzoyl peroxide, tretinoin has also been combined with clindamycin, in a 0.025% tretinoin/1% clindamycin formulation (Velac gel, currently under development by Connetics Corporation and probably available by late 2005).

Table 8-6. Cost of common acne medications

Drug	Formulation	Cost to patient
Oral antibiotics		
Tetracycline	500 mg PO b.i.d.	$ 8.29 (100, 250-mg capsules)
Doxycycline	100 mg PO b.i.d.	$12.69 (50)
Minocycline	100 mg PO b.i.d.	$47.79 (50)
Topical antibiotics		
Clindamycin		
Cleocin T (Upjohn)	1% solution (gel, lotion)	$51.99 (60 cc)
Erythromycin		
T-Stat (Westwood)	2% solution	$26.39 (60 cc)
Erycette (Ortho)	2% pledgets	$33.39 (60 pads)
Clindamycin +		
Benzoyl peroxide =		
BenzaClin (Dermik)	1%/5%	$72.99 (25 g)
Duac (Stiefel)	1%/5%	$135.99 (45 g)
Erythromycin +		
Benzoyl peroxide =		
Benzamycin (Dermik)	3%/5%	$137.27 (46.6 g)
Benzoyl peroxide		
Benzoyl peroxide (Glades)	2.5% aqueous gel	$14.99 (60 g)
Tretinoin		
Retin-A (Ortho)	0.025% cream	$84.59 (45 g)
Retin-A Micro (Ortho)	0.1% gel	$50.67 (20 g)
Adapalene		
Differin (Galderma)	0.1% gel	$41.99 (15 g)
Azelaic acid		
Azelex (Allergan)	20% cream	$52.29 (30 g)
Isotretinoin		
Accutane	40 mg PO b.i.d.	$917.98 (60)

Data from www.costco.com and www.walgreens.com (accessed 7/7/04).

2. Other drugs

Azelex. Azelex is 20% azelaic acid, which was approved for use by the Federal Drug Administration (FDA) in 1996. Azelex is an interesting drug in that it is a "natural" product, derived from wheat. It is comedolytic and may be useful in helping the violaceous hue of pustules and scars to fade. However, it takes several months to achieve this effect, and some patients find it unacceptably greasy. The cream is used twice a day and comes in 30-g tubes.

Differin. Differin is 0.1% adapalene gel, the first new topical retinoid in 25 years. As effective as 0.025% Retin-A gel, it is less irritating. If it is on the formulary, it may be preferable.

Tazorac. Tazorac is an acetylinic retinoid originally developed for treatment of psoriasis. It is available as a 0.1% gel or cream for treatment of acne; however, it may be more irritating than either Retin-A or Adapalene and is more expensive (Table 8-6).

3. Topical antibiotics:

For inflammatory acne, patients should use an antibiotic in conjunction with either benzoyl peroxide or Retin-A. Topical antibiotics include **clindamycin** and **erythromycin** (Table 8-7), which have the equivalent effect of 500 mg of their oral counterparts. They have the advantage of getting the medicine to the problem area immediately and so it is not necessary to wait for tissue levels to build up from an orally administered antibiotic. Topical solutions (or pads) are preferable, because they are less drying than gels. Both topicals inhibit the growth of *P. acnes* and decrease chemotaxis. Although a few cases of pseudomembranous colitis have been reported with the use of topical clindamycin, less than 5% of the drug is absorbed systemically; and Cleocin-T has now been used in millions of doses.

Some concern exists regarding drug-resistant strains of *P. acnes*. With erythromycin particularly, resistant strains may exceed 50% and are multiply resistant. For this reason, some dermatologists avoid the use of topical erythromycin except in combination with benzoyl peroxide (Benzamycin), or use short bursts of benzoyl peroxide to try to diminish resistance. Clindamycin seems to cause less resistance. Topical fluoroquinolones (1% nadifloxacin) and nicotinamines are being developed that may help with this problem.

As mentioned, benzoyl peroxide can be combined with topical antibiotics in formulations that are actually *less* irritating than benzoyl peroxide alone. Clindamycin and benzoyl peroxide are found in Duac and in BenzaClin. Erythromycin and benzoyl peroxide are in Benzamycin (Table 8-6). Benzamycin requires ethyl alcohol to compound it and must be kept refrigerated, so it is a little more difficult to use.

Recently, the complete genome of *P. acnes* was sequenced. This should allow the development of designer drugs for targeting the bacterium and could represent a major advance in combating acne.

Table 8-7. Topical antibiotics

Clindamycin
Cleocin-T 1% solution, gel, lotion, solution, pledgets
(Upjohn, Fougera, Greenstone, Clay Park Lab, Alpharma)
BenzaClin 1% gel with 5% benzoyl peroxide (Dermik)
Duac 1% gel with 5% benzoyl peroxide (Stiefel)

Erythromycin
T-Stat 2% solution, pads (Westwood)
T-Stat 2% solution (Barre-National, Fougera)
T-Stat 2% pledgets (Glaxo, Goldline, Glades)
Staticin 1.5% solution (Westwood)
Erycette 2% solution, pledgets (Ortho)
Eryderm 2% solution, gel (Abbott)
Erymax 2% solution, gel (Allergan)
Erygel 2% gel (Merz)
Emgel 2% gel (Glaxo)
A/T/S 1% and 2% solution, gel, lotion (Upjohn)
Aknemycin 2% ointment (HPM)
Benzamycin 3% gel with 5% benzoyl peroxide (Dermik)

4. **Systemic antibiotics:** If more than four pustules exist, a systemic antibiotic should be considered *in addition to* a topical antibiotic. Once the inflammation has been calmed, the oral dose can be tapered or eliminated if possible.

   For decades, **tetracycline** has been the mainstay of systemic treatment. Other antibiotics are active against *P. acnes* but are not nearly as well tolerated (e.g., erythromycin) or as safe (e.g., clindamycin). Even with long-term use, tetracycline remains one of the safest drugs in the formulary. It has been studied repeatedly, and no routine laboratory tests are required. Commonly, patients may experience an upset stomach. Tetracycline should be taken on an empty stomach (it is bound by milk or milk products). For these reasons, some dermatologists prefer **doxycycline**, although it is more photosensitizing. Occasionally, **candidal vaginitis results because of the impact of this broad-spectrum antibiotic on the normal vaginal lactobacilli**; but most patients seem to accommodate to long-term usage. Serious side effects are rare but include pseudotumor cerebri and erythema multiforme. Tetracycline is used in a dosage of 500 mg to 1,000 mg twice a day for 4 to 6 months and then gradually tapered to the lowest possible dose, often 250 mg to 500 mg once daily. Doxycycline is used in a dosage of 100 mg twice a day. Some dermatologists use a sub-antimicrobial dose of 20 mg twice a day to prevent resistance.

   Minocycline (Minocin) is an alternative that may penetrate the sebaceous follicle better and does not need to be taken on an empty stomach. It is used at a dose of 100 mg per day to 200 mg per day. However, it is considerably more expensive and has been associated with autoimmune hepatitis, a systemic lupus erythematosus-like syndrome, and increased skin pigmentation.

   If patients experience treatment failures with tetracycline, then erythromycin can be tried in a dosage of 500 mg twice a day with clindamycin (150 mg twice a day) or minocycline as back-ups.

5. **Hormonal therapy:** The use of oral contraceptives (OCPs) is now approved in the treatment of acne in female teenagers. OCPs affect acne by increasing levels of sex hormone-binding globulin, thereby decreasing free testosterone levels, and by suppressing gonadotropin secretion, thus reducing ovarian androgen production. The use of OCPs has the additional advantage of protecting teens against pregnancy if they are sexually active. In addition, OCPs often can diminish or even eliminate the need for topical medications.

   Since acne is exacerbated by androgens, the clinician needs to select an OCP that is predominantly estrogenic in effect (e.g., Desogen, Ortho Cyclen, Ortho Tri-Cyclen, Demulen). These pills contain weakly androgenic progestins (e.g., norethindrone, norgestimate), which allow the estrogen component to dominate. Although placebo-controlled studies have been done only with Ortho Tri-Cyclen according to all of the TV ads (Alesse has been studied but the results haven't yet been published), *any* estrogen-dominant/weak progestin pill can be used successfully. On the other hand, OCPs such as Ovral and Lo/Ovral with more androgenic progestins may worsen acne.

   OCPs are generally viewed as adjunctive therapy for acne, not as the primary drug of choice. However, in a patient who is noncompliant with topical medications or who is already sexually active, OCPs can be an excellent first-line drug. Combining OCPs with tetracycline is an ongoing dilemma: does tetracycline use make OCPs less effective in preventing pregnancy? Good data are not available so good counseling is essential.

   The contraceptive patch (Ortho Evra) uses norelgestromin, a weak progestin, but also has relatively low levels of estrogen, 20 mcg., compared with OCPs.

   Progestin-based contraceptives—Depo-Provera or Norplant—may worsen acne. Occasionally, girls with hyperandrogenic disorders may require treatment with agents such as spironolactone (an androgen antagonist). Spironolactone can be used in doses of 100 mg to 200 mg per day but may be effective in doses as low as 25 mg to 50 mg. Several months' worth of usage is required, however, to achieve an effect on acne; and teenagers must avoid pregnancy while taking the drug.

6. **Oral isotretinoin (Accutane):** Accutane, or 13-cis retinoic acid, is a vitamin A derivative that is indicated for the treatment of nodulo-cystic acne. Accutane totally obliterates the sebaceous gland's production of sebum for the duration of treatment. Originally approved in 1982 by the FDA, it was nearly removed from the market several years ago because isotretinoin is the most potent teratogen ever available as a prescription drug, and physicians were not prescribing it carefully.

In addition, there have been recent concerns about whether it causes or worsens depression. Given all of this, Accutane needs to be prescribed by dermatologists.

Accutane typically is prescribed for a 16 to 20 week course of treatment, at a cost of approximately $500 to $700. Even after the patient's sebum excretion rate returns to normal, his or her acne remains quiescent. Virtually all patients experience moderate to severe dryness of the face, lips, nasal mucosa, and conjunctivae. Epistaxis is common. Bone pain or chronic fatigue also is an occasional side effect (15% of patients). Blood tests, including a complete blood count (CBC), liver function tests, cholesterol, and triglycerides must be done periodically. Women require two negative pregnancy tests before beginning the drug and a monthly test thereafter. Accutane can cause extremely high levels of serum lipids, although no liver damage occurs and levels revert to normal once the Accutane is discontinued.

For most patients, an initial dose of 0.5 mg/kg/d to 1.0 mg/kg/d is used (40–80 mg/d). Lower doses can be effective and cause fewer side effects but may require repeat courses of treatment. Approximately 90% of patients will respond to an initial course but 10% to 25% may relapse and require re-treatment. Patients will require lip balm and an emollient and baking soda toothpaste.

Due to its teratogenicity, patients must sign a packet of forms attesting to their use of two forms of effective birth control (one medical and one barrier) during treatment and for at least 1 month before and after treatment. No teratogenic effects have ever been described for boys who go on to father children.

In regard to depression and suicide, only one study has examined this problem: no difference was found between controls and users in psychiatric diagnoses or suicide. Severe acne sufferers might experience *less* depression after their skin is effectively treated since many studies have found that severe acne in teens is strongly associated with depression.

   C. Acne surgery: In general, any patient with significant scarring, or with nodular cystic acne, warrants referral to a dermatologist. Dermatologists have experience in using intralesional corticosteroid injections to reduce the inflammation in nodules or cysts; nevertheless, patients sometimes develop scars from acne. A number of treatment options are available, but none are ideal and all usually require retreatment.

III.   **Clinical pearls and pitfalls:** Clinicians need to differentiate between noninflammatory and inflammatory acne, since the latter will require oral and/or topical antibiotics. If a teen has only comedonal or papular acne, offer him or her a choice between benzoyl peroxide (easier to use) and Retin-A (more difficult to use, with more side effects). The other can then be added at a later time, if needed. Avoid common mistakes in treating acne (Table 8-8). Other tips include

- Reassure the teenager that acne is very common and very treatable.
- Explain that prescription medications far exceed over-the-counter medications in efficacy.
- Explain that acne cannot be scrubbed away, nor are blackheads black because of dirt. Intense scrubbing may disrupt microcomedones. Care should be taken in washing the face, and gentle soaps should be used.
- Simplify the treatment regimen, especially at the first visit. More medications can always be added at a later date.
- Allow teenagers time to ask questions.
- Reassure teens that acne is not "their fault." It is not caused by too much fast food, chocolate, too much sex, or not enough sex.
- Remember to check and treat a teenager's back and chest.
- Give teenagers choices in medications and regimens, if possible.
- Be aware of the cost of medications (Table 8-6).

Table 8-8. Common mistakes in treating acne

1. Too little explanation and counseling
2. Too little concern
3. Too complex a medication regimen
4. Inappropriate use of:
   - X-ray treatment
   - Vaccines
   - Dietary manipulation

BIBLIOGRAPHY

For the clinician

Halder RM, Brooks HL, Callender VD. Acne in ethnic skin. *Dermatol Clin* 2003;21:609–615.

Hanna S, Sharma J, Klotz J. Acne vulgaris: more than skin deep. *Dermatol Online J* 2003;9(3):8. Available at www.dermatology.cdlib.org.

Institute for Clinical Systems Improvement (ICSI). *Acne management.* Bloomington, MN: Institute for Clinical Systems Improvement, 2003: Available at www.guildeline.gov or www.icsi.org.

James WD. Acne. *New Engl J Med* 2005;352:1463–1472.

Krowchuk DP, Luck AW. Managing adolescent acne. *Adolesc Med Clin* 2001;12:355–374.

Lee DJ, VanDyke GS, Kim J. Update on pathogenesis and treatment of acne. *Curr Opin Pediatr* 2003;15:405–410.

Leyden JJ. A review of the use of combination therapies for the treatment of acne vulgaris. *J Am Acad Dermatol* 2003;49(Suppl 3):S200–S210.

Sanfilippo AM, Barrio V, Kulp-Shorten C, et al. Common pediatric and adolescent skin conditions. *J Pediatr Adolesc Gynecol* 2003;16:269–283.

Stashwick C. Amenorrhea and acne in the adolescent girl: is it polycystic ovary syndrome? *Contemp Pediatr* 2000;17:118–129.

WEB SITES

www.aad.org American Academy of Dermatology
www.dermatology.cdlib.org Dermatology Online Journal

9

Infectious Mononucleosis

I. Description of the condition: Infectious mononucleosis (IM) is one of the most common and significant infections seen during adolescence. Clinicians often have misconceptions about how to diagnose and treat IM.

Not until 1968 was the Epstein-Barr virus (EBV) identified as the cause of IM. Because it is a protean viral infection, mono can have a bewildering array of presentations. The classic triad of fever, pharyngitis, and lymphadenopathy is well known, but patients do not always read the textbooks to see how they should present! Nor is EBV the only cause of an infectious mono-like syndrome (Table 9-1).

A. Epidemiology: EBV is a member of the Herpesviridae family, one which also includes herpes simplex, varicella zoster-virus, cytomegalovirus, and human herpes viruses 6 and 7. These are large DNA-containing enveloped viruses with the unique potential to become latent following primary infection and to immortalize the B-cells that they infect.

Incidence and prevalence. By adulthood, nearly 100% of adults possess antibodies to EBV. The majority of children in lower socioeconomic classes in the United States have experienced asymptomatic (or alternatively diagnosed) EBV infection by age 5. In middle- and upper-classes, the infection is often delayed until adolescence or young adulthood and is more likely to be symptomatic. The incidence of EBV-associated IM in the United States is estimated to be six to eight cases per 1,000 per year among teenagers and as high as 11 to 48 cases per 1,000 per year among college students. College freshmen who have not yet had EBV infection display a seroconversion rate of approximately 12% to 15% per year.

B. Etiology:

1. Transmission: EBV is not a very contagious virus because it is fragile and requires exposure to fresh bodily fluids. Thus, there are no confirmed epidemics of mono. Infection usually occurs by contact with oral secretions: nearly everyone who is seropositive is shedding the virus in their saliva, hence the moniker **"the kissing disease."** However, no evidence of aerosol transmission has ever been found.

2. Incubation period: Conventional wisdom is that the incubation period for EBV is 4 to 6 weeks.

3. Pathogenesis: EBV first infects and replicates in the oropharynx. There, the virus infects B-lymphocytes, which then disseminate the infection throughout the lymphoreticular system. Infected B-cells next induce proliferation of reactive T-cells, the so-called **atypical lymphocytes** seen in a peripheral blood smear. Enlarged lymph nodes, liver, and spleen are the result of increased numbers of both infected B cells and reactive T cells.

II. Making the diagnosis:

A. Signs and symptoms: Infectious mono is a common, benign, self-limited disease in 99% of adolescents. Typically, a viral prodrome appears, with gradual onset of:

- Headache
- Chills
- Sweating
- Malaise
- Anorexia
- Inability to concentrate
- Fever is often present and may remain for up to 5 weeks, with afternoon or evening peaks to 37.8°C to 39.5°C (100°F–103°F).

The "classic" presentation is the triad of fever, sore throat, and lymphadenopathy, but this description requires some elaboration. Any pharyngitis will usually involve the **anterior cervical nodes;** however, the lymph nodes that characterize infectious mono are the **posterior cervical nodes.** Other nodal groups can be involved in infectious mono, including hilar nodes and mesenteric nodes. The one nodal group *not* associated with EBV infection is the supraclavicular group: enlarged nodes here

63

Table 9-1. Differential diagnosis of mono syndromes

Etiology	Age group	Features
EBV	Mostly <25 yr	Persistent sore throat; lymphadenopathy, esp. post. cervical nodes, fever, hepatosplenomegaly, malaise; heterophil may be negative—do EBV-IGM antibody test if necessary.
Cytomegalovirus	Mostly >25 yr	Sore throat rare; minimal adenopathy; hepatosplenomegaly common
Toxoplasmosis	Any age	Sore throat rare; some lymphocytosis; exposure to cats or raw meat
Hepatitis A	Young adult	Sore throat, adenopathy, splenomegaly rare; fever before jaundice
Herpesvirus-6	Any age	EBV-like illness with atypical lymphs
Adenovirus	Child/Young adult	Respiratory symptoms usually prominent
Rubella	Childhood	With or without rash
HIV	Young adult	EBV-like prodrome

EBV, Epstein-Barr virus; HIV, human immunodeficiency virus; IGM, Immunoglobulin M.

indicate lymphoma until proven otherwise. Rarely, atypical lymphs on a peripheral smear will be so concerning that leukemia is considered as a diagnosis.

Besides the classic triad, other common presentations include:
- A persistent sore throat, especially one that seems unresponsive to antibiotics.
- Severe fatigue in the context of a preceding viral illness.
- Dysphagia.
- Prolonged high fever with mild pharyngitis and a delay in appearance of lymphadenopathy (typhoidal IM).
- Mild pharyngitis, low-grade fever, and lymphadenopathy disproportionate to the degree of pharyngitis (glandular IM).
- In one large, prospective study of 200 young adults, most patients had 1 to 2 days of malaise before the onset of a high fever. The symptoms continued until the fifth day of the illness, when sore throat and headache developed.

Because of its protean nature, IM can also present in a variety of unusual ways:
- Mesenteric adenopathy can cause abdominal pain.
- Axillary adenopathy can cause shoulder pain.
- Jaundice may occur in up to 5% of patients because of liver inflammation.
- Hemolytic anemia, aplastic anemia, or thrombocytopenia may be present.
- There are a wide variety of neurologic complications, including:
  - Encephalitis
  - Seizures
  - Guillain-Barre syndrome
  - Acute hallucinations ("Alice in Wonderland" syndrome, in which shapes and sizes are distorted)
  - Coma.

B. Examination: Clinicians who see a lot of teenage patients should always maintain a high index of suspicion for IM. The disease is somewhat milder in younger patients and in those with negative heterophil titers. Ideally, the diagnostic criteria include (Table 9-2):
- **Clinical:** Common symptoms include sore throat, posterior cervical lymphadenopathy, and fever. Significant physical findings include periorbital edema, splenomegaly, and palatal petechiae.
- **Laboratory:** Complete blood count shows at least 50% lymphocytes and monocytes (a **"right shift"**), with at least 10% atypical lymphocytes. Liver function tests are abnormal 80% to 90% of the time.
- **Serologic:** Monospot, heterophil antibody, or specific EBV antibody tests should be positive.

Diagnostic errors are common, especially because IM is a dynamic disease, with a changing clinical and laboratory pattern, and because the serologic tests are frequently misunderstood. Some helpful hints include:
- Understand the Monospot! It is a rapid slide test, designed to assess the presence of heterophil antibody. Meanwhile, heterophil antibody is *not specific for EBV infection, nor is it predictable* (Figure 9-1). It is an IgM antibody that the body manufactures

Table 9-2. Making the diagnosis of mono

Clinical:	
Maintain high index of suspicion in teenagers	Fever, sore throat, malaise
	Tonsillopharyngitis **80%**
	Lymphadenopathy, esp. posterior cervical
	Other findings:
	• Splenomegaly
	• Periorbital edema
	• Soft palate petechiae
Laboratory:	Lymphocytosis: >50% in differential WBC count, >4,500/mm^3 total
	Atypical lymphocytes: ≥10% total WBC count, >1,000/mm^3 total
	Mildly elevated liver function tests (80%–90% of patients)
Serologic:	Positive monospot or heterophil antibody
	Positive Epstein-Barr virus antibody test

WBC, white blood cell.

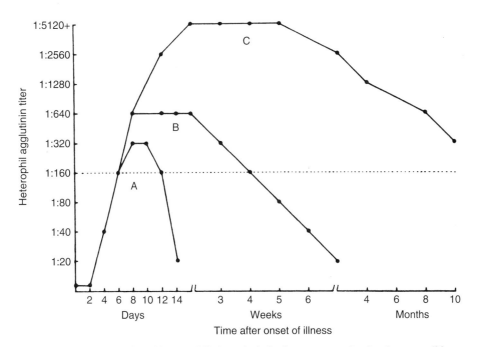

Figure 9-1. The rise and fall of heterophil titers in infectious mononucleosis: three possible patterns. Titers above the horizontal line are considered significant. Because of these varying patterns, physicians should not be misled by one negative value. Heterophil antibodies are more likely to be present in adolescents than in younger children, and usually peak *after* the first week of the illness. If an absolute serologic diagnosis must be reached and the heterophil titer remains negative, then specific anti-Epstein-Barr virus IgG and IgM titers should be obtained. (From Krugman S, Katz SL, Gerson AA, Wilfert CM. *Infectious diseases of children,* 8th ed. St. Louis: Mosby, 1985, with permission.)

against a variety of different antigens, and it can agglutinate the red blood cells from other species—hence, the name "heterophil." Heterophil antibody is a qualitative test; the Monospot is a qualitative test. The latter requires only 2 minutes to perform and is 96% to 99% accurate. But neither one is specific for EBV infection, nor does it necessarily turn positive at all in certain situations. Children younger than 3 years of age do not ordinarily mount any heterophil response to EBV infection. In teenagers, the heterophil response *usually* peaks in the second week of the illness, but many different possibilities exist (Figure 9-1).

- A Monospot test should be performed during the second week of the illness, not after just a few days. Heterophil titers are only necessary if a clinician wants to try to make a retrospective diagnosis, and specific EBV tests are preferable in that case. A heterophil titer greater than 1:40 is considered positive. A variety of diseases can produce weak titers (less than 1:40), including mumps, rubella, and lymphoma. The antibody can remain elevated for up to a year in 75% of patients, and an anamnestic response can be generated by subsequent viral infections.
- Understand that the most common cause of heterophil- or Monospot-negative IM is still EBV infection. In that case, specific anti-EBV antibodies can be measured (Table 9-3, Figure 9-2). Anti-EBV immunoglobulin G (IgG) and immunoglobulin M (IgM) antibodies cost $35 to $50 apiece but are specific for EBV infection. As with other viral infections, an elevated IgM antibody but negative IgG antibody indicates acute infection; a negative IgM but positive IgG indicates past infection.
- Remember that EBV produces a dynamic infection. Early on, the white blood count (WBC) is low, but it may rise to 20,000/mm^3 or more by the end of the first week. Mild thrombocytopenia is common (100,000 to 140,000/mm^3). Atypical lymphocytes may occasionally be labeled as lymphoblasts, but the former are far more pleomorphic.

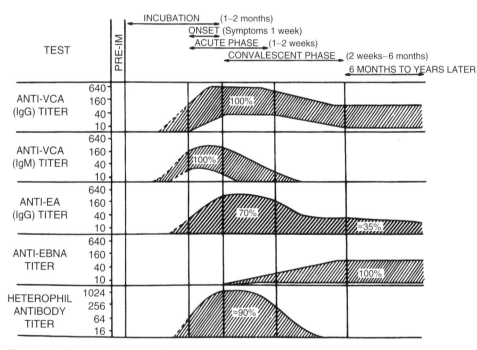

Figure 9-2. Pattern of specific Epstein-Barr virus antibodies in infectious mononucleosis (IM), compared with heterophil response. ANTI-VCA, viral capsid antigen; IgG, immunoglobulin G; IgM, immunoglobulin M; ANTI-EA, early antigens; ANTI-EBNA: Epstein-Barr nuclear antigens. Percentage in shaded area indicates frequency of detection in acute IM. (From Durbin WA, Sullivan JL. Epstein-Barr virus infection. *Pediatr Rev* 1994;15:63. Copyright © American Academy of Pediatrics, with permission.)

Table 9-3. Interpretation of specific EBV antibodies

	IgM capsid antigen	IgG capsid antigen	Early antigen (IgG)	Antinuclear antigen
Susceptible to IM infection	–	–	– –	–
Acute primary infection (IM)	+	+	+ –	–
Acute infection, asymptomatic	+	+	– +	–
Old, quiescent infection	–	+	– –	+
Reactivated infection	±	+	+ or –	+

IgM, immunoglobulin M; IM, infectious mononucleosis.
From Sumaya CV. Epstein-Barr virus infections in children. *Curr Probl Pediatr* 1987;17:1. Copyright © American Academy of Pediatrics. Reprinted with permission.

- Use liver function tests when necessary. Serum levels of liver enzymes (lactate dehydrogenase and serum glutamic transaminases) are mildly elevated in 80% to 90% of patients and usually return to normal within 3 to 5 weeks. Elevations of bilirubin occur less commonly.

C. **Complications:** The most feared complication of IM is splenic rupture, yet it is exceedingly rare—less than 2 per 1,000 cases, and 90% in male patients. In many cases, a ruptured spleen is the presenting sign of IM. Rupture occurs most often during the second or third week of the illness; half occur spontaneously, and another 30% follow minimal exertion. Increasingly, conservative medical management is being used.

Although clinically, splenomegaly is reported only 50% of the time, by ultrasound all IM patients have splenic enlargement.

Deaths among IM patients are rare (only several hundred cases can be found in the literature), but the leading cause of death is not splenic rupture but neurologic involvement. The incidence of CNS involvement in IM ranges from 1% to 8%, with half of those patients presenting with encephalitis or meningoencephalitis. Airway obstruction is the third leading cause of death, either from extreme tonsillar enlargement, glottic edema, or peritonsillar abscess. Rarely, fatal immunoproliferative disorders can occur in predisposed individuals. Overall, the estimated case fatality rate is no higher than 1 in 3,000.

III. **Management:**

A. **Treatment:** There is no specific therapy for the treatment of IM. Appropriate counseling and supportive treatment is all that is necessary in the majority of cases. A vaccine that would not prevent EBV infection but might prevent both the clinical disease and possibly the later complications is currently being investigated in Europe.

B. **Medications:** Antibiotics are indicated only if a throat culture or rapid test for group A Streptococcus is positive. Steroids are indicated only if there is impending airway obstruction. Antiviral agents like acyclovir and interferon have been tried, without much success.

Although a variety of complications of IM have been treated with steroids, impending airway obstruction remains the only proven indication. Such patients can be treated with 2 to 4 mg/kg/day of steroids for 5 to 7 days, with no need to taper off the drug. *Use of steroids in the patient without complications is probably unwise because there are significant theoretical contraindications.* Glucocorticoids are immunosuppressive, specifically diminishing T-cell-mediated immunity. Because IM represents an infection of B cells, with T cells mobilized to help clear the infection, it may be unwise to suppress the latter. Studies have shown diminished levels of T-helper and T-suppressor cells in IM patients treated with steroids. Although uncontrolled trials have documented that students with IM and treated with steroids show a decreased duration of fever and infirmary stay by a few days, and an increased sense of well-being, such symptomatic relief does not justify their routine use. In double-blind, placebo-controlled trials, even these minor improvements cannot be demonstrated.

Acyclovir—a deoxyguanosine analog, with limited activity against herpesviruses—has been shown to decrease oropharyngeal shedding of EBV, but no clinical improvement has been demonstrated in multiple trials, including a meta-analysis of five randomized controlled studies (*Scand J Infect Dis* 1999;31:543–547). Intravenous gamma-globulin may be effective in severe thrombocytopenia.

   C. **Supportive treatment and appropriate counseling:** What is good supportive treatment and appropriate counseling? Supportive measures include:
   - Limiting activity to what is tolerated by the patient during the febrile stage of the illness.
   - Administering antipyretics or analgesics for relief of fever, sore throat, or headache. Liquid codeine preparations may help ease dysphagia, and saline irrigants may help to relieve pain from membranous tonsillitis.
   - Avoiding strenuous exercise and contact sports for the duration of splenomegaly, usually 4 to 6 weeks.
   - Considering dietary changes or the use of a mild laxative to avoid straining to pass stool.

   In counseling patients and their parents, the following points should be stressed:
   - IM is nearly always a self-limited viral disease that teenagers will recover from without difficulty. Often, they feel ill for a week or two and then gradually resume their former level of activity over the next 2 to 4 weeks. Emphasizing the complications or talking about "chronic fatigue" will only result in a self-fulfilling prophecy.
   - Bed rest is indicated only during the febrile period. After that, patients should seek their own individual level of activity.
   - Whether or not the spleen is palpable, patients should be strongly cautioned against any activity that results in increased intra-abdominal pressure or the risk of blunt trauma to the abdomen. This includes activities such as jogging, swimming, roughhousing with friends, and contact sports, as well as straining to pass stool.
   - Teenagers should never be told that they have "hepatitis." Invariably, they later report this to other health care workers as Hepatitis A or B.
   - Although clinicians have routinely cautioned patients with IM to avoid alcoholic beverages (because of the chemical hepatitis), there is no scientific evidence to support this recommendation. Ideally, teenagers should not be consuming alcohol anyway.
   - IM can best be explained as being a viral disease, like the common cold. As such, it is self-limited. Patients can be told that the spleen functions like the oil filter in a car, filtering out the infected white blood cells. Eye-rolling or hand-wringing on the part of the clinician or the parent about what a devastating illness IM is should be discouraged.

IV.   **Clinical pearls and pitfalls:** Several aspects of IM in teenagers are worth re-emphasizing:
   - Splenomegaly that can be palpated occurs in only half of patients, usually in the second or third week of their illness. It is usually subtle, detectable only on deep inspiration. Clinicians should exercise care when examining for splenomegaly. Gross enlargement warrants a reconsideration of the diagnosis.
   - Periorbital edema is nearly as common as splenomegaly and is a frequently neglected sign of IM. Often, parents are first to report this.
   - Petechiae on the soft palate are also frequently overlooked as a sign of IM.
   - A variety of rashes has been described in patients with IM: macular, maculopapular, scarlatiniform, petechial, urticarial, or erythema multiforme. Most often, the rash of IM is faint and best seen on the neck and upper chest.
   - Streptococcal infection occurs as frequently in IM patients as in other teens with acute pharyngitis, between 15% and 25% of the time. Although the posterior pharynx of patients with IM may be covered with grayish-white membranes and exudate, most of the time the etiology is viral, not bacterial.
   - Nearly 100% of patients given amoxicillin or ampicillin will develop a dramatic, maculopapular rash, resembling measles. This *does not represent a true allergy, and it is safe to continue the drug.* The rash is not immunoglobulin (IgE)-mediated and probably represents an interaction between a by-product of the drug and the virus. Onset is usually 5 to 9 days after administration of the antibiotic, whereas an acute allergic reaction is more likely to occur within 24 to 48 hours and be urticarial. Other antibiotics, especially penicillin, can produce this picture as well.
   - Primary EBV infection can present solely with neurological manifestations, without any clinical evidence of IM.

BIBLIOGRAPHY

For the clinician

Bazemore AW, Smucker DR. Lymphadenopathy and malignancy. *Am Fam Physician* 2002;66: 2103–2110.

Cohen JI. Epstein-Barr infection. *N Engl J Med* 2000;343:481–492.

Ebell MH. Epstein-Barr virus infectious mononucleosis. *Am Fam Physician* 2004;70:1279–1287.

Hickey SM, Strasburger VC. What every pediatrician should know about infectious mononucleosis in adolescents. *Pediatr Clin North Am* 1997;44:1541–1556.

Jenson HB. Acute complications of Epstein-Barr virus infectious mononucleosis. *Curr Opin Pediatr* 2000;12:263–268.

Junker AK. Epstein-Barr virus. *Pediatr Rev* 2005;26:79–85.

WEB SITES

familydoctor.org/handouts/077.html   Handout on IM from American Academy of Family Physicians

www.emedicine.com/EMERG/topic319.htm   E-medicine review article on IM

For patients and parents

www.nlm.nih.gov/medlineplus/infectiousmononucleosis.html   National Library of Medicine Web site for parents and teenagers

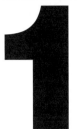

Chronic Fatigue

I. **Description of the condition:**
A. **Introduction:** Fatigue is a relatively common complaint among adolescents. In this chapter we will review the various reasons for persistent, recurrent, prolonged, or chronic fatigue, and offer diagnosis and management tips.
B. **Definitions:** The feeling of fatigue, that is, not having had enough sleep, can be confused with weakness or with easy fatigability. Therefore some definitions are needed:
 • **Fatigue:** feeling of not having had enough sleep
 • **Easy fatigability:** rapid tiring with minimal exertion
 • **Weakness:** lack of ability of muscles to do their usual amount of work
 • **Chronic fatigue:** unremitting fatigue that lasts for at least 6 months
 • **Prolonged fatigue:** unremitting fatigue of at least 2 to 3 months but less than 6 months
   Chronic Fatigue Syndrome: Chronic Fatigue Syndrome (CFS) is one cause of unremitting fatigue. CFS has an accepted set of criteria that must be met for diagnosis. Fewer adolescents than adults have this. Adolescents also do not always meet full criteria for CFS, so we use the term Chronic Fatigue of Adolescents (CFA) rather than CFS.
   These criteria are listed in Table 10-1.
   In addition to the Centers for Disease Control and Prevention (CDC) criteria, there are United Kingdom criteria and Australian criteria for CFS. Each of these sets of criteria is similar.
C. **Epidemiology:** CFA affects anywhere from 0.04% to 2.9% of adolescents at any one time. These rates are difficult to compare, however, because of differing criteria for inclusion in the category of chronic fatigue. There is a female predominance, as is seen in adults, and no racial/ethnic preponderance.
D. **Characteristics of CFA:**
 • Onset of fatigue dates to a viral illness whose symptoms never completely resolve
 • Fatigue is unremitting
 • Increasing exhaustion after seemingly limited physical activity or emotional stress
 • Sleep is nonrestorative
 • Fatigue worsens to a point at which the adolescent may be unable to do any activities or go to school
 • Sore throats, headaches, adenopathy, inability to concentrate, myalgias, and arthralgias all can occur, albeit without the consistency of CFS in adults.
   In adolescents, the length of time to recovery seems to correlate with the severity of the fatigue, a factor best measured by time needed to be absent from school. For example, if a teenager needs to miss a month of school, the time course of the condition will be shorter than with a teen who needs to miss a semester or a whole year of school (i.e., actually going to school physically, not home-tutoring).
   Most adolescents with CFA require from 1 to 4 years to fully recover. About 75% have a good recovery, about 20% partially recover, and about 5% continue with significant debility.
E. **Etiology:** No etiology has been detected for CFA or for CFS in adults. Possible etiologies include immune dysfunction, aberrant response to viral infection, problems with regulation of the hypothalamic-pituitary-adrenal axis, and psychological issues. No evidence supports any of these possibilities, and, indeed, there is some evidence to rule out most of them.
II. **Making the diagnosis:**
A. **Why do adolescents get tired?**
 1. The **most common reason** is *lack of sleep*. Adolescents require from 8 to 10 hours per night of sleep, less as they age. Many adolescents do not get this much sleep, especially during the school week. Teens tend to stay up later at night and

Table 10-1. 1994 International case definition of chronic fatigue syndrome

CFS is a syndrome characterized by fatigue that is:	• Medically unexplained • Of new onset • Of at least 6 months' duration • Not the result of ongoing exertion • Not substantially relieved by rest • Causes a substantial reduction in previous levels of occupational, educational, social, or personal activities
In addition, there must be 4 or more of the following symptoms:	• Impaired memory or concentration • Sore throat • Tender neck (cervical) or armpit (axillary) lymph nodes • Muscle pain (myalgia) • Headaches of a new type, pattern, or severity • Unrefreshing sleep • Postexertional malaise (lasting more than 24 hours) • Multijoint pain (arthralgia without swelling or redness)

Chronic Fatigue Syndrome (CFS) can be excluded by other medical disorders known to cause fatigue, major depressive illness, medication that causes fatigue as a side effect, and alcohol or substance abuse.

Adapted from Fukuda K, Straus SE, Sharpe MC, et al. The chronic fatigue syndrome: a comprehensive approach to its definition and study. *Ann Intern Med* 1994;121:953–959.

wake up later in the morning than do adults, a true reflection of differing circadian rhythms. In spite of this, school hours in the typical community reflect more closely the sleep needs of adults than the sleep needs of adolescents.

2. **Adolescents are also very busy.** Many of them have "too much to do," that is, they are over-programmed. They have school and homework; they may have after school jobs; many have extracurricular activities, lessons, etc.; and teens want a social life.

3. The **sleep habits/hygiene** of adolescents frequently are poor. Many teens use their bedrooms as recreation/communication centers. They may have their own phones, and they may have computers, televisions, music centers, and radios where they sleep. So bedtime may not equate with sleep time. Many teens also ingest a lot of caffeine, which may induce insomnia.

Once these reasons for fatigue are considered the clinician needs to review all the possible pathologic reasons for fatigue (Table 10-2). First, fatigue must be differentiated from weakness and/or easy fatigability. Then the **differential diagnosis of CFA** must be considered.

Table 10-2. Causes of fatigue in adolescents

• Too little sleep
• Too much to do
• Poor sleep hygiene
• Different circadian rhythm
• Depression
• Stress
• Sleep disorder
• Anemia
• Thyroid dysfunction
• Chronic infection
• Inflammatory bowel disease
• Autoimmune disease
• Neuromuscular disease
• Cancer
• Eating disorder
• Pregnancy
• Medication side effects
• Substance abuse

Table 10-3. Symptoms of 58 children and adolescents with CFS

Symptom	Number
Fatigue	58 (100%)
Headache	43 (74%)
Sore throat	34 (59%)
Abdominal pain	28 (48%)
Fever	21 (36%)
Impaired cognition	19 (33%)
Myalgia	19 (31%)
Diarrhea	17 (29%)
Adenopathy	17 (29%)
Anorexia	16 (28%)
Nausea or vomiting	15 (26%)
Dizziness	10 (17%)
Arthralgia	10 (17%)
Sweating	5 (9%)
Chills	4 (7%)
Depression	4 (7%)

CFS, Chronic Fatigue Syndrome.
Adapted from Krilov LR, Fisher M, Friedman SB, et al. Course and outcome of chronic fatigue in children and adolescents. *Pediatrics* 1998;102:360.

    B. Differential diagnosis: Chronic fatigue differs in adolescents. Most adolescents who suffer from prolonged or chronic fatigue do not have the requisite symptom complex to qualify for the diagnosis of CFS. Table 10-3 shows the most common symptoms in adolescents with CFA in one study.

    C. Evaluation: The key component of evaluation is the initial history and physical examination.

        1. History. When asking about fatigue, the clinician must differentiate fatigue from weakness and from easy fatigability. Onset usually is after a viral illness. One must inquire about fevers, weight loss or gain, odd rashes or skin pigment changes, lumps that are abnormal, gastrointestinal (GI) symptoms, and so on. In girls, a detailed menstrual history is very important. A family history, social history, and inquiry into possible stresses is mandatory. Individual interviews with the teen and parent alone garners important information. Questions about substance abuse, eating disorders, and sexual activity are all important. In addition, a history of recent travel is needed, as is history of drinking unclean water or of hunting and preparing wild animals. A chronic fatigue checklist filled out by the patient and family can be helpful.

        2. The **physical examination** must be thorough with attention to general appearance, possible pallor, adenopathy, abdominal masses, signs of eating disorders (lanugo, calluses on knuckles, etc.), skin tone, and palpation of the fibromyalgia tender points.

        3. Laboratory tests can be helpful initially in ruling out organic causes of fatigue. A complete blood count, a thyroid-stimulating hormone (TSH) analysis, and an erythrocyte sedimentation rate should be ordered along with a urine analysis, Epstein-Barr virus (EBV) titers, an antinuclear antibody (ANA), a purified protein derivative (PPD), and possibly stool studies for ova and parasites. Imaging studies are rarely helpful.

III.   **Management: Management really begins with:**

    A. The initial evaluation: In addition to a thorough review of the history and a complete physical examination, the initial evaluation gives the clinician the chance to convince the patient and the family that the **patient is valued,** that the **symptoms are believed,** and that the clinician feels **the problem is significant** and **worthy of considerable attention.**

        Certainly, if the investigation reveals a diagnosable cause of the fatigue, that dictates the direction of further interventions. However, if the investigation leads to the diagnosis of CFA, then the **following approaches to treatment** can be helpful.

First, the clinician must reframe the discussion of fatigue from general statements of being tired to having the adolescent and the family think of the adolescent as having so many **"bad" days** and so many **"good" days.** That is, **how many days per week is the adolescent severely fatigued and how many days does the adolescent feel relatively energetic.** At the nadir of the disease course, the adolescent may feel severely fatigued every day of the week. As the severity wanes, the adolescent may feel fatigued on a few days per week but not on the others. As further resolution occurs, the adolescent then can track the days per week of feeling good and see that progress is being made.

The adolescent and family need to be educated about true CFA facts. The **time course of the condition should be explained,** and the adolescent and parents need to be cautioned about assigning significance to what they hear from friends, from the media, and from the Internet. The family should be directed to **check out any rumors with the clinician before believing what they hear or read.**

B. **Treatment: Two treatments that have been shown to be successful in adults** with CFS are a **graded exercise program (GEP)** and **cognitive behavioral therapy (CBT).** The exercise program needs to start slowly and build up very gradually, with caution about doing too much, since overdoing it might produce a severe setback. This GEP should be supervised by a physical therapist or a trainer. CBT can help the adolescent learn to manage stress more effectively and better cope with the relatively long course of the condition. No other treatment method has been shown conclusively to help. Some possibly helpful treatments are muscle relaxants for patients with significant musculoskeletal pain, sedative antidepressants for fitful sleep, and selective serotonin reuptake inhibitor (SSRI) antidepressants where depression is present. Some patients seem to benefit from a stimulant such as methylphenidate, but that is by no means a proven treatment.

C. **Working with the school:** Finally, **the clinician must work closely with the patient's school** to make sure that the condition is given the credence it deserves. CFA can be a very stressful and debilitating condition, but with astute evaluation and firm management sufferers can go on to recovery.

IV. **Clinical pearls and pitfalls:**
   - Most commonly, adolescents are tired because they get too little sleep.
   - Fatigue must be differentiated from just tiredness and weakness.
   - The key to diagnosis and management is the history.
   - Chronic fatigue syndrome in adolescents is NOT the same as in adults.
   - The ONLY proven treatments are graded aerobic exercise and cognitive behavioral therapy.

BIBLIOGRAPHY

For the clinician

Cavanaugh RM Jr. Evaluating adolescents with chronic fatigue: ever get tired of it? *Pediatr Rev* 2002;23:337–348.

Gill AC, Dosen A, Ziegler JB. Chronic fatigue syndrome in adolescents: a follow-up study. *Arch Pediatr Adolesc Med* 2004;158:225–229.

Jones JF, Nisenbaum R, Solomon L, et al. Chronic fatigue syndrome and other fatiguing illnesses in adolescents: a population-based study. *J Adolesc Health* 2004;35:34–40.

Millman RP, et al. Excessive sleepiness in adolescents and young adults: causes, consequences, and treatment strategies. *Pediatrics* 2005;115:1774–1786.

Rangel L. Family health and characteristics in chronic fatigue syndrome, juvenile rheumatoid arthritis, and emotional disorders of childhood. *J Am Acad Child Adolesc Psychiatry* 2005;44(2):150–158.

For patients and parents

Schiff D, Shelov SP. *The American Academy of Pediatrics guide to your child's symptoms: The official, complete home reference, birth through adolescence (guide to your child's symptoms).* Elk Grove Village, IL: American Academy of Pediatrics, 1997.

WEB SITES

www.cfids.org/resources/pediatric-CFIDS.asp

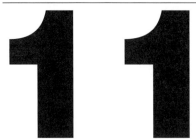

Hepatitis

Hepatitis is an uncommon problem in adolescents, but when it occurs it can cause significant morbidity. There are many forms of adolescent hepatitis: infectious, autoimmune, toxic, and those entities due to genetic defects. **Most commonly, the clinician will encounter hepatitis of infectious etiology.** This category includes hepatitis A, B, and C, the hepatitis that is part of infectious mononucleosis, and, in the developing world, hepatitis due to parasites and protozoans. The salient points of hepatitis A, B, and C will be reviewed and highlighted in this chapter.

HEPATITIS A

I. **Description of the condition:**
   A. **Etiology:** Hepatitis A virus (HAV), an RNA virus belonging to the picornavirus family, genus Hepatovirus, is the cause of this infection. The disease is usually **transmitted via the fecal–oral route**, and has an **incubation period** (time of exposure to the onset of symptoms) of **about 4 weeks, with a range of 15 to 50 days.** HAV replicates in the liver and is shed in the feces in high concentrations from 2 weeks prior to the infection to about 1 week after the disease becomes clinically apparent.
   B. **Clinical course:** The **course is usually self-limited** with symptoms that last approximately 2 weeks in most patients, with possible relapse in 6 months in 10% to 15% of patients. Acute liver failure occurs ~0.3% of the time and is more frequent in the elderly and in patients with preexisting liver disease. **The older the patient, the worse the symptoms,** with children usually showing no overt disease. Lifelong antibodies confer permanent immunity after the first infection.
   C. **Epidemiology and disease acquisition:** Most cases in the United States occur in community outbreaks. The **most common source is person-to-person transmission in households or among sexual contacts.** Outbreaks also are common among injection drug users and among men having sex with men (MSM). Up to 50% of infected persons do not have an identified source of infection. Infection can also be spread through contact with impure water, especially during travel in developing countries.
II. **Diagnosis:** The diagnosis cannot be made solely on clinical grounds, therefore it is **necessary to obtain serological testing.** The presence of IgM to HAV is diagnostic of acute HAV infection; positive tests for HAV antibody alone only indicate a previous infection.
III. **Treatment:**
   A. **Supportive care** is usually sufficient. Medications that are liver-metabolized or possibly liver-toxic should be avoided during the acute illness.
   B. **Prevention:** There are **two methods of prevention,** hepatitis A vaccine and intramuscular (IM) immune globulin.

   The **vaccine** is an inactivated hepatitis A product and has been available in the United States since 1995 for people older than 2 years old. It is given in a 2-dose series with doses at least 6 months apart. Table 11-1 gives the recommended vaccine regimens. The vaccine is 94% to 100% effective in preventing clinical disease and lasts at least 20 years.

   There is a combination hepatitis A and B vaccine for adults that is given on a 0, 1, 6 month schedule. Immunoglobulin (Ig) derived from pooled human plasma that (in the USA) has tested negative for HBV, anti-HIV, anti-HCV, and HCV-RNA is given 0 to 2 weeks after exposure and is at least 85% effective. Prevaccination testing for previous infection is prudent when considering immunization of large populations. There is no harm in vaccinating a person who has already been immunized. There is no need to do postvaccine serologic testing, due to the excellent effectiveness of the vaccine.
   C. **Postexposure prophylaxis:** Unvaccinated people who have been exposed to HAV should be given a single IM dose of Ig as soon as possible, but not more than 2 weeks after exposure. The hepatitis A vaccine can be administered at the same time as the Ig when indicated.

Table 11-1. Recommended regimens: dose and schedule for hepatitis A vaccines

Vaccine	Age (years)	Dose	Volume (mL)	Two-dose schedule (months)[a]
HAVRIX[b]	2–18	720 (EL.U)	.05	0, 6–12
	>18	1,440 (EL.U)	1.0	0, 6–12
VAQTA[c]	2–18	25 (U)	0.5	0, 6–18
	>18	50 (U)	1.0	0, 6–12

EL.U, enzyme-linked immunosorbent assay (ELISA) units; U, units.
[a]0 months represents timing of the initial dose; subsequent numbers represent months after the initial dose.
[b]Hepatitis A vaccine, inactivated, SmithKline Beecham Biologicals.
[c]Hepatitis A vaccine, inactivated, Merck & Co., Inc.

IV.   **Clinical pearls and pitfalls:**
   • Hepatitis A is most usually acquired via the fecal–oral route.
   • Hepatitis A is NOT a cause of chronic hepatitis.
   • HAV vaccine provides excellent protection and should be used freely.

HEPATITIS B

I.   **Description of the condition:**
   A. **Etiology:** Hepatitis B is caused by the hepatitis B virus (HBV), a 42nm double-stranded DNA virus from the hepadnavirus family that has multiple genotypes and serotypes capable of causing chronic disease. The **incubation period** (time of exposure to onset of clinical disease) is 6 weeks to 6 months. HBV is found primarily in blood and liver tissue. Hepatitis B can be self-limited or chronic, but only 50% of acute infections are symptomatic. One percent of cases result in liver failure and death. **Young children are much more likely (60% for those under 5 years old) to become chronically infected than are adults (2%–6%).** With chronic HBV infection, risk of death from cirrhosis or hepatocellular carcinoma is 15% to 25%.
   B. **Epidemiology:** In the United States in 1998, 181,000 people became infected, and about 5,000 people died from HBV-related cirrhosis or hepatocellular carcinoma. Estimates are that **1.25 million people are chronically infected with HBV.** These people serve as a **reservoir for infection** and are at increased risk for further disease and death.
   C. **Disease acquisition:** HBV is transmitted by percutaneous or mucous membrane exposure to infectious body fluids. **In the United States, sexual transmission accounts for most adult infection,** 40% from heterosexual contacts and about 15% from MSM. The **most common risk factors for heterosexual infection** are as follows:
   • Multiple sex partners
   • Recent history of a sexually transmitted infection (STI)
   The **most common risk factors for MSM infection** are as follows:
   • Multiple sex partners
   • Unprotected receptive anal intercourse
   • Having a history of other STIs.
   Among 15- to 22-year-old MSM, 6% to 13% show evidence of HBV infection while 3% to 27% show evidence of being immunized for HBV. Up to 70% of persons with acute hepatitis B have previously received care in settings where they could have been vaccinated.

II.   **Diagnosis and clinical course:**
   A. **Serologic markers:** Diagnosis of HBV infection is via serologic markers (listed in Table 11-2). From this table, one can glean the antigen and antibody markers that delineate hepatitis B status.
   When symptomatic, HBV infection presents a prodrome of malaise, fatigue, anorexia, nausea, and low-grade fever following an incubation period of 45 to 160 days. Jaundice then develops while aminotransferase levels rise. Occasionally, one finds clinical features such as papular acrodermatitis (Gianotti-Crosti syndrome) and acute glomerulonephritis. Rarely, fulminant liver failure may ensue. Alanine transaminase and aspartate aminotransferase (ALT/AST) reach peak levels at about 16 weeks after acquisition; IgM Anti-HBc lasts from about 16 to 36 weeks; Anti-HBs starts rising at 24 weeks and stays elevated. Convalescence usually begins around 30 weeks post infection.

Table 11-2. Serologic markers of hepatitis B infection

Tests for HBV	Description	Presence Indicates
HBsAg	Surface antigen of HBV	Acute or chronic infection
Anti-HBs	Antibody to surface antigen	Immunity due to viral clearance or immunization
HBeAg	Hepatitis Be antigen	Active viral replication and increased infectivity
Anti-HBe	Antibody to HBeAg	Low risk of transmitting virus; asymptomatic carrier in those who have HBsAg
IgM Anti-HBc	IgM antibody to HBV core antigen	Acute HBV infection
Anti-HBc	Total antibody to HBV core antigen (IgG and IgM)	Present or past HBV infection
HBV DNA	Quantitates HBV viremia level by PCR	Active replication of HBV

    B. Chronic disease: Not all of those infected with HBV clear the infection. Some become **carriers** with normal aminotransferase levels or clinical features of infection while others develop **chronic disease** with elevated aminotransferase levels and abnormal hepatic histology. It is important to remember that **more than 95% of those infected after the age of 5 clear HBV and recover without any lingering infection. In those who are chronically infected, the major potential sequelae** are **cirrhosis** and **hepatocellular carcinoma (HCC).** Age at infection seems to be important in determining who is at greatest risk for the latter complication. HCC is more likely the earlier one acquires the infection. Without vaccination or treatment, where HBV is endemic, HCC occurs in 20% to 50% of those infected by age 72 years.

III. Monitoring and treatment:
    A. Goals of treatment, or general guidelines:
- Patients with chronic hepatitis B (i.e., HBeAg-positive, elevated liver enzymes), and compensated liver disease should be observed for 3 to 6 months for spontaneous seroconversion from HBeAg to HBe antibody prior to any treatment.
- Patients who meet the criteria for chronic hepatitis B (i.e., serum HBV DNA $>10^5$ copies/mL and persistent or intermittent elevation in liver enzymes), should have a liver biopsy.
- Patients who are inactive carriers (HBsAg) should be monitored by checking liver enzyme levels every 6 to 12 months.

    B. Medications: Recommendations for treating hepatitis B are listed in Table 11-3. The mainstay of treatment has been interferon, but recently new drugs have been found to be beneficial. However, current therapies all have limited long-term efficacy. It is important to balance patient age, disease severity, chances of response, and potential adverse events and complications before deciding how to treat.

        Current drugs for HBV infection are **interferon ἀ(IFN), lamivudine, and adefovir.**
        1. IFN's advantages are finite duration of treatment, more durable response, and lack of resistant mutants. **IFN's disadvantages** are cost and side effects.
        2. Lamivudine is more economical and better tolerated than IFN, but the durability of response to it seems lower, and long-term treatment increases the risk of developing drug-resistant mutants that may negate positive treatment effects and possibly result in worsening of the disease.
        3. Adefovir is active against lamivudine-resistant mutants and evokes little resistance to itself during initial therapy, but it is significantly more costly than lamivudine, and we do not as yet know its long-term safety profile and risk of resistance to it by HBV. For adolescents, treatment decisions should be determined by hepatologists versed in the most recent treatment recommendations.
    C. Prevention: Hepatitis B is prevented by avoiding practices that spread the disease and by vaccination. The current vaccine recommendations for hepatitis B are listed in Table 11-4.

IV. Clinical pearls and pitfalls:
- Hepatitis B is preventable.
- Chronic disease is more likely the younger one is when the virus is acquired.
- Treatment is less than optimal, but it can work.

Table 11-3. Recommendations for treatment of chronic hepatitis B

HBeAg	HBV DNA^a	ALT	Treatment Strategy
+	+	≤2 × ULN	Low efficacy with current treatment. Observe; consider treatment when ALT becomes elevated.
+	+	>2 × ULN	IFN-Interferon, LAM, or ADV may be used as initial therapy. End point of treatment-seroconversion from HBeAg to anti-HBe. Duration of therapy: • IFN-Interferon: 16 weeks • Lamivudine: minimum 1 year, continue for 3–6 months after HBeAg seroconversion • Adefovir: minimum 1 year IFN-Interferon Nonresponders/contraindications to IFN-Interferon → LAM or ADV. LAM resistance → ADV.
−	+	>2 × ULN	IFN-Interferon, LAM or ADV may be used as initial therapy, IFN-Interferon or ADV is preferred because of the need for long-term therapy. End point of treatment—sustained normalization of ALT and undetectable HBV DNA by PCR assay. Duration of therapy • IFN-Interferon: 1 year • Lamivudine: >1 year • Adefovir: >1 year IFN-Interferon Nonresponders/contraindications to IFN-Interferon → LAM or ADV. LAM resistance → ADV.
−	−	≤2 × ULN	No treatment required.
±	+	Cirrhosis	Compensated: LAM or ADV. Decompensated: LAM (or ADV); coordinate treatment with transplant center. Refer for liver transplant. IFN-Interferon contraindicated.
±	−	Cirrhosis	Compensated: Observe. Decompensated: Refer for liver transplant.

HBeAg, hepatitis Be antigen; HBV, hepatitis B virus; ALT, alanine aminotransferase; ULN, upper limit of normal; IFN-Interferon, interferon alfa; LAM, lamivudine; ADV, adefovir; PCR, polymerase chain reaction.
^{a}HBV DNA >10^5 copies/mL; this value is arbitrarily chosen.

Table 11-4. Current vaccine recommendations for hepatitis B

• All infants
• Adolescents who were not immunized during childhood
• Injection drug users
• Sexually active heterosexual men and women with more than one sex partner during the previous 6 months
• Men who have sex with men
• Contacts and sexual partners of HBsAg-positive people
• Health care personnel
• Residents and staff of institutions for developmentally disabled persons
• Patients on hemodialysis
• Patients who receive clotting factor concentrate
• International travelers to areas in which hepatitis B virus infection is endemic
• Inmates of correctional facilities

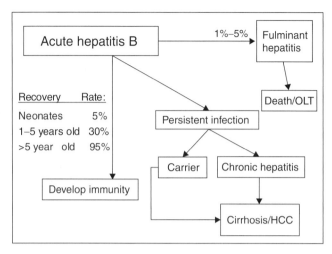

Figure 11-1. Clinical sequelae of HBV infection. The sequelae of HBV are age-related. Among neonates born to HbsAg + mothers who do not receive HBV prophylaxis, approximately 5% clear HBV and recover completely. Most develop a persistent infection. Between 1 and 5 years of age, only 30% of affected children recover completely. After age 5, approximately 95% of affected children clear acute HBV and recover without sequelae. In all age groups, a small percentage develop fulminant hepatic failure.

HEPATITIS C

I.   **Description of the condition:**
A.   **Etiology:** Hepatitis C is caused by HCV, a single-strand RNA virus of the Flavivirus family. There are 9 known serotypes. with type 1 being most prevalent in the United States. **HCV has the ability to mutate rapidly.** This makes it **very difficult to treat,** since rapid mutation in defiance of the host immune response causes great difficulty in eliminating the virus, which leads to chronic infection. Within each infected person, therefore, the virus exists as the heterogenous mixture of closely related viruses called "quasi-species." The viremia continues, as does the inflammatory process with the emergence of resistant strains. This then makes treatment and vaccine development difficult.
B.   **Epidemiology:** The overall prevalence worldwide is about 2% in adults, but this varies widely. In the United States, the prevalence is 0.2% in children under 12 years old and 0.4% in adolescents. Two percent of incarcerated teens are HCV positive.
C.   **Disease acquisition:**
1.   **The primary method of acquiring HCV is via direct percutaneous exposure to blood or blood products.** Intravenous drug users, persons who are tattooed or pierced under less than sterile conditions, those who received transfusion prior to 1991, and hemophiliacs treated with clotting products prior to 1987 have HCV prevalence rates of 60% to 90%. Hemodialysis patients have prevalence rates of 10% to 20%.
2.   **There is some maternal–fetal transmission of the virus.** The infection is present in 5% of the infants born to HCV positive mothers, but the rate is 14% if the mother is coinfected with HIV. Transmission via breast milk has never been detected.
3.   **Sexual transmission,** while **not common** at all, does occur. There is a reported 5% transmission rate to sexual partners, with the rate being higher in male-to-female transmission. Risks include multiple sexual partners and non-use of condoms. Monogamous partners with no other risk factors have a transmission rate of 1.5%. Nonsexual household contact rate is 4%.

II.   **Clinical course and diagnosis:** Hepatitis C has an **incubation period of about 6 to 7 weeks** with a range of 2 weeks to 6 months. The **acute illness, if any, is mild. Persistent infection** develops in 60% to 80% of those infected. Less than 1% have a fulminant course. Chronic infection increases the risk of cirrhosis and HCC. Figures 11-1 and 11-2 show what happens when a person is infected.

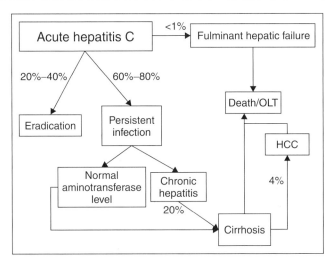

Figure 11-2. Clinical sequelae of HCV. Acute HCV infection is generally benign; only 20% of affected patients have symptomatic infection, and fulminant hepatic failure is exceedingly rare. However, approximately 60% to 80% develop persistent infection that results in chronic hepatitis in most affected patients. Serious sequelae, including cirrhosis and HCC, may develop over many years in about 20% of infected patients. The time course for these varies. Typically, cirrhosis is seen 20 years or more following acquisition of HCV; the time course is even longer in patients who have normal aminotransferase levels. For this reason, the incidence of cirrhosis among pediatric patients is less than 5%. Cirrhosis most often precedes HCC by several years.

Diagnosis is made serologically. Table 11-5 shows how to interpret HCV test results. The anti-HCV immunoassay should be obtained in persons suspected of having hepatitis C. If positive, detection and quantification of HCV RNA is done. For infants of infected mothers, HCV antibody testing is recommended after 18 months of age, since it may take that long for maternal HCV in the infant to dissipate. Table 11-6 lists persons for whom HCV testing is recommended. When HCV infection is diagnosed, liver biopsy was previously recommended uniformly. At present the utility of this procedure is being reviewed.

III.   **Management and treatment:**

   A. Identification of primary goals: Patients with recently acquired hepatitis C should be treated as soon as possible, because 42 of 43 patients in a small study showed elimination of the virus when treatment was initiated within 89 days of infection or within 1 month of the onset of the illness. **For those with more chronic infection there are two primary treatment options:** observe or treat.

   The decision in adolescents is not at all clear. If an adolescent has tested positive for HCV and has mildly elevated liver enzymes, the clinician may decide to either observe or treat. One should be aware that as of the time of this book's publication, there are no large-scale, multicenter, prospective, placebo-controlled, randomized pediatric studies of HCV treatment. Moreover, the adverse effects of the drugs that are used may dissuade the clinician from treating adolescents.

Table 11-5. Interpretation of HCV test results

Anti-HCV	HCV RNA	Interpretation of diagnostic tests
Negative	Negative	No infection
Positive	Positive	Acute or chronic infection
Negative	Positive	Early infection or chronic infection in an immunosuppressed host
Positive	Negative	Resolved infection, chronic infection, or false-positive antibody test

Table 11-6. Persons for whom HCV testing is recommended

- Persons who have injected illicit drugs in the recent and remote past, including those who injected only once and do not consider themselves to be drug users
- Persons with conditions associated with a high prevalence of HCV infection, including:
  - Persons with HIV infection
  - Persons with hemophilia who received clotting factor concentrates before 1987
  - Persons who were ever on hemodialysis
  - Persons with unexplained abnormal aminotransferase levels
- Prior recipients of transfusions or organ transplants, including:
  - Persons who were notified that they had received blood from a donor who later tested positive for HCV infection
  - Persons who received a transfusion of blood or blood products before July 1992
  - Persons who received an organ transplant before July 1992
- Children born to HCV-infected mothers
- Health care, emergency medical and public safety workers after a needle stick injury or mucosal exposure to HCV-positive blood
- Current sexual partners of HCV-infected persons

B. **Medications:** The **current treatment** for hepatitis C is a combination of **pegylated interferon (PEG-IFN) and ribavirin.** This combination has been shown to be superior to other regimens. Treatment is given for 6 months with weekly injections of PEG-IFN and daily oral ribavirin. Side effects include those associated with IFN (e.g., malaise, muscle aches, weight loss, and depression). Ribavirin is teratogenic, a factor when treating female adolescents. It can cause hematologic problems, especially early in the treatment, so monitoring blood counts is important.

The combined treatment, while effective, is not perfect. In those infected with **HCV type 1, the major viral type in the United States,** combined treatment has a chance of totally eradicating the virus in about 35% of patients. **Eradication is called a sustained virologic response (SVR),** which means that there is no detectable virus at the end of treatment and at 6 months post treatment. The SVR is higher with types 2 and 3.

Given that an adult with chronic hepatitis C has a reported 5% to 20% chance of developing cirrhosis over a 20 to 25 year period, and given that there is a risk for development of HCC, the patient with this disease has a choice. When treatment has been tried in children and adolescents, an SVR was obtained in 36% compared to 5% in those not treated. With genotype 1, SVR was achieved in 27%.

C. **Additional information for the patient:** Patients should be counseled to maintain liver health by not using liver-toxic substances or drugs. They should also be counseled about avoiding practices that could transmit the virus. These recommendations are listed in Table 11-7.

Table 11-7. Counseling to avoid transmission of HCV

- HCV-infected persons should be counseled to avoid sharing toothbrushes and dental or shaving equipment and be cautioned to cover any bleeding wound in order to keep their blood away from others.
- HCV-infected persons should be counseled to stop using illicit drugs. Those who continue to inject drugs should be counseled to avoid reusing or sharing syringes, needles, water, and cotton or other paraphernalia; to clean the injection site with a new alcohol swab; and to dispose safely of syringes and needles after one use.
- HCV-infected persons should be counseled that the risk of sexual transmission is low and that the infection itself is not a reason to change sexual practices (i.e., those in long-term relationships need not start using barrier precautions, and others should always practice "safer" sex).
- HCV-infected persons should be advised to not donate blood, body organs, other tissues, or semen.

Adapted from Recommendations for prevention and control of hepatitis C virus (HCV) infection and HCV-related chronic disease. Centers for Disease Control and Prevention. *MMWR Recomm Rep 1998*;47(RR-19):1–39.

IV. **Clinical pearls and pitfalls:**
- The cause of most cases of Hepatitis C is unknown.
- Few cases are caused by sexual transmission.
- Acute hepatitis C is curable.
- Treatment for chronic disease can work, but in only a minority of cases.

BIBLIOGRAPHY

For the clinician

Giboney PT. Mildly elevated liver transaminase levels in the asymptomatic patient. *Am Fam Physician* 2005;71:1105–1110.

Hochman JA, Balistreri WF. Chronic viral hepatitis: always be current! *Pediatr Rev* 2003;24: 399–410.

Joffe A, Blythe MJ. Handbook of adolescent medicine. *Adolesc Med State Art Rev* 2003;14:360.

For patients and parents

Berkman A, Bakalar, N. *Hepatitis A to G: The facts you need to know about all the forms of this dangerous disease.* New York: Warner Books, 2000.

WEB SITES

www.cdc.gov/ncidod/diseases/hepatitis/
www.hepfi.org

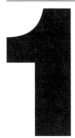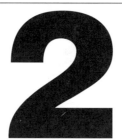

Abdominal Pain

I. **Description of the condition:**
   A. **Epidemiology: Recurrent abdominal pain (RAP)** affects between 7% and 25% of school children and accounts for 2% to 4% of pediatric office visits. About 8% of adolescents in one community-focused study reported going to the doctor for abdominal pain in the past year. Females are more commonly affected in adolescence than are males. Gynecological causes of pain will be mentioned here, but will be more fully discussed in Chapter 26, on gynecologic problems.

   Chronic abdominal pain is defined as:
   - at least 3 episodes of pain
   - that occur within 3 months and
   - that are severe enough to affect the adolescent's normal activities.

   B. **Etiology:** Most commonly RAP is not found to have obvious organic origins. Other causes are:
   - Inflammatory bowel disease (IBD)
   - Gastritis, peptic ulcer disease
   - Gastroesophageal reflux disease (GERD)
   - Constipation
   - Celiac disease
   - Lactose intolerance
   - Gallbladder disease
   - Kidney stones
   - Ureteropelvic obstruction
   - Gynecologic disease, for example, endometriosis
   - Congenital abnormalities
   - Psychiatric disease
   - Musculoskeletal conditions
   - Mittelschmerz
   - Sexual abuse

   C. **Types: Functional abdominal pain,** as defined by the Rome II criteria, can be of the **following types:**
   - **Functional dyspepsia:** epigastric pain or discomfort that is often associated with nausea, bloating, belching, and vomiting, but is not associated with changes in bowel habits.
   - **Irritable bowel syndrome (IBS):** pain relieved with defecation and/or associated with a change in bowel habits.
   - **Functional abdominal pain:** often periumbilical, but not related to physiologic events where no other pathologic cause can be found.

Table 12-1. Factors that differentiate functional from organic RAP

Organic	Functional
Consistently localized	Periumbilical or diffuse
Awakens patient from sleep	Variable locations
Precipitated by eating	Exacerbated by stress
Recent onset	Present for months before seeking medical attention
	Effects of pain out of proportion to findings
Systemic symptoms consistent with a single disease process	Systemic symptoms NOT consistent with a single disease process
	Normal lab/imaging exams

- **Abdominal migraine:** recurrent abdominal pain often associated with headaches, photophobia, family history of migraines, and/or aura.
- **Aerophagia:** air swallowing, abdominal distention, and belching or flatus.

    Depression, anxiety, psychosomatic dynamics, and life stressors are all sometimes associated with functional causes of chronic pain. Specifically, in one recent study, about 80% of adolescents with RAP had an anxiety disorder and about 40% suffered from depression.

II.   **Making the diagnosis:**

   A. **History:** Most important in the exploration of RAP is a detailed history with attention to activity limitation and to physical findings such as weight loss, fever, vomiting, diarrhea, dysuria, menstrual problems, vaginal discharge, sexual history, history of abuse, musculoskeletal activities, travel, and substance use. Symptoms of **anxiety and depression** need to be sought. Bowel movement pattern is important to discern. Simply asking if a patient is constipated is not enough.

   B. **Differential diagnosis:** Historical factors that might help differentiate functional from organic causes of RAP are shown in Table 12-1.

   C. **Physical examination:** A careful physical examination is mandatory, with a rectal or pelvic examination as needed based on the history and other physical findings. Pay attention to the abdominal wall and its skeletal attachments, since adolescents frequently strain these structures and do not recall the inciting incidents. Musculoskeletal palpation with tensing of affected muscles will, in these cases, frequently reproduce the pain.

   D. **Laboratory evaluation:** Laboratory studies need to be selected carefully. Begin with a complete blood count, an erythrocyte sedimentation rate, liver function studies, and a test for occult blood in the stool.

    A urine analysis with possible culture can be helpful, as can studies to detect sexually transmitted diseases. Obtaining pancreatic enzyme levels might help when there is substernal pain.

   E. **Imaging studies:** With guidance from the history and physical examination, appropriate imaging studies might assist in diagnosing abdominal pain. Usually a pelvic/abdominal ultrasound is most useful, since it can reveal obvious masses and congenital anomalies. Ultrasound of the gall bladder occasionally can help, as can a CT or MRI in selected instances. Helicobacter titers and breath hydrogen tests for lactose intolerance are rarely any good, but in selected cases they can make the diagnosis.

III. **Management:**

   A. **Management begins with the initial interview:** One should always begin the evaluation of a patient with RAP by stating clearly to the patient and the family that there are many causes for RAP, some organic and some functional, and that you will explore both areas. When something positive is revealed in one area, then the workup in the other area will stop while the more likely cause is explored further. If the symptoms persist, there is always an opportunity to renew exploration in the area that has been set aside.

    It is essential that you convey to the patient and parents your conviction that the pain is real. Reassurance that no serious disease, such as cancer, is the cause of the pain also is mandatory.

   B. **Treatment:** Management then proceeds with:
   - treatment of psychosocial problems that have been detected,
   - instruction (by the clinician or a psychosocial colleague) on stress management techniques,
   - cognitive behavioral therapy (if necessary), and
   - **most immediately,** symptom relief.

    It is always good to offer such simple things as use of a heating pad, a bowel regulating regimen, or massage as initial treatments. Frequent visits for reassurance and to head off crises are often helpful. Finally, some adolescents respond well to the task of keeping a treatment diary.

    RAP in adolescents is common, and the care and management of it does not have to be unduly stressful for either the patient or the clinician.

   C. **When to refer:** When the patient's pain seems more likely to stem from an identifiable organic cause, when the patient does not respond to the treatment approach outlined above, or when the parent just will not rest until a "specialist" has been consulted, a referral to a pediatric gastroenterologist is indicated. Frequently, such a referral results in confirmation of the primary care clinician's impression, and then management ensues as outlined in B. above.

IV. **Clinical pearls and pitfalls:**
- Chronic abdominal pain in adolescents is common.
- Pain that emanates from the mid-abdomen is more likely to be from a less serious organic cause.
- Look out for possible psychosomatic causes related to the family, that is, enmeshment between one parent and the child, distancing of the other parent, problems between the parents.
- Do the minimal necessary laboratory/imaging workup.
- Musculoskeletal causes of pain are relatively common in adolescents.
- Do not forget about gynecologic causes of pain, especially in female adolescents.
- Management begins with the initial evaluation.

BIBLIOGRAPHY

For the clinician

American Academy of Pediatrics, North American Society for Pediatric Gastroenterology, Hepatology, and Nutrition. Chronic abdominal pain in children. *Pediatrics* 2005;115:812–815.
Brown RT, Hewitt GD. Chronic pelvic pain and recurrent abdominal pain in female adolescents. In: Sultan C, ed. *The adolescent girl, pediatric and adolescent gynecology.* Basel: Karger, 2004.
Crandall W. Gastroenterology. In: Holland-Hall C, Brown RT, eds. *Adolescent medicine secrets.* Philadelphia, PA: Hanley & Belfus, 2002:101–107.
Holland-Hall C, Brown RT. Evaluation of the adolescent with chronic abdominal or pelvic pain. *J Pediatr Adolesc Gynecol* 2004;17:23–27.
Hyams JS. Irritable bowel syndrome, functional dyspepsia, and functional abdominal pain syndrome. *Adolesc Med Clin* 2004;15:1–15.

For patients and parents

Van Vorous H, Posner DB (forward). *The first year–IBS (Irritable Bowel Syndrome): An essential guide for the newly diagnosed.* New York: Marlowe, 2001.

WEB SITES

www.aafp.org/afp/990401ap/1823.html

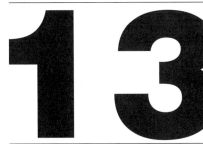

Musculoskeletal Problems

No area of the adolescent's body goes through more changes during puberty and adolescence than the musculoskeletal system. We will review some of the more common problems. Those due to sports and sports injuries will be presented in Chapter 28, on sports medicine.

SCOLIOSIS

I. **Description of the condition:**
A. **Clinical features:** Scoliosis is a lateral curvature of the spine of greater than 10 degrees. The curve or curves can occur in the lumbar or thoracic spine (or in both) and are associated with rotation of the vertebrae and sometimes with excessive kyphosis or lordosis. Scoliosis typically involves a **three-dimensional deformity of the spinal column and rib cage.** In adolescents, idiopathic scoliosis is most common, but this condition can be secondary to other conditions.
B. **Epidemiology:** While as many as one in 25 children has some degree of scoliosis, **only 4 in 1000 people in the United States have moderate to severe curves beyond 20 degrees.** (Degrees indicate the angle of curve, that is, the angle formed from perpendiculars dropped from lines parallel to the top and bottom of the curve on A-P spine radiographs). Idiopathic scoliosis usually develops in early adolescence. The ratio of males:females with curves less than 20 degrees is nearly equal (nearly 80% of the cases), but curves whose Cobb angle is greater than that (Figure 13-1) occur 5 to 7 times more often in females. These curves can be progressive and require treatment. Curves that progress usually do so while a female is going through the period of peak height velocity, prior to menarche.
C. **Etiology:** Most scoliosis in adolescents is idiopathic. Table 13-1 lists the types and possible causes.
   Particular attention should be paid to whether or not the curve noted is structural or functional. Functional curves can be from poor posture or from other musculoskeletal causes such as leg length discrepancy.
II. **Screening:** Screening adolescents for idiopathic scoliosis is usually done by visual inspection of the spine to detect asymmetry of the shoulders, scapulae, and hips. While the adolescent is bent over at the waist, the examiner, from behind the patient, looks for a unilateral rib hump.
   Screening programs are held in many schools, particularly for children in grades 5 to 9. The ideal screening test is low cost, easy to do, has a high sensitivity, has a high positive predictive value (PPV) (i.e., prevalence in the population in question is high enough to diminish chance of false positives), and is intended to detect a problem for which there is effective treatment.
   The **sensitivity of scoliosis screening** programs is high. Specificity is high since those children without the problem are readily identified. The PPV varies widely between finding scoliosis which does *not* require treatment and finding that which does. So while those adolescents in whom scoliosis is detected do have the condition, fewer than 5% of them require treatment.
III. **Management:**
A. **Criteria for referral:** Once a sign of scoliosis is detected in a screening program, the child should be referred to their clinician for confirmation of the finding and for the decision of whether further evaluation is needed. If the scoliosis is detected during a primary care visit, the assessment proceeds. Radiographs to measure the angle of curve are the next step.
B. **Identification:** Primary Goals. Management depends on several **factors**, but as a rule:
   • Females who are relatively immature and who have curves of 20 degrees to 29 degrees are at highest risk for progression. They should be referred to a pediatric orthopaedist for further management.

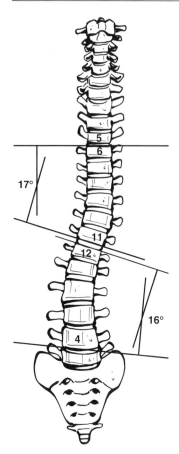

Figure 13-1. Cobb angle for measuring degree of curve in scoliosis.

Table 13-1. Etiologic classification of structural scoliosis

Type	Possible cause
Idiopathic	
Congenital	Failure of formation—hemivertebra
	Failure of segmentation—bony bar joining one side of two or more adjacent vertebrae
Neuromuscular	Cerebral palsy
	Muscular dystrophy
	Myelomeningocele
	Spinal muscular atrophy
	Friedreich ataxia (spinocerebellar degeneration)
Vertebral disease	Tumor
	Infection
	Metabolic bone disease
Spinal cord disease or anomaly	Tumor
	Syringomyelia
Disease associated	Neurofibromatosis
	Marfan syndrome
	Connective tissue disorders

From Green, WB, ed., *Essentials of musculoskeletal care.* 2nd ed. Rosemont, IL: American Academy of Orthopaedic Surgeons, 2001, 696, with permission.

- If the curve is less than 20 degrees in a female who is Tanner stage 1 to 3, the clinician should follow with another examination and radiograph in 6 months.
- If the curve has progressed at least 3 degrees to 5 degrees, referral to an orthopaedist is indicated.

  In the adolescent who is more mature, that is, Tanner stage 4 or 5, and who has achieved menarche, curves up to 30 degrees have little risk of significant progression.
- Still, with significant curves, referral to the specialist is often prudent.
- Curves of less than 50 degrees at full maturity have little risk of further progression.

  Pain is not a usual symptom for curves less than 50 degrees. Pulmonary compromise does not occur unless the curve is at least 90 degrees.

C. **Braces: Bracing treatment** for curves is used for patients with progressing curves of 20 degrees to 45 degrees. The goal of bracing is to stop the progression of the curve until bony maturity is achieved, at which time further progression of a curve less than 50 degrees is unlikely. Bracing is not always effective, especially with patients who do not comply well with the requirements of treatment.

D. **Surgery: Surgery** is indicated for curves 50 degrees or greater or for curves of 40 degrees to 50 degrees that are likely to progress.

E. **Exercise: Exercise as a treatment** for scoliosis has traditionally been said to be of no use, but there are some studies that suggest that it might have a role.

IV. **Clinical pearls and pitfalls:** Patients with an obvious curve or one of more than 5 degrees with a scoliometer should have the degree of curve documented radiographically with an estimate of the likelihood of progression.

Patients with **unusual findings,** such as convex left thoracic curves, pain, abnormal neurologic findings, bladder or bowel dysfunction, or deformities of the feet, **need to be investigated** for causes other than idiopathic scoliosis.

OTHER BACK PROBLEMS

Kyphosis is an accentuated forward, anterior–posterior curve of the spine. The normal kyphotic curve is less than 40 degrees. Any larger curve in a relatively immature adolescent may require bracing, and surgical fusion might be needed if bracing is not successful. It is **important** to note that **95% of teens with apparent kyphosis** have a **postural** problem, **not a structural** one.

One condition that can lead to structural kyphosis is **Scheuermann's Disease.** This condition accounts for a large proportion of adolescents who have kyphosis needing treatment. The key finding is irregularity of the apophyseal growing areas of the thoracic vertebrae on radiograph.

Back Pain

Back pain in older adolescents is usually due to muscular spasm, as in adults. The causes of back pain in one study comparing adults to children and adolescents is shown in Table 13-2.

Table 13-2. Low back pain comparison between adults and children participating in sports

	Adult	Child	P value
Ankylosing spondylitis	1	0	–
Discogenic	48	11	0.05
• Degenerated	22	1	–
• Herniated	24	9	–
• Both	2	1	–
Hamstring strain	0	1	–
Hyperlordotic mechanical back pain	0		26
Lumbosacral strain	27	6	0.05
Neoplasm	2	0	–
Osteoarthritis	4	0	–
Scoliosis	7	8	–
Spinal stenosis	6	0	–
Spondyloysis/-isthesis	5	47	0.05
Trochanteric bursitis	0	1	–
Total	100	100	

Adapted from Micheli LJ, Wood R. Back pain in young athletes. *Arch Pediatr Adolesc Med* 1995;149:15.

Younger adolescents and athletes in certain sports should be examined radiographically for spondylolysis and spondylolisthesis. These topics are covered in Chapter 28, on Sports Medicine.

SLIPPED CAPITAL FEMORAL EPIPHYSIS (SCFE)

I. **Description of the problem:**
   A. **Definition and etiology:** SCFE is displacement of the femoral head through the physis during the adolescent growth spurt. During adolescence, the orientation of the **physis (growth plate) of the femoral head** changes from horizontal to oblique. That, plus increasing body size, may cause excessive shear at the physis with resultant microscopic fractures and gradual **slippage** of the femoral head posteriorly and usually also medially. Sometimes there is an acute slippage, i.e. an acute fracture.
   B. **Epidemiology:** SCFE occurs in 3 to 10 of 100,000 pubertal adolescents. **Obese, male, African American adolescents who are involved in sports are at increased risk for this problem, particularly between Tanner stages 2 and 3.** The male to female ratio is between 2 and 4:1. SCFE is unilateral 3 times more often than bilateral. About 40% to 50% of teens with SCFE will have the other hip involved prior to closure of the growth plates.

II. **Making the diagnosis:**
   A. **Presentation and assessment:** SCFE usually presents with a complaint of pain in or around the affected hip. This pain may be perceived as coming from the ipsilateral knee or lower thigh. Physical examination shows that the patient has a limp with a characteristic gait in which the leg is externally rotated at the hip. There is limited passive range of motion of the affected hip, especially with internal rotation, flexion, and abduction. **Assessing internal rotation with the hip flexed at 90 degrees is an effective screening maneuver,** and is done easily on all adolescents who have lower-extremity pain. Systemic signs are absent. Tanner stage is usually 3 or 4.
   B. **Radiographs: Diagnosis is confirmed** by anteroposterior and frogleg hip radiographs.

III. **Management:**
   A. **Goals of treatment:** Stabilization of a mild to moderate slippage provides good long-term function with symptomatic arthritis not a significant future problem. The same cannot be said for severe SCFE, **making the diagnosis and treating the condition as early as possible very important.**
      The goals of treatment are to prevent further slippage of the femoral head, to promote closure of the physis, and to avoid osteonecrosis and chondrolysis.
   B. **Surgery:** Most patients are treated by surgical stabilization of the femoral head with bone pegs.

IV. **Clinical pearls and pitfalls:**
   • Think of SCFE when seeing **any adolescent who has an unexplained limp** so that detection and treatment are not delayed.

KNEE PAIN

I. **Description of the condition:** Knee pain can be due to several conditions during adolescence.
   A. **Athletics:** Obviously, knee injury is a frequent cause of pain in athletes. Those entities more associated with sports participation are discussed thoroughly in Chapter 28, on Sports Medicine. In addition, patellofemoral pain is common in both athletes and non-athletes. This condition, too, is discussed in Chapter 28.
   B. **Osteochondritis dissecans:** Another cause of knee pain in the adolescent can be **osteochondritis dissecans.** This is due to repetitive stress that causes osteonecrosis of the underlying bone and, ultimately, subchondral stress fracture. The most common site of this condition is the medial femoral condyle. This type of lesion can heal, or progress to a fissure or separation in the articular cartilage, and can ultimately result in a loose piece of bone in the joint. Although symptoms usually present in late adolescence or in adulthood, the condition starts in childhood.
      1. **Presentation and findings:** Making the diagnosis of osteochondritis dissecans during the growing years is important because at this stage healing is possible.
         a. **Physical examination: Pain and stiffness after running or athletic activities is the usual presentation.** The examination is usually non-revealing, although there may be some swelling or quadricep atrophy.
         b. **Imaging:** Radiographs are needed to make the diagnosis.

2. **Prognosis:** Prognosis depends on the size of the lesion and the physical maturity of the adolescent. After the distal femoral physis closes there is little chance of healing. Activity modification is needed, with no sports participation for 3 to 12 months. **Indications for surgery** include:
    - a loose body,
    - an unstable lesion, or
    - persistent symptoms despite compliant nonoperative treatment.

FOOT PROBLEMS

Two foot conditions that can bring the adolescent to the clinician are **pes cavus (high arched foot)** and **pes planus (flat feet).**

I. **Pes cavus:**

A. **Description of the condition:** A cavus foot frequently accompanies **some other neuromuscular disorder** with associated spasticity or muscle weakness. The presence of this condition should prompt an investigation of other conditions that are not known to be present. **Unilateral pes cavus** is associated with localized disorders of the lumbosacral spinal cord. There can be difficulty in fitting shoes, and there can be repeated ankle sprains. Over time, painful calluses can develop over the prominent metatarsal heads. Some causes are familial.

B. **Examination** of pes cavus includes a thorough neurological examination and radiographs of the feet and of the spine. There is an extensive differential diagnostic list for this condition.

C. **Treatment** is dictated by the cause. Shoe modifications can be used early on, but **progressive deformity requires operative intervention.**

II. **Pes planus:**

A. **Description of the condition: Pes planus**, or flat foot, is due to an abnormally low or absent longitudinal arch. **Flexible flat feet** are **more common** than fixed, and is considered **normal** in infants and **in up to 20% of adults**. Rigid flat foot is uncommon. **Flexible flat foot is usually asymptomatic.** Occasionally activity-related pain is noted as well as aching at night. Adolescents with this condition have an abnormally short Achilles tendon and may report focal pain with redness and callosities under the bony prominence beneath the sagging arches.

B. **Examination** shows the foot to be rotated outward in relation to the leg, and the heel to be in valgus alignment. This gives the medial malleolus a prominent appearance. In flexible flat foot, the arch is present when the adolescent is sitting and when the patient stands on tiptoes. The arch cannot be created with rigid flat feet. Radiographs are indicated only with rigid flat foot.

C. **Treatment** is not indicated unless there is pain. Occasionally there is heel pain due to a contracted Achilles tendon, so **stretching exercises** are helpful. Rigid orthotics are not helpful, but **soft orthotics** such as those which come with running shoes can help ease the pain and prolong the life of running shoes. Surgery is rarely indicated for flexible flat foot. The adolescent with persistent Achilles pain and tightness and callosities under the sagging arch requires orthopedic referral.

III. **Clinical pearls and pitfalls:**
    - Flat feet usually do not require treatment.

CHEST PROBLEMS

I. **Pectus deformities of the chest,** that is, pectus excavatum and pectus carinatum, can be significant cosmetic problems, and they can cause respiratory and circulatory problems as well. Recent studies have demonstrated that affected patients have **true physiologic respiratory and circulatory impairment** that is corrected by surgical repair. Therefore clinicians and third party payers should be reminded that the deformities are not just cosmetic.

   These two deformities occur in 1 in 300 men and 1 in 1,500 women. While both deformities may be somewhat apparent in children, they **worsen significantly during the period of rapid adolescent growth.** The **optimum age for repair** of both deformities is between **11 and 18 years.** There was extensive removal of sternal and chondral segments in earlier years, but this has been shown to be unnecessary. Minimal removal of tissue along with implants, particularly in pectus excavatum, is the most common current approach.

II. **Chest pain/costochondritis**

A. **Description of the condition:** Most chest pain in adolescents is of **musculoskeletal** origin. The various causes of chest pain in this age group are listed in Table 13-3. Several studies have confirmed this impression. The major differential diagnosis of chest pain in adolescents other than chest wall causes include gastroesophageal reflux, pulmonary problems such as pneumonia or psychosomatic conditions, and, when sudden, pneumothorax. Compared to adults, adolescents have little de novo cardiac disease, so **the heart is rarely the cause of any significant chest pain.**

B. **Physical examination:** Adolescents have a preoccupation with their bodies and a blossoming awareness of their own mortality. This combination makes teenagers acutely aware of persistent chest pain, especially when the pain is on the left side of the chest, since they know that the heart is on that side. When these teens are seen by clinicians, it is to be expected, then, that they will appear somewhat psychologically distressed. This distress can easily be mistaken for the cause of the pain rather than a response to it. A **meticulous examination of the chest wall with single digit palpation of the costal cartilages** is needed in order to find the source of the pain in many cases.

   Costochondritis is defined as pain that is reproducible by palpation of the affected chest cartilage when no signs or symptoms of other abnormalities are present. The pain is usually sharp, may radiate laterally from the sternal area or down into the upper abdomen, is frequently associated with a particular movement or position, and the patients often report a history of upper respiratory infection, vomiting, or heavy exercise in the weeks preceding the onset of the pain.

   When the pain is unilateral, more adolescents (and adults) report it as coming from the left side. This may be because of the position of the heart. More women see doctors for this than do men. **Costochondritis can only be diagnosed once other possible causes of chest pain have been ruled out.** If they have not been ruled out, more information must be obtained.

C. **Management:** Management of costochondritis is fairly simple. After the possibility of other causes has been considered and a single digit palpation of sternocostal cartilages has reproduced the pain, **simple education and reassurance** as to the cause and the benign nature of the pain is usually sufficient. The patient must be told that the pain may persist for many weeks due to the constant movement of the rib cage. Then all that is needed is the occasional analgesic.

III. **Hyperventilation** is another cause of chest pain that must be considered. In adolescents, this is a relatively common manifestation of anxiety that frequently causes chest pain.

Table 13-3. Causes of chest pain in adolescents

Musculoskeletal
   Costochondritis
   Traumatic injury
   Muscle strain
   Rib cage anomaly
Infectious or inflammatory
   Pleurisy
   Pneumonitis
   Bronchitis
   Herpes zoster
   Esophagitis or esophageal reflux
   Pericarditis
Mitral valve prolapse
Arrhythmia
Hyperventilation
Psychosomatic
Idiopathic

From Strasburger VC, Brown RT. *Adolescent medicine: A practical guide.* 2nd ed. Philadelphia, PA: Lippincott Williams & Wilkins, 1998, p. 96, with permission.

On the other hand, the presence of chest pain may cause the patient to become anxious and hyperventilate. When there is
- light-headedness,
- difficulty "catching" one's breath, and
- tingling in fingers, toes, or lips,

hyperventilation is the likely culprit. Education, and having the patient reproduce the symptoms in the controlled environment of the office (pointing out that they can be in control of their breathing), are usually sufficient to abort the symptoms.

IV. Finally, it has been thought that **mitral valve prolapse (MVP)** can be a cause of chest pain. While that may be true when there is an associated arrhythmia, studies show no increase in chest pain in patients with MVP.

ARTHRITIS

I. **Description of the condition:** The **major causes** of arthritis are collagen-vascular diseases such as juvenile rheumatoid arthritis (JRA), spondyloarthropathies (including Reiter syndrome), and systemic lupus erythematosus. Other significant causes include rheumatic fever, gonococcal arthritis, and Lyme Disease.

  A. JRA is arthritis that:
  - is objectively present in one or more joints for at least 6 weeks,
  - has its onset prior to age 17, and
  - for which other causes of joint inflammation have been excluded.
  - There are 3 types of JRA:

    1. Systemic: this can begin at any age with equal distribution among females and males. Joint destruction occurs, and there are:
    - fevers
    - a characteristic rash
    - polyserositis
    - adenopathy/hepatosplenomegaly
    - arthritis
    - anemia/elevated white blood cell (WBC) count
    - elevated erythrocyte sedimentation rate (ESR)/C-reactive protein (CRP)
    - negative rheumatoid factor (RF) and antinuclear antibody (ANA)

    2. Polyarticular: This can be diagnosed when there are **5 or more joints involved in the absence of systemic signs.** There are two types:
    - RF-negative (type 1): this occurs in younger children and primarily in females. Many joints, including small ones in the hands and feet can be involved. It is less associated with iridocyclitis, and the laboratory profile includes elevated ESR/CRP, negative RF, and positive ANA in 40%.
    - RF-positive (type 2): this type is more common in older children and adolescents with more females than males. This is where adult type disease begins in childhood/adolescence. Rheumatoid nodules are present in 50% of patients, and there can be vasculitis, lung disease, and adult type deformities. Laboratory profile includes elevated ESR/CRP, positive RF, and positive ANA in 50%.

    3. Pauciarticular: This can be diagnosed when there are fewer than **5 joints involved, without systemic signs.** There are two types:
    - Type I: this occurs mostly in young females (2–5 years old), mainly in the knees and ankles but also in arm and hand joints and in the cervical spine. There can be flexion contractures and limb length discrepancies, and 20% have iridocyclitis. The laboratory profile includes elevated ESR/CRP, negative RF, and positive ANA in 90%.
    - Type II: This occurs primarily in children older than 8, and is found mainly in lower extremity joints. Enthesitis can occur. Laboratory profile includes elevated ESR/CRP, and negative RF and ANA.

  B. The **spondyloarthropathies** all have arthritis of the spine and axial joints with or without peripheral arthritis. These include:
  - Ankylosing spondylitis
  - Reiter syndrome
  - Spondylitis of inflammatory bowel disease
  - Spondylitis of psoriasis
  - Reactive arthritis
  - Enthesopathy syndromes
  - Pauciarticular RF type II
  - Acute iritis

Table 13-4. Differential diagnosis of arthritis in adolescents

Collagen vascular disorder
Juvenile rheumatoid arthritis
Ankylosing spondylitis
Systemic lupus erythematosus
Dermatomyositis
Scleroderma
Polyarteritis nodosa
Psoriasis
Sjogren syndrome
Henoch-Schonlein syndrome
Infectious or parainfectious process
Gonococcal disease
Reiter syndrome
Rheumatic fever
Lyme arthritis
Traumatic injury
Slipped capital femoral epiphysis
Legg-Calve-Perthe disease
Chondromalacia patellae
Other conditions with arthritis as a feature
Hemophilia
Sickle cell disease
Serum sickness
Inflammatory bowel disease
Sarcoidosis

From Strasburger VC, Brown RT. *Adolescent medicine: A practical guide.* 2nd ed. Common musculoskeletal problems. Philadelphia, PA: Lippincott Williams & Wilkins, 1998, p. 98, with permission.

People with these syndromes are usually seronegative. More males than females have these, there is familial clustering, and there is an association with HLA-B27. The most common one of these that affects adolescents is **Ankylosing Spondylitis (AS).** This affects mostly male teens and young adults, and the **characteristic presenting symptom is lower back stiffness and pain.** The axial skeleton is most heavily involved, and enthesitis is a feature. AS is often associated with HLA-B27 tissue type.

II.   **Diagnosis: Diagnosis** is made when there is **limitation of lumbosacral mobility** and **radiographic evidence of sacroiliitis.** The **natural course** is one of progressive lordosis, limitation of chest excursions leading to respiratory compromise, aortic valve insufficiency, and aortitis.

The differential diagnosis of arthritis in adolescents is extensive as shown in Table 13-4.

Reiter Syndrome is a reactive arthritis and sacroiliitis with conjunctivitis, urethritis, and skin rash. Many organisms are associated with this syndrome, but one thinks most often of the association with STIs such as *chlamydia trachomatis.*

The other major collagen vascular syndrome seen in adolescence is **systemic lupus erythematosus (SLE).** A disease of unknown etiology, SLE involves production of autoantibodies with consequent formation of IgG-containing immune complexes that have the ability to activate the complement pathways and induce vasculitis when deposited in small blood vessels. Inflammation occurs and exacerbates the problems. Table 13-5 shows the criteria for diagnosis of SLE, and Table 13-6 shows the pathogenesis of the various clinical features.

About **15% of patients present during adolescence,** and females, particularly African American females, are affected more frequently. There is no curative treatment.

CHRONIC MUSCULOSKELETAL PAIN

I.   **Description of the condition:** Another musculoskeletal (MS) problem is **chronic musculoskeletal pain (CMSP).** The most well known of these chronic pain syndromes is

Table 13-5. The 1982 revised criteria for the diagnosis of systemic lupus erythematosus (SLE)

1. Malar rash
   Fixed erythema, flat or raised, over the malar eminences, tending to spare the nasolabial folds.
2. Discoid lupus
   Erythematous raised patches with adherent keratotic scaling and follicular plugging; atrophic scarring may occur in older lesions.
3. Photosensitivity
   Skin rash as a result of unusual reaction to sunlight, by patient history or physician observation.
4. Oral ulcers
   Oral or nasopharyngeal ulceration, usually painless, observed by a physician.
5. Arthritis
   Nonerosive arthritis involving one or more peripheral joints, characterized by tenderness, swelling, or effusion.
6. Serositis
   Pleuritis—convincing history of pleuritic pain or rub heard by physician, or evidence of pleural effusion.
7. Renal disorder
   - Persistent proteinuria >0.5 g/d or >3+.
   - Cellular casts may be red blood cell, hemoglobin, granular, tubular, or mixed.
8. Neurologic disorder
   - Seizures in the absence of offending drugs or known metabolic derangements; for example, uremia, ketoacidosis, or electrolyte imbalance.
   - Psychosis in the absence of offending drugs.
9. Hematologic disorder
   - Hemolytic anemia with reticulocytosis.
   - Leukopenia <4,000/mm^3 total on two or more occasions.
   - Lymphopenia <1,500 mm^3 on two or more occasions.
   - Thrombocytopenia <100,000/mm^3 in the absence of offending drugs.
10. Immunologic disorder
    - Positive LE cell preparation.
    - Anti-DNA-presence of antibody to native DNA in abnormal titer.
    - Anti-Sm-presence of antibody to the Sm nuclear antigen.
    - False-positive serologic test for syphilis; known to be positive for at least 6 months and confirmed by fluorescent treponemal antibody tests.
11. Antinuclear antibody
    An abnormal titer of antinuclear antibody on immunofluorescence or equivalent assay at any point, in the absence of drugs known to be associated with drug-induced lupus syndrome.

From Tucker LB. Caring for the adolescent with systemic lupus erythematosus. *Adolesc Med* 1998 Feb;9(1):61, with permission.

fibromyalgia (FM), but many patients who do not meet all the criteria for FM suffer from CMSP. Adolescents are more likely to have CMSP without all the FM criteria. One should be hesitant to diagnose an adolescent with FM, since once so labeled the adolescent might expect to have a lifelong condition. However, once in a while that diagnosis has to be made.

Eighty to ninety percent of FM cases are found in white females, and the **peak age of diagnosis** is late adolescence to mid-adulthood. FM has widespread MS pain with no objective evidence of arthritis. It is frequently associated with fatigue, and, indeed, some feel that there is a spectrum of conditions involving fatigue and CMSP, ranging from fatigue only to CMSP only, with all gradations in between.

II. **Diagnosis:** To **diagnose** FM, the patient needs to have **unremitting pain for at least 3 months** and **specific areas of tenderness on the body known as tender points.** There are 18 points, and tenderness in 11 is needed for diagnosis (Figure 13-2).

All laboratory tests are normal. Table 13-7 lists the prevalence of symptoms and signs of FM in adolescence, and Table 13-8 lists the features of FM that help exclude other diagnoses.

Table 13-6. Pathogenesis of manifestations of systemic lupus erythematosus (SLE)

Manifestation	Serologic marker	Pathogenic mechanism
Anemia	Coomb's test positive	Complement-fixing IgG antibody to erythrocytes
Leukopenia	Anti-Neutrophil antibodies	Enhanced phagocytosis by RES
Thrombocytopenia	Anti-platelet antibodies	Enhanced phagocytosis by RES
Glomerulonephritis	Anti-dsDNA	Immune complex deposition with complement activation
Photosensitive rash	Anti-Ro	UV light increases antigenicity of DNA; increases expression of RO
Arthritis	?	Immune complexes autoreactive T-cells
Encephalopathy	Anticardiolipin; antineuronal	Thrombosis, cytotoxic antibodies
Pleuropericardial inflammation	?	Inflammatory mediators
Antiphospholipid syndrome	Antibody to SS/A, SS/B	Cytotoxic; binding to antigen on surface of myocardial cells, skin

RES, reticuloendothelial system; dsDNA, double-stranded DNA.
From Petty RE. Etiology and pathogenesis of rheumatic diseases in adolescence. *Adolesc Med* 1998;9:19, with permission.

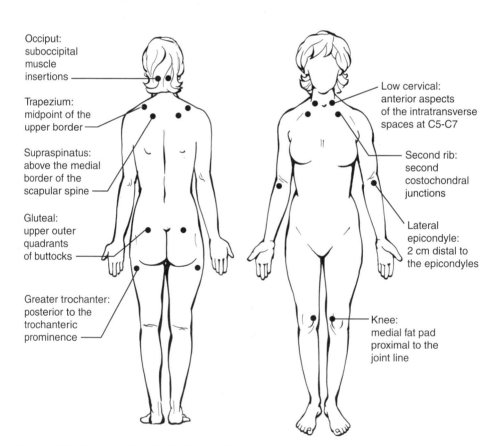

Figure 13-2. Tender point sites in fibromyalgia.

Table 13-7. Prevalence of symptoms and signs in adolescents with fibromyalgia syndrome (FS)

Symptom/Sign	Percentage of patients at initial presentation	Percentage of patients over time
Sleep disturbance	96	94
Diffuse pain	93	94
Headache	71	82
Fatigue	62	97
Morning stiffness	53	88
Morning fatigue	49	82
Depression	43	61
Subjective swelling[a]	40	59
Irritable bowel	38	46
Dysmenorrhea	36	42
Paresthesias	24	36
Anxiety	22	58
Raynaud phenomenon	13	30

[a]Swelling reported by the patient (typically in the hands and fingers) but not confirmed by physician examination (e.g., "My rings are tighter than they used to be").
From Siegel DM. Fibromyalgia syndrome. *Adoles Health Update* 2003;15(2):1–8, with permission.

III. **Clinical pearls and pitfalls:**
  • Make sure that when adolescents and their parents complain of arthritis, it is truly arthritis and not just arthralgia.
  • SLE can start very slowly and mimic other conditions, so suspicion needs to be high.
  • The most common cause of infectious arthritis in adolescents is gonorrhea.
  • The only proven treatments for fibromyalgia are aerobic exercise and cognitive behavioral therapy.

Table 13-8. Features of fibromyalgia syndrome (FS) that help exclude other diagnoses

Diagnosis	Clinical features *not* seen in FS	Laboratory results *not* seen in FS
Infectious Mononucleosis	Fever Enlarged tonsils Adenopathy Hepatosplenomegaly	Epstein-Barr viral titers Elevated LFTs
Chronic Lyme disease	History of tick bite with typical cutaneous eruption Erythema migraines	Positive Lyme antibody with confirmatory test
Juvenile rheumatoid arthritis (systemic or polyarticular)	Fever Rash Swollen, red, warm joints Hepatosplenomegaly	Elevated ESR Elevated WBC Anemia
Systemic lupus erythematosus	Fever Rash Oral lesions Alopecia Serositis Renal disease	Positive ANA Positive anti-dsDNA Positive anti-Smith Leukopenia Anemia Thrombocytopenia
Obstructive sleep apnea	Snoring Apnea	Diagnostic sleep study

LFTs, liver function tests; ESR, erythrocyte sedimentation rate; WBC, white blood cell count; ANA, antinuclear antibody; dsDNA, double-stranded DNA.
Adapted from Siegel DM. Fibromyalgia syndrome. *Adolesc Health Update* 2003;15(2):5.

BIBLIOGRAPHY

For the clinician

Fonkalsrud EW. Management of pectus chest deformities in female patients. *Am J Surg* 2004; 187:2:192–197.

Greene WB, ed. *Essentials of musculoskeletal care*, 2nd ed. Rosemount, IL: American Academy of Orthopaedic Surgeons, American Academy of Pediatrics, 2001.

Joffe A, Blythe MJ, eds. Handbook of adolescent medicine. *Adoles Med State Art Rev* 2003;14: 407–430, 14:505–507.

Scoliosis. MDConsult.com, 2004.

US Preventative Services Task Force. Screening for idiopathic scoliosis in adolescents: recommendation statement. *Am Fam Physician* 2005;71:1975–1976.

Wall E, Von Stein, D. Juvenile osteochondritis dissecans. *Orthop Clin North Am* 2003;34:3.

For patients and parents

Lehman TJA. *It's not just growing pains: A guide to childhood muscle, bone and joint pain, rheumatic diseases, and the latest treatments.* New York: Oxford University Press, 2004.

WEB SITES

www.orthoinfo.aaos.org/brochure
www.scoliosis.org
www.fmnetnews.com

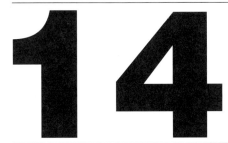

Urinary Tract Infection

I. **Description of the condition: Urinary tract infection (UTI)** is the term used to describe the growth of bacteria in the urinary tract with infection occurring anywhere from the urethral meatus to the renal cortex. UTI is a common clinical problem that affects 11% of women annually and more than 50% of all women during their lifetime. UTIs result in more than 3.5 million office visits per year, at a cost of more than 1.5 billion dollars. There is an increase in the rate of UTI during puberty, related in part to the onset of sexual activity and pregnancy. This problem affects primarily adolescent females; adolescent males have very low rates of infection. The diagnosis in women is further complicated because the symptoms of UTI can be similar to those of vaginitis or a sexually transmitted infection (STI).

A. **Epidemiology and classification: The epidemiology of UTI changes throughout life.** While 1% to 3% of school-age females experience UTI, the incidence is less than 1% in school-age males. The rates increase among females during adolescence to 0.5 episodes per year, possibly related to the onset of sexual activity, while the rates remain low in males. A study of university students found rates of only 5 UTI per 10,000 males per year in the absence of an anatomic abnormality.

Symptomatic UTI is divided into:
- **Acute cystitis,** in which the infection is only located in the lower urinary tract.
- **Acute pyelonephritis,** in which the infection involves the kidney (upper tract disease).
- **Acute urethral syndrome,** representing inflammation that is limited to the urethra.

Recurrent infections are those that occur after resolution of the previous episode. **Reinfection** occurs with introduction of a new organism. **Bacterial relapse** is infection that reemerges because it was not completely eradicated. Relapse is uncommon, but urea-splitting organisms such as *Proteus mirabilis* can be associated with infected renal stones, which may be curable only by surgery.

Infections can be classified as **uncomplicated** or **complicated.** Determining the type of infection has important implications for the risk of recurrent infection or the failure of therapy. Factors that make a UTI complicated are listed in Table 14-1.
- UTI is a particular problem during **pregnancy** because the hormonal changes cause decreased ureteral peristalsis and dilation of the renal calices and ureters. As the pregnancy progresses, complete emptying of the bladder also becomes more difficult. The incidence of acute pyelonephritis in pregnant patients with untreated cystitis is 25% to 35%.
- Diabetic women, but not men, have increased incidence of symptomatic UTI, and overall more severe infections appear to occur in **diabetics.**
- Diseases that cause chronic interstitial nephritis and primary renal papillary damage, such as diabetes and sickle cell disorders, have a higher incidence of renal scarring with infection.

B. **Etiology and contributing factors:**
1. **The urinary tract is normally kept sterile by local host defense mechanisms including:**
   - Free unobstructed flow of urine from the bladder
   - Complete evacuation of the bladder
   - Local antibacterial properties of the bladder mucosa
   - In males, a long urethra and bactericidal properties of prostatic secretions

   Retrograde ascent from the fecal reservoir, through the urethra, into the bladder, and then to the kidney via the ureter is the most common mechanism for infection. The same strains of bacteria found in the urine of patients with UTI are found in the stool. In addition, the endotoxins of gram-negative bacteria, as well as pregnancy and ureteral obstruction, can negatively affect the normal antiperistalic effects that protect the urinary tract from infection. Reflux may factilitate retrograde flow, and the edema of cystitis may cause changes in the ureterovesical

Table 14-1. Factors associated with complicated UTI

- Functional or anatomic abnormality of the urinary tract, including neurogenic bladder
- Pregnancy
- Being male
- Diabetes
- Sickle-cell disease
- Kidney stones
- Indwelling catheter
- Immunosuppression
- Instrumentation
- History of UTI as a child
- Hospital acquired infection

junction that facilitate this process. **Hematogenous and lymphatic routes do not play significant roles in otherwise healthy individuals.**

2. **Independent risk factors for UTI include:**
   - Sexual intercourse: Bacteriuria increases in the 24 hours after sexual intercourse, and the use of antibiotics coincident with sexual intercourse reduces the number of episodes of symptomatic infection. Individuals who have more frequent sexual intercourse are at higher risk for UTI. Local trauma during intercourse may be a contributing factor.
   - Use of a contraceptive spermicide with or without a diaphragm: Spermicide has antibacterial properties that can alter the normal population of bacterial flora in the genital area resulting in an increase in the uropathogens that cause UTI. The diaphragm further contributes to the problem by creating obstruction within the urethra.
   - History of recurrent UTI: Women with UTI tend to have recurrences—10% to 20% of women experience a repeat infection within a few months.

3. **Uroepithelial adherence, colonization, and familial or inherited factors:**
   a. **Virulence factors:** Certain strains of organisms have **virulence factors** that allow them to adhere to the mucosa and cause an inflammatory response. Examples of these factors are P-fimbriae and F-adhesins. Half of the recurrent episodes of UTI in women are caused by the same strain of bacteria with the same virulence factors as the original infection. Men with UTI also have organisms with these same virulence factors. Patients with pyelonephritis in the absence of reflux have been found to have bacterial strains with high adhesive properties 70% to 80% of the time. A specific association has been found between P-fimbriated *E. Coli* and acute pyelonephritis.
   b. **Colonization:** The organisms that cause UTI have been found to colonize the perineum including the vaginal introitus and periurethral areas. Individuals with recurrent infection are more likely to be colonized between symptomatic infections and to have a higher density of organisms than healthy controls. Estrogen levels also appear to play a role in colonization, since estrogen replacement in postmenopausal women decreases colonization with uropathogens, as well as the incidence of UTI.
   c. **Genetic susceptibility:** There is evidence that there may be a genetic susceptibility to recurrent UTI. Females who are nonsecretors of blood group antigens and those with certain blood group antigen phenotypes are more likely to have recurrent UTI.

4. **Microbiology:** Women and men have similar patterns of microbes causing UTI. *Escherichia coli* **is found in 85% to 90% of community-acquired acute UTI.** *Staphylococcus saprophyticus* **is present in 10 to 20% of cases of UTI in adolescent females** and is a common cause of UTI in sexually active women. This organism has also been found in men, and is a known cause of pyelonephritis. Other common UTI organisms include *Klebsiella*, *Enterococcus fecalis*, and Proteus. Other organisms include *Citrobacter*, *Serratia*, *Enterobacter*, *Pseudomonas*, *Providencia*, *S. epidermidis*, and *S. aureus*, although these are much less prevalent and are frequently associated with nosocomial infections or catheters. Nonbacterial causes of UTI include fungi (*Candida* species) and viruses. Specifically, adenovirus is a known cause of hemorrhagic cystitis.

II. **Making the diagnosis:**
   A. **Signs and symptoms/physical exam:**
      1. **Lower tract disease:** Symptoms of **lower tract infection** include:
         * Dysuria
         * Frequency
         * Urgency
         * Suprapubic pain
         * Hematuria
      2. **Upper tract disease:** Symptoms of **upper tract infection** also include systemic symptoms, although patients with upper tract disease may not have lower tract symptoms. Systemic symptoms include:
         * Fever
         * Flank pain
         * Costovertebral angle tenderness
   B. **Differential diagnosis:**
      1. **Lower tract disease: The differential diagnosis of lower tract disease includes:**
         * Urethritis
         * Vaginitis
         * Noninfectious causes of urethral discomfort
         In sexually active adolescent males, symptoms of dysuria may actually represent urethritis from an STI rather than a UTI, and dysuria may be accompanied by urethral discharge. **Acute urethral syndrome** occurs in females and is characterized by pyuria, dysuria, frequency, and nocturia. This syndrome can be caused by low colony counts of organisms that cause UTI as well as those associated with STI pathogens and vaginitis (e.g. *Chlamydia trachomatis, Neisseria gonorrhoeae, Trichomonas vaginalis* and *Candida* species.) Symptoms of lower tract infection in females may be the result of vaginitis or noninfectious causes of urethral irritation such as trauma from sexual intercourse or chemical irritants. **It is important to keep in mind that concurrent UTI and vaginitis or STI is not uncommon, particularly among sexually active females.**
      2. **Upper tract disease: The differential diagnosis of upper tract disease includes:**
         * Appendicitis
         * Pancreatitis
         * Diverticulitis
         * Gastroenteritis
         * Cholecystitis
         * Hepatitis
         * Pelvic inflammatory disease
         * Inflammatory bowel disease
         * Renal stone
         * Renal abscess
   C. **Laboratory evaluation:**
      1. **Urine:**
         a. **Urinalysis:** Presumptive diagnosis of UTI can be made on the basis of a urinalysis. Specific findings suggestive of UTI are pyuria, bacteriuria, and hematuria. **Proteinuria is not predictive.**
            * **Pyuria** is 95% sensitive and 71% specific for infection. It can represent both inflammation and infection, and most patients with symptomatic UTI have pyuria. Ten or more leukocytes per high-powered field (HPF) of unspun urine, which is equivalent to 1 to 2 white blood cells (WBCs) per HPF of spun urine, is significant. However, finding pyuria does not indicate the source of the infection. This is particularly relevant in females, where vaginal infection can be the source of WBCs in urine. Furthermore, WBCs in urine do not necessarily represent bacterial infection. **Sterile pyuria** can be seen with renal calculi, renal tuberculosis, neoplasia of the renal tract, prostatitis, urethritis, and appendicitis. **WBC casts** can be found in patients with pyelonephritis, but the absence of casts does not rule out upper tract disease. Finally, **the absence of pyuria does not exclude infection.** Patients with neutropenia may not mount a response and WBCs can disintegrate, especially in alkaline urine, prior to examination in the laboratory.
            * **Visible bacteria** has a sensitivity of 40% to 70% and specificity of 85% to 95%. Microscopy of unspun and unstained urine can detect bacteriuria with

10^5 bacteria per mL. 1 to 2 organisms in an unspun urine specimen is consistent with this concentration and is equivalent to 10 or more organisms in a spun specimen. Bacteria in the urine may be the result of urethritis alone.

- **Hematuria,** usually gross hematuria, can be seen in acute cystitis. However, this is not diagnostic since hematuria can also be found in other clinical entities, such as renal stones, renal neoplasia, or in noninfectious renal disease such as glomerulonephritis.

b. **Urine dipstick:** Urine dipstick can quickly give information suggestive of UTI in the office setting. Although positive results for nitrite or leukocyte esterase are less sensitive than microscopic examination, they are easier to perform. The use of nitrite and leukocyte esterase together has a sensitivity of 70% to 100% for predicting UTI.

- Nitrite is found in urine when bacteria using the enzyme nitrate reductase convert nitrate to nitrite. This test has high specificity with a sensitivity of 35% to 85%, and yields the best results when it is performed on an early morning specimen. This test has limitations since it is only positive with certain gram-negative organisms and will miss enterococcus and *S. saprophyticus*. Furthermore, a positive test result depends on the patient having nitrate in his or her diet, as well as there having been enough time for the bacteria in the bladder to produce nitrite. A negative test does not rule out infection.
- Leukocyte esterase measures esterase contained in WBCs. The test will be positive even when the cells have lysed, which is an advantage over microscopy. Leukocyte esterase has a sensitivity of 72% to 97% with a high specificity. False negatives are possible with ascorbic acid, glycosuria, urobilinogen, significant proteinuria, and certain antibiotics such as doxycycline and cephalexin. False positives are possible with clavulanic acid and in contaminated specimens.

c. **Urine culture:** Some clinicians treat uncomplicated UTI without performing a culture if the patient has classic symptoms and the findings of a urinalysis or urine dipstick are consistent with UTI. In those cases, culture is reserved for those who do not respond to the first course of antibiotic therapy. Other clinicians, however, perform a culture on all patients. Because UTI is uncommon in males and would warrant further investigation, any male suspected of having UTI should have a urine culture prior to initiating treatment. It is important to remember that sensitivity of the organism can only be determined if a culture is performed.

Urine culture is usually obtained as a **clean catch specimen.** The first morning urine is most accurate because the bacteria have had time to incubate. The perineal area or glans are washed with water or saline-soaked swabs. Soaps and antiseptics should be avoided because they can cause false negative results. Females should be instructed to wipe from front to back and males should retract the foreskin, if present, and wipe in only one direction. The urine collected should be **a mid-stream specimen** in a sterile container and plated within two hours, or kept refrigerated for plating within 24 to 48 hours.

Traditionally, a positive urine culture has been defined as greater than 10^5 organisms per mL. Although using this definition results in a high specificity, the sensitivity is only 50%. In symptomatic women, cultures with **"low count" bacteriuria** (10^2–10^4 organisms per mL) have been found to grow the same organisms, and many patients respond to antibiotics with resolution of symptoms (counts of 10^3 are the lower limit in men). *S. saprophyticus* is one of the common UTI pathogens which presents with lower counts. A pure culture with low organism counts should be considered as a possible significant specimen in a symptomatic individual with pyuria. Some authors have suggested that these lower-count infections may represent an early phase of UTI.

Polymicrobial infection usually represents contamination and rarely indicates true infection, except in patients with complicated anatomy such as an ileal conduit, neurogenic bladder, stones, or a long-term indwelling catheter. Polymicrobial results should be evaluated for a dominant organism and for the presence of WBCs.

Asymptomatic bacteriuria is not significant and should not be treated unless there are complicating circumstances such as pregnancy. Pregnancy is the exception because of the changes that occur in the urinary tract which make it more likely for these patients to develop pyelonephritis.

2. **Blood:** Patients with upper tract disease can have leukocytosis on a complete blood count and an elevated C reactive protein or erythrocyte sedimentation rate. These findings are not seen in lower tract disease.

3. **Testing for sexually transmitted infections and vaginitis:** Patients who are sexually active and those who have signs and symptoms of vaginitis regardless of sexual activity should be evaluated for STIs and organisms that cause non-STI vaginitis. External examination of the genitalia should be performed to look for trauma or other diseases such as *Herpes simplex* virus and other causes of vulvar ulcers. Specific testing should be performed to detect *C. trachomatis, N. gonorrhoeae, T. vaginalis,* bacterial vaginosis, and yeast.

4. **Radiologic studies: Radiologic studies are not usually necessary.** Finding abnormalities is uncommon, even in women with recurrent UTI or patients with pyelonephritis who respond promptly to therapy. Radiologic studies are indicated when there is:
   - Recurrent pyelonephritis
   - Lack of response to therapy
   - Male gender
   - Suspicion of an underlying abnormality

   Examples of underlying abnormalities include obstructive uropathy, urolithiasis (particularly if Proteus is cultured), an underlying anatomic abnormality, or a complication of infection such as a renal or perinephric abscess.

   a. **Choosing a study: Renal ultrasound or computed tomography (CT)** will demonstrate nephrolithiais, obstructive uropathy, and complicated renal and perirenal infections. Spiral CT may be superior for identification of stones. Ultrasound is frequently a first line modality because it is readily available and is noninvasive.

   DMSA scanning (technetium-99m) can demonstrate inflammation in the kidney with areas of uptake defects. Clinicians may find it useful to demonstrate upper tract disease if there is diagnostic confusion. However, DMSA cannot distinguish between acute inflammatory changes and renal scars. The acute changes may persist for 4 to 5 months while renal scars persist 6 months after the infection is treated.

   Voiding cystourethrogram can demonstrate vesicoureteral reflux and infravesical obstruction (posterior urethral valves). Use of isotope cystography is good for reflux but is not adequate for demonstrating anatomy of the urethra. These abnormalities usually first present in childhood and are unlikely to be new diagnoses in an adolescent.

   Cystoscopy and excretory urography are indicated if there is persistent hematuria after treatment.

III. **Management:**
   A. **Goals of treatment:**
      - Eliminate symptomatic infection
      - Prevent permanent damage to the upper urinary tract
   B. **Treatment:**
      1. **Lower tract infection: Three-day regimens** are preferred in uncomplicated cystitis in women. They are as effective as 7- to 10-day regimens and cause fewer side effects. One-day regimens are not as effective and are not recommended. **Seven-day regimens** are recommended for women with symptoms lasting for more than 1 week, for pregnant women, for men, and for patients with complicated UTI including diabetes. **Choice of antibiotic should be guided by local resistance patterns and final sensitivity results on the urine culture.** See Table 14-2 for examples of medications and doses.

Table 14-2. Treatment of acute uncomplicated UTI

Medication	Dose
Trimethoprim-sulfamethoxazole (160/800 mg)	1 tablet twice a day × 3 days
Trimethoprim	100 mg twice a day × 3 days
Norfloxacin	400 mg twice a day × 3 days
Ciprofloxacin	250 mg twice a day × 3 days
Levofloxacin	250 mg twice a day × 3 days
Ofloxacin	200 mg twice a day × 3 days
Amoxicillin	500 mg three times a day × 3 days
Nitrofurantoin macrocrystals	50–100 mg four times a day × 7 days
Nitrofurantoin monohydrate macrocrystals	100 mg twice a day × 7 days

TMP-SMX and fluoroquinolones are usually recommended as first choices when considering cost and sensitivity patterns of UTI organisms. It is important to note that quinolones are not currently approved for individuals younger than 18 and only cure 67% to 70% of enterococci. Nitrofurantoin requires a 7-day regimen and is inactive against Proteus and Pseudomonas. Futhermore, except for *E. coli,* nitrofurantoin is less active against aerobic gram-negative rods compared to TMP-SMX. Amoxicillin is not recommended as a first line therapy because of low cure rates and frequent resistance. During pregnancy, quinolones would be contraindicated. However, cephalosporins, such as cephalexin and nitrofurantoin, and amoxicillin are acceptable. Most women with uncomplicated infection have clinical improvement in 72 hours. Phenazopyrindine can be used for 1 to 2 days to reduce symptoms of UTI.

2. **Upper tract infection:** If the patient is toxic or cannot tolerate oral medications, therapy with broad spectrum antibiotics should be administered intravenously for several days at a minimum. Once there is clinical improvement, oral medication can be substituted to complete a 10- to 14-day course of therapy. Intravenous medications include parenteral fluoroquinolones, aminoglycoside with or without ampicillin, or an extended spectrum cephalosporin (ceftriaxone). Some studies have found fluoroquinolones to be superior to other medication regimens. Patients with mild illness of upper tract disease can be treated as outpatients for 10 to 14 days. Sensitivity testing from urine culture results should guide choice of an effective medication with the fewest side effects.

3. **Recurrent UTI:** Several therapeutic options are available for patients with recurrent UTI.

   a. **Antimicrobial prophylaxis: Low dose continuous prophylaxis** at night should be considered for those patients with two or more symptomatic UTIs in 6 months or three or more in 12 months. Breakthrough infections are treated with full dose therapy. Some clinicians monitor patients with urine cultures every 1 to 3 months. There is general agreement that therapy should be discontinued after 6 months to evaluate for remission. Medications and doses include:
      • Nitrofurantoin macrocrystals, 50–100 mg
      • TMP-SMX, 40/200 mg
      • TMP, 100 mg
      • Norfloxacin, 200 mg
      • Cephalexin, 250 mg

   b. **Self-start intermittent therapy:** The patient performs a urine culture and then empirically self starts a full dose 3-day regimen. Fluroquinolones are an excellent choice because of their broad spectrum. Nitrofurantoin and TMP-SMX are less effective but have the advantage of not being contraindicated for patients under age 18. Tetracycline, ampicillin, and cephalexin should not be used because of potential bacterial resistance. Many clinicians repeat the urine culture 7 to 10 days after therapy to ensure adequate treatment.

   c. **Postcoital therapy:** To reduce infection which is clearly related to coitus, the patients can take a single dose of nitrofurantoin macrocrystal (50–100 mg), cephalexin (250 mg), TMP-SMX (40/200 mg), or a fluoroquinolone.

C. **Follow up:**
   • Lower tract disease: repeat urine culture should be performed if symptoms do not resolve or recur shortly after appropriate treatment.
   • Upper tract disease: repeat urine culture should be performed after completion of treatment (1–2 weeks). Some authors advocate culture 5 to 7 days into the course of treatment to demonstrate clearance of the organism.

D. **Prevention strategies:**
   • Eliminate use of spermicidal agents.
   • Consider use of a contraceptive method other than a diaphragm.
   • **Cranberry juice** has been shown to decrease UTI possibly by inhibiting adherence of uropathogens to uroepithelial cells.
   • Postcoital voiding and increased fluid intake **have not** been effective in reducing UTI in controlled studies.

IV.   **Clinical pearls and pitfalls:**
- UTI is common in adolescent women particularly those who are sexually active.
- UTI in adolescent males is rare, and when documented should prompt urologic evaluation.
- Symptoms of UTI in females may represent STI or vaginitis rather than UTI. There may also be STI or vaginitis concurrent with a UTI.
- Symptoms of UTI in males commonly represent STI.
- Cases of uncomplicated UTI in females that respond promptly to therapy do not require further urologic evaluation.

BIBLIOGRAPY

For the clinician

Avner ED, Harmon WE, Niaudet P, eds. *Pedatric nephrology*, 5th ed. Philadelphia, PA: Lippincott Williams & Wilkins, 2004.

Bonny AE, Brouhard BH. Urinary tract infections among adolescents. *Adol Med Clinc N Am* 2005;16:149–161.

Fihn SD. Acute uncomplicated urinary tract infection in women. *N Engl J Med* 2003;349:259–266.

Gearhart JP, Rink RC, Moriquand PD, eds. *Pediatric urology*. Philadelphia, PA: WB Saunders, 2001.

Gillenwater JY, Grayhack JT, Howard SS, et al., eds. *Adult and pediatric urology*, 4th ed. Philadelphia, PA: Lippincott Williams & Wilkins, 2002.

Graham JC, Galloway A. The laboratory diagnosis of urinary tract infection. *J Clin Pathol* 2001;54:911–919.

Libecco JA, Powell KR. Trimethoprim/sulfamethoxazole: clinical update. *Pediatr Rev* 2004;25: 375–380.

WEB SITES

www.mayohealth.org   Mayo clinic site

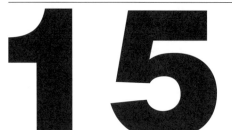

Diabetes Mellitus

Diabetes mellitus (DM) is a group of metabolic diseases characterized by hyperglycemia resulting from defects in insulin secretion, insulin action, or both. DM is also characterized by increased lipid and protein utilization.

Chronic hyperglycemia is associated with long term microvascular (retinopathy, nephropathy, and neuropathy) and accelerated macrovascular (coronary artery disease and stroke) complications.

DM can be classified into type 1 (DM1) and type 2 (DM2), gestational diabetes (GDM), maturity onset diabetes of the young (MODY), and other specific, less common types. Five and possibly six subtypes of MODY have been described in the literature with mutations in proteins that control insulin secretion.

DIABETES MELLITUS, TYPE 1

I. **Description of the condition:**
   A. **Epidemiology and classification:** Type 1 diabetes (DM1) is characterized by the development of a state of complete insulin deficiency. In its fully developed form, patients will, if deprived of insulin, develop ketoacidosis, coma, and death.

   The incidence of DM1 in the United States is estimated to be approximately 30,000 new cases per year. Although the peak incidence occurs in childhood and early adolescence, this form of diabetes can occur at any age.

   Recent epidemiologic and immunologic research has lead to the recognition of two major forms of type 1 diabetes, based on the presence or absence of certain immunologic markers.

   1. **Autoimmune type 1 diabetes:** This form of diabetes accounts for 5% to 10% of those individuals with diabetes.

      Autoimmune type 1 diabetes is a prototype autoimmune disorder. Individuals who develop this form of diabetes are born with a genetic predisposition to autoimmune dysfunction, which may manifest itself in the development of other autoimmune conditions such as Addison disease, Hashimoto thyroiditis, Graves disease, vitiligo, myasthenia gravis, and autoimmune hepatitis. Markers of the immune destruction of the B-cell include islet cell autoantibodies, autoantibodies to insulin, autoantibodies to glutamine and decarboxylase (GAD 65) and autoantibodies to the tyrosine phosphatase IA-2 and IA-2B. One, and usually more, of these autoantibodies are present in 85% to 90% of individuals with autoimmune diabetes when fasting hyperglycemia is initially detected.

      In this form of diabetes, the rate of B-cell destruction is variable, being rapid in some individuals (mainly infants and children) and slow in others (mainly adults).

      Some patients, particularly children and adolescents, may present with ketoacidosis as the first manifestation of the disease. Others have modest fasting hyperglycemia that can rapidly change to severe hyperglycemia and/or ketoacidosis.

   2. **Idiopathic type 1 diabetes:** Idiopathic type 1 diabetes has no known etiology, with no evidence of autoimmunity. Some of these patients have permanent insulopenia and are prone to ketoacidosis. This form of diabetes is strongly inherited. Only a minority of patients with type 1 diabetes have this form, and most are of African or Asian ancestry.

II. **Making the diagnosis:**
   A. **Diagnostic features:** The American Diabetes Association (ADA) diagnostic criteria for the diagnosis of diabetes are shown in Table 15-1. There are three ways to diagnose diabetes and each, in the absence of unequivocal hyperglycemia, must be confirmed on a subsequent day by any of the three methods. The use of hemoglobin A_{1c}

Table 15-1. American Diabetes Association (ADA) criteria for diagnosis of diabetes mellitus

1. Symptoms of diabetes plus casual plasma glucose concentration ≥200 mg/dL.
   • Casual is defined as any time of day without regard to time since last meal.
   • Classic symptoms of diabetes include polyuria, polydipsia, and unexplained weight loss.

or

2. FPG ≥126 mg/dL. Fasting is defined as no caloric intake for at least 8 hours.

or

3. 2-hour post load glucose ≥200 mg/dL during an OGTT. The test should be performed using a glucose load containing the equivalent of 75 g anhydrous glucose dissolved in water.

FPG, fasting plasma glucose; OGTT, Oral Glucose Tolerance Test.
From American Diabetes Association. Diagnosis and classification of diabetes mellitus. *Diabetes Care* 2004;17(Suppl. 1), with permission.

(HbA$_{1c}$) for the diagnosis of diabetes is not recommended at this time. Glycosolated hemoglobin reported in values equivalent to HbA$_{1c}$ reflects the average blood glucose (BG) over the previous 6 to 8 weeks.

Diabetic dyslipidemia is a term loosely used to describe a constellation of abnormalities characteristically observed in those with both type 1 and type 2 diabetes. The most common features are:
• hypertriglyceridemia
• low levels of high density lipoprotein (HDL) cholesterol
• elevated low-density lipoprotein (LDL)

The dyslipidemia seen in both DM1 and DM2 is believed to increase the risk of cardiovascular disease two- to four-fold and reflects various degrees of insulin resistance, obesity, diet, and poor glycemic control.

   B. Clinical presentation: Diabetic ketoacidosis (DKA) is the leading cause of hospitalization among adolescents and children with DM1. Sixty-five percent of all patients admitted with DKA are younger than 19. The triad of symptoms of DKA consists of:
   1. hyperglycemia
   2. ketosis
   3. metabolic acidosis

   Stress is the usual trigger for DKA in a person deprived of adequate insulin. Without the insulin to counteract the increased activity of the counter-regulatory hormones (such as growth hormone, epinephrine, glucagon, and cortisol), ketosis and metabolic acidosis ensue. The stress that precipitates ketoacidosis can be anything from a minor medical illness to the emotional stress of breaking up with a boyfriend or girlfriend.

   Hyperglycemia causes an osmotic diuresis that leads to dehydration, electrolyte depletion, and hypertonicity. Metabolic acidosis, secondary to ketosis, causes compensatory hyperventilation and hypocapnia, which causes changes in renal, central nervous system, cardiovascular, bowel, and blood oxygen transport functions.

III. **Management of diabetic ketoacidosis:**
   A. Home: Diabetic ketoacidosis can be managed on an outpatient basis if detected early, or an inpatient basis otherwise. Development of DKA is slow; therefore, assiduous monitoring of BG at home should detect persistent hyperglycemia and allow time for the patient to seek outpatient management of the problem.

   Educating the patient about checking for ketonuria is the key to home management of DKA. If the teenager falls ill or is vomiting, or if the BG exceeds 240 mg per dL, then urine ketones should be measured. If the ketone level is "moderate" or "large," the physician should be called. Supplements of regular subcutaneous insulin are given, approximately 5% to 10% of the total daily dose for "moderate" ketonuria and 10% to 20% for "large" ketonuria.

   The blood sugar checks, urine ketone checks, telephone calls, and regular insulin supplements are repeated every 3 hours until the urine ketone measurement is "small" or "negative." Phone contact with a member of the care team is vital. Liquids are begun slowly in the form of fruit juices, and when BG is lower than 120 mg per dL sugar-containing fluids are begun. If the vomiting persists, the parents are instructed to bring the adolescent to the emergency room. If there are deep (Kussmaul) respirations, sunken eyes, and more than mild lethargy, the adolescent must be admitted.

B. Hospital: When home management fails or DKA is not detected early enough, hospital management is indicated. See Table 15-2 for the hospital management of the adolescent with ketoacidosis.

Table 15-2. Management of the adolescent with diabetic ketoacidosis

I. Initial Management
  A. Physical examination:
    1. Assess hydration, pulse, blood pressure, skin temperature
    2. Assess respiratory status: Kussmaul breathing
    3. Search for signs of an infection
    4. Assess mental status: document current status and provide baseline for future
  B. Laboratory assessment:
    1. CBC with differential, electrolytes, BUN, creatinine, glucose, Ca^{2+}, PO_4
    2. Blood gas (arterial or venous), HbA_{1c}
    3. Diabetes antibody panel for new diabetic patient:
      a. Anti-insulin antibodies
      b. Anticytoplasmic islet cell antibodies
      c. Glutamic acid decarboxylase antibodies
  C. Fluids: 0.9% NS, 10 mL/kg over 30–60 minutes as a bolus, once
  D. Insulin
    1. If serum bicarbonate is <15 mEq/L, use insulin drip:
      a. After fluid bolus, insulin drip should be started (1 unit insulin/1 mL)
      b. Start 0.1 unit/kg/h (hourly rate = 0.1 mL × weight in kg)
      c. Ideally, blood sugar should drop 80–100 mg% per hour
    2. If serum bicarbonate is ~15 mEq/L, start or use insulin subcutaneously rather than intravenously

II. Treatment
  A. Exam
    1. Observe for neurologic changes and document mental status changes at least every 2 hours
    2. Abdominal pain should resolve when bicarbonate is >10 mEq/L; consider pancreatitis for severe, unrelenting pain
  B. Labs
    1. Every hour: BG by meter
    2. Every 2 hours: electrolytes, BUN, creatinine, glucose
    3. Every 8 hours: Ca^{2+}, PO_4
    4. Arterial blood gases necessary only for severe acidosis or neurologic compromise
  C. Fluids after initial bolus
    1. Rate: 3,000–3,500 mL/m^2/24 h, or 2 × maintenance until IV fluids are no longer necessary; do not use urinary output as a guide for replacement of fluids
    2. Maintenance fluids:
      a. 100 mL/kg/d for the first 10 kg of weight
      b. 50 mL/kg/d for the second 10 kg of weight
      c. 20 mL/kg/d for each additional kg of weight above 20 kg
    3. Fluids
      a. Use 0.9% NS for the first 4–6 hours and then switch to 0.45% NS
      b. Serum Na artificially low with elevated glucose: Corrected Na = [(serum glucose −100) × 0.016] + measured Na
    4. Glucose
      a. Ideally, blood sugar should drop 80–100 mg% per hour
      b. As glucose begins to approach 300 mg/dL, add 5% dextrose to the IV fluids
      c. If glucose falls below 200 mg/dL while acidosis persists, use 10% dextrose so the insulin drip may continue
      d. Glucose should be maintained between 180 and 250 mg%

(continued)

Table 15-2. *(Continued)*

    5. Potassium
      a. Intracellular K^+ stores are always low
      b. Once insulin and fluids are started, serum K^+ will fall rapidly
        (1) If serum $K^+ >6$ mEq/L, wait to add K^+ to IV fluids
        (2) If serum $K^+<4.5$ mEq/L, add 20 mEq/L of KCl and 20 mEq/L of KPO_4 to each 1,000 mL of initial fluids administered
        (3) If serum K^+ is >4.5 mEq/L, add 15 mEq/L of KCl and 15 mEq of KPO_4 to each 1,000 mL of initial fluids administered
  D. Patient intake-should be NPO except for ice chips until acidosis improves significantly
  E. Insulin
    1. Maintain insulin drip until acidosis resolves as measured by serum bicarbonate or serum pH
    2. Serum bicarbonate will often stabilize around 15 mEq/L until large amounts of Cl^- administered during initial therapy are excreted
    3. Once the patient's bicarbonate is above 15 mEq/L, and the adolescent has eaten, insulin may be switched to subcutaneous
    4. Anion gap = $Na^+K^-Cl^-HCO_3$ (normal = 13–16)
  F. Cerebral edema
    1. Usually occurs early in treatment within the first 24 hours
    2. Decline in neurologic status appears similar to hypoglycemia. Check blood sugars
    3. For declining neurologic status, 1 g/kg of mannitol given rapidly over 15–20 minutes should result in rapid improvement
    4. Mannitol may need to be repeated in another 1–3 hours

CBC, complete blood count; BUN, blood urea nitrogen; IV, intravenous; NS, normal saline; NPO, nothing by mouth. Adapted from Department of Pediatrics, Indiana University School of Medicine: endocrinology. In *Pocket Pediatric Manual*. Indianapolis, Indiana University School of Medicine, 2001–2002, p. 17.

    C. Follow up office visits: Adolescents with DM1 should be seen frequently by the physician in the first few months after diagnosis and then on a regular schedule of three to four times yearly. At these sessions a physical exam should be done with attention to blood pressure, growth and development, eyes, skin, and joints. If limitations of joint mobility are present, this may be a sign that other microvascular complications may be present.
    Table 15-3 lists the elements of the minimal annual evaluation for an adolescent with DM1.

Table 15-3. Elements of minimum annual evaluation of adolescents with insulin-dependent diabetes mellitus

A. Height, weight, growth percentile, and maturation.
B. Blood urea nitrogen, creatinine and microalbumin levels, and creatinine clearance. Urine cultures should be considered for all females.
C. Antimicrosomal and antithyroglobulin antibodies at onset. If positive, annual thyroxine, thyroxine-binding globulin, and thyroid-stimulating hormone levels. If initially negative, reevaluate if thyroid is enlarged or growth rate changes. All females should be reevaluated at puberty.
D. Cholesterol and triglyceride levels and high- and low-density lipoprotein fractions.
E. Blood pressure.
F. Peripheral pulses.
G. Deep-tendon reflexes.
H. Neurologic examination (sensory nerves, touch and position sense). If abnormal, nerve conduction velocities should be measured.
I. Ophthalmologic examination with dilation by certified ophthalmologist every other year for prepubertal children and yearly for postpubertal adolescents.
J. Gynecologic and urologic evaluations when indicated.
K. Psychosocial assessment of teenager and family.

From Ginsberg-Fellner F. Insulin-dependent diabetes. *Pediatr Rev* 1990;11:239, with permission.

Table 15-4. Summary of recommendations for adults (non-pregnant) with diabetes

Glycemic control	
A_{1c}	<7.0% I
Prepared capillary plasma glucose	90–130 mg/dL (5.0–7.2 mmol/l)
Peak postprandial capillary plasma glucose[a]	<180 mg/dL (<10.0 mmol/l)
Blood pressure	<130/80 mmHG
Lipids[b]	
LDL	<100 mg/dL (<2.6 mmol/l)
Triglycerides	<150 mg/dL (<1.7 mmol/l)
HDL	>40 mg/dL (>1.1 mmol/l)[c]

Key concepts in setting glycemic goals:
- A_{1c} is the primary target for glycemic control
- Goals should be individualized
- Certain populations (children, pregnant women, and elderly) require special considerations
- Less intensive glycemic goals may be indicated in patients with severe or frequent hypoglycemia.
- More stringent glycemic goals (i.e., a normal A_{1c}, <6%) may further reduce complications at the cost of increased risk of hypoglycemia (particularly in those with type 1 diabetes)
- Postprandial glucose may be targeted if A_{1c} goals are not met despite reaching preprandial glucose goals

Referenced to a nondiabetic range of 4.0%–6.0% using a DCCT-based assay.
[a]Postprandial glucose measurements should be made 1–2 h after the beginning of the meal, generally peak levels in patients with diabetes.
[b]Current NCEP/ATP III guidelines suggest that in patients with triglycerides ≥200 mg/dL, the "non-HDL cholesterol" (total cholesterol minus HDL) be used. The goal is ≤130 mg/dL (31).
[c]For women, it has been suggested that the HDL goal be increased by 10 mg/dL.
Adapted from American Diabetes Association. Standards of medical care in diabetes. *Diabetes Care* 2005;28(Suppl 1).

       Table 15-4 lists the glycemic control targets as established by the American Diabetes Association.

       Table 15-5 lists the characteristics of the common human insulin preparations.

IV.   Clinical pearls and pitfalls:
- Good glycemic control significantly reduces the risk of progressive microvascular complications. Diabetes regimens that target normalization of BG are the standard of care.
- Children and adolescents with DM1 are generally symptomatic (polyuria, polydipsia, polyphagia, weight loss), not overweight, and often at least mildly ketotic at the time of diagnosis.
- Dosage Hints: For the average adolescent with total daily insulin dose of about 1 unit per kg, 1 unit short/rapid acting insulin will usually lower BG by 50 to 100 mg per dL.

Table 15-5. Characteristics of human insulin preparations

Informal description	Proprietary or other name	Onset (hours)	Peak (hours)	Effective duration (hours)	Maximum duration (hours)	Technical description
Rapid-acting	lispro	0.25	1–2	2–3	4	Insulin analog
Rapid-acting	aspart[a]	0.25	1–2	2–3	4	Insulin analog
Short-acting	Regular	0.5–1	2–3	3–6	4–6	Insulin
Intermediate-acting	NPH	2–4	4–10	10–16	14–18	Insulin isophane (suspension)
Intermediate-acting	Lente	3–4	4–12	12–18	16–20	Insulin zinc (suspension)
Long-acting	Ultralente	6–10	12–18	18–20	20–30	Insulin zinc (suspension) extended

[a]New drug application on file with the FDA.
Not yet available is insulin glargine, a long-acting insulin analog providing basal insulin with once-daily injection; new drug application on file with FDA.

Eight to fifteen grams of carbohydrates will require about 1 unit of short/rapid acting insulin. Ten to fifteen grams of dietary carbohydrates will usually change BG by about 40 to 60 mg.
- Alcohol cannot be converted to glucose, and it tends to inhibit gluconeogenesis. Severe hypoglycemia may result many hours after as little as 2 ounces of alcohol unless additional carbohydrates were eaten at the time of alcohol consumption.
- Elevated blood pressure significantly increases the risk and progression of all complications of DM1. Sustained elevation of diastolic pressure greater than 85 or systolic pressure greater than 135 should be treated with an angiotensin converting enzyme inhibitor.
- Sustained microalbuminuria is an indication of nephropathy.

DIABETES MELLITUS, TYPE 2

I. **Description of the condition:**
   A. **Epidemiology:** The incidence of type 2 diabetes (DM2) is increasing in dramatic fashion among young adolescents. The population at greatest risk is the 10- to 16-year-old age group. Up to 46% of newly diagnosed cases of DM in children are type 2. Before 1990, fewer than 4% of children with diabetes mellitus had type 2.

   The rate of DM2 has increased especially among African Americans, Hispanic Americans, Asian/Pacific Islanders, and Native Americans who have evidence of insulin resistance (e.g., hypertension, dyslipidemia, polycystic ovarian syndrome, acanthosis nigricans).

   Obesity is a well-recognized finding in children with DM2. The coincident epidemic of childhood obesity provides one theory as to why there has been such a dramatic increase in DM2.

   A family history of DM2 in first- and second-degree relatives is found in 75% to 100% of children (and adults) with DM2. Even in children without diabetes, a family history of DM2 is associated with a decline of 20% in insulin sensitivity, suggesting that such children already require more insulin for a given glucose lead than those without a history. Thus, a genetic predisposition to insulin resistance exists.
   B. **Etiology:** DM2 is a complex metabolic disease of altered carbohydrate utilization and metabolism. Dyslipidemias are common in DM2 and thus increase the risk for cardiovascular disease two to four fold and reflect various degrees of insulin resistance, obesity, diet, and poor glycemic control. The typical pattern is an elevated triglyceride (TG) and decreased HDL.

   Maintenance of normal glucose levels depends on coordination of insulin secretion by the β cells of the pancreas, suppression of hepatic glucose production and insulin action at peripheral tissues such as muscle. The characteristic abnormalities of DM2 are impaired insulin secretion from the β cells of the pancreas and impaired insulin action. The epidemiology of early-onset DM2 suggests that puberty may play a role in its pathogenesis. It has been shown that adolescents with normal β-cell activity increase insulin secretion to counteract the affects of growth hormone (GH). (Increased GH levels decrease insulin sensitivity.) However, adolescents with impaired β-cell secretion or pre-existing insulin insensitivity are unable to respond adequately to counteract the effects of GH.

II. **Making the diagnosis:**
   A. **Laboratory evaluation and tests:** Annual screening may be considered for members of high risk groups, including youth who are obese, have a parent with DM2, are African American, Asian/Pacific Islander, or Native American, *and* have evidence of insulin resistance (e.g., hypertension, dyslipidemia, polycystic ovarian syndrome, acanthosis nigricans).

   As the ADA consensus committee observed, fasting plasma glucose (FPG) and 2 hour postload glucose (2-h PG) are suitable screening tests for DM2. The FPG is preferred because of convenience and cost. As with any screening test, abnormal results must be confirmed at another time. No data exist on the use of random levels of 2-h PG, BG, insulin, or C-peptide as screening tests. HbA$_{1c}$ is currently not recommended for diagnosis but is recommended for monitoring glycemia.
   B. **Clinical presentation:** Table 15-6 presents an overview of the characteristics of the common types of diabetes. DM2 refers to individuals who have insulin resistance and relative (rather than absolute) insulin deficiency. Although still primarily a diagnosis of adults, DM2 does occur among children, most commonly during adolescence. Individuals with DM2 are usually obese, and if not obese may have an increased predominance of abdominal fat (central adiposity), which is causally related in insulin resistance.

Table 15-6. Testing for type 2 diabetes in children

Criteria[a]

Overweight (BMI >85th percentile for age and sex, weight for height >85th percentile, or weight >120% of ideal for height)

plus

Any two of the following risk factors:

Family history of DM2 in first- or second-degree relative

Race/ethnicity (African American, Hispanic, Asian/Pacific Islander, American Indian)

Signs of insulin resistance or conditions associated with insulin resistance (hypertension, dyslipidemia, polycystic ovarian syndrome, acanthosis nigricans)

- *Age of initiation:* Age 10, or at onset of puberty if puberty occurs at a younger age.
- *Frequency:* Every 2 years.
- *Test:* FPG preferred.

BMI, body mass index; FPG, fasting plasma glucose.
[a]Clinical judgment should be used to test for diabetes in high-risk patients who do not meet these criteria.
From American Diabetes Association. Type 2 diabetes in children and adolescents. *Diabetes Care.* 2000;23:381–389 (Table 4, 386) Copyright 2000, American Diabetes Assn, with permission.

Acanthosis nigricans, hyperpigmentation with thickening of the skin into velvety, irregular folds in flexural or redundant skin areas (neck, axilla, area beneath breasts and elbow), is common in youth with DM2 (86% in one series). Obese individuals with insidious onset of hyperglycemia and those who present with non-ketosis severe hyperglycemia (BG >750 mg/dL) usually have DM2, and additional testing for classification is generally not useful.

Other types of diabetes

1. **Atypical DM2 of African Americans (DM2-A):** These patients are African American youth who may not be obese, do not have acanthosis nigricans, and may present acutely with ketoacidosis. These patients appear to have normal insulin sensitivity but moderately low insulin secretion. Insulin can usually be withdrawn

Table 15-7. Characteristics of common types of diabetes

	Type 1	Type 2	DM2-A	MODY
Age	Childhood	Adolescent—adult	Pubertal	Pubertal
Onset	Acute-severe	Mild-severe;	Acute-severe	Mild-insidious
Insulin secretion	Very low	Variable	Moderately low	Variable
Insulin sensitivity	Normal	Decreased	Normal	Normal
Insulin dependence	Permanent	Not until late	Variable	Not until late
Racial/ethnic groups at increased risk	All (low in Asians)	African Americans, Hispanics, Asian/ Pacific Islanders, Native Americans	African Americans	All
Genetics	Polygenic	Polygenic	Autosomal dominant	Autosomal dominant
Proportion of those with diabetes	~80%	10%–20%	5%–10%	Rare
Association:				
Obesity	No	Strong	Variable	No
Acanthosis Nigricans	No	Yes	No	No
Autoimmune etiology	Yes	No	No	No

DM2-A, atypical DM2; MODY, maturity onset diabetes of youth.
From Rosenbloom et al. Emerging epidemic of type 2 diabetes in youth. *Diabetes Care* 1999;22:345–354, with permission.

after recovery from the acute episode, and patients can be managed with traditional regimens for DM2.

2. **Maturity onset diabetes of youth (MODY):** MODY (an autosomal dominant condition) occurs rarely, is an entity distinct from DM2, and is characterized by impaired insulin secretion with minimal or no defects in insulin action (resistance) and insidious presentation before age 25. Patients with MODY can usually be managed initially with oral hypoglycemic agents. The clinical presentation appears to vary broadly from asymptomatic hyperglycemia to weight loss and dehydration (see Table 15-7).

III.   **Treatment, intervention, and management of patients with DM2:**

A. **Identification:** Acutely ill adolescents and those who have significant hyperglycemia (≥300 mg/dL) require simultaneous management with insulin and intravenous fluids if dehydrated or ketoacidotic. Insulin therapy may later be withdrawn and traditional DM2 treatment instituted. The initial use of insulin does not commit the physician to long term use of insulin when subsequent evidence (such as family history, presence of insulin resistance, or failure to develop ketonemia in the absence of exogenous insulin) suggests that the diagnosis is not DM2.

B. **Clinical treatment goals:** BG, lipid profile, blood pressure, and signs of complication are monitored in DM2. DM2 is *not* an autoimmune process and it is not necessary to screen for thyroiditis. Goals in treating adolescents with DM2 are weight loss, continued normal linear growth, normalization of BG and HbA_{1c} levels, and control of hypertension and abnormal lipid levels, if present.

Fasting blood glucose (FBG) level is the major determinant of mean day-long BG level reflected in HbA_{1c} levels. Postprandial BG contributes less to glycohemoglobin levels. (Target levels of BG and HbA_{1c} were detailed in Table 15-4.)

Dyslipidemias are common in DM2 and reflect various degrees of insulin resistance, obesity, diet, and poor glycemic control. The typical pattern is an elevated triglyceride (TG) and decreased high density lipoprotein (HDL) cholesterol. Although all hypoglycemic agents improve glycemic control, weight loss (if appropriate) and reduced intake of saturated fat are fundamental goals. Yearly measurement of fasting lipid profiles is recommended among those with previously abnormal profiles or ongoing poor glycemic control. Measurement every other year is probably sufficient among the remainder of children and adolescents with DM2.

DM2 is a progressive disease that appears eventually to require the use of exogenous insulin. Treatment goals are the same as for DM1 (described in Table 15-4). Plan to reevaluate progress every 4 to 6 weeks, making necessary changes until the adolescent achieves the target level of control of HbA_{1c}. The ADA recommends that adolescents with DM2 participate in diabetes self-management education. Diabetes self-management includes basic knowledge about pathophysiology, short and long-term complications, medication, meal planning, exercise guidelines, and SMBG.

1. **Nutrition management and exercise:** Modification of diet and exercise are the mainstay of treatment. There is no longer a standard ADA diet. Rather the distribution of carbohydrates (CHO), protein, and fat is individualized by patient needs. The goals are:

a. near normal BG levels

b. normal serum lipid levels

c. weight loss when indicated

d. normal growth and development

The ADA recommends that adolescents with diabetes be referred to a dietitian for help with a weight reduction program, when necessary, and exercise program independent of weight loss. Exercise is important because it increases the glucose transport into skeletal muscle resulting in lower levels of BG. The goal should be at least 150 minutes per week of brisk walking.

Organized diet and exercise programs may prove beneficial for adolescents who prefer group support and activities. Recruiting the family to exercise may improve the patient's likelihood of exercising if other members of the family also exercise. Failure to see improvement in the FBG in the face of substantial weight loss suggests that diet and exercise alone will be insufficient to achieve satisfactory control.

2. **Pharmacotherapy:** If, despite dietary and activity modifications, significant improvement in BG control (manifested as levels of HbA_{1c} dropping to 8% or less) has not been attained after 3 months, an oral hypoglycemic agent or insulin should be added. When using oral agents, it is important to remember that:

a. The response to oral agents follows a sigmoid curve with a rapid rise in therapeutic activity, leveling off and gradually tapering to maximal therapeutic effect.

Table 15-8. Comparison of oral hypoglycemic agents prescribed for adolescents

Effect	Biguanides[1]	Sulfonylureas[2]	Glucosidase inhibitors[3]
Mechanism of action	Decrease hepatic glucose production; increase muscle insulin sensitivity	Increase insulin secretion	Decrease GI absorption
Duration of action	>3–4 weeks	12–24 hours	~4 hours (postprandial period)
Decrease in FPG (mg/dL)	60–70	60–70	20–30
Decrease in HbA$_{1c}$ (%)	1.5–2.0	1.2–2.0	0.7–1.0
Triglyceride level	Decrease	No effect[a]	No effect[a]
HDL cholesterol level	Slight increase	No effect[a]	No effect[a]
Body weight	No effect or decrease	Increase	No effect[a]
Plasma insulin	Decrease	Increase	No effect[a]
Adverse effects	GI disturbance; lactic Acidosis[4] rare	Hypoglycemia	GI disturbance

[1]Metformin is the only current agent in this class.
[2]Commonly prescribed second generation sulfonylurea drugs include glyburide, glipizide, and glimepiride. Closely related to these is repaglinide, similar to sulfonylurea drugs in most respect, but with a duration of action of 4–6 hours.
[3]This class includes acarbose and miglitol.
[4]Incidence of 0.03 cases per 1,000 patient years (see text).
[a] Independent of effect due to lowered BG
From American Diabetes Association. Type 2 diabetes in children and adolescents. *Pediatrics* 2000;105:671–680, with permission.

       b. Half the maximal dosage yields more than half the maximal effect (60%–80%).
       c. Side effects increase slowly at low dosages and then more rapidly at higher dose.
          Table 15-8 lists and compares the oral hypoglycemic agents prescribed for adolescents. Depending upon the level of clinical comfort a physician has with using oral hypoglycemic agents in adolescents, a pediatric endocrinologist's involvement at this level of treatment may be warranted. Follow up of teenagers with DM2 is virtually the same as for those with DM1 with the exception that there is no need to test for autoimmune complications in DM2. Considerations include monitoring to ensure proper control, the role of the multidisciplinary diabetes team in education and encouraging adherence, and scheduling screenings for common complications.

IV.   **Clinical pearls and pitfalls:** The pediatrician or specialist in adolescent medicine who is interested in diabetes can play an integral role in the care of patients with DM. However:
- Specialty consultation when indicated and collaboration with a multidisciplinary team is crucial in the management of the patient with DM2.
- Early recognition, consistent follow-up and aggressive treatment will increase the likelihood of achieving improved control of hyperglycemia and reducing the risks of long-term complications.
- It has been estimated that the prevalence of DM2 would double if all those who met the criteria were diagnosed.
- Those not diagnosed are at risk for long-term sequelae.
- Children of a parent with DM2 become more insulin resistant with additional weight gain.
- It is recommended that adolescents at risk for DM2 be screened every 2 years beginning at age 10 or at puberty if puberty begins at a younger age.
- An FPG greater than 126 mg per dL is considered to be impaired fasting glucose.
- Acanthosis nigricans is present in more than 80% of adolescents with DM2. Acanthosis nigricans is associated with obesity, hyperinsulinemia, and insular resistance.
- A normal BG level is an important goal when treating adolescents with DM2, because any reduction in HbA$_{1c}$ will translate to decreased risk of complications.
- If, despite dietary and activity modifications, significant improvement in blood glucose control (manifest as levels of HbA$_{1c}$ dropping to 8% or less) has not been attained after 3 months, an oral hypoglycemic agent or insulin should be added.

BIBLIOGRAPHY

For the clinician

American Diabetes Association. Criteria for diagnosis of diabetes mellitus. *Diabetes Care* 2004; 17(Suppl. 1):S9.

American Diabetes Association. *Endocrinology*. Indianapolis, In: Deptartment of Pediatrics. Indiana University School of Medicine. Pocket Pediatric Manual, 2001–2002:17.

American Diabetes Association. Standards of medical care in diabetes. *Diabetes Care* 2005; (Suppl. 1).

American Diabetes Association. Type 2 diabetes in children and adolescents. *Pediatrics* 2000; 105:671–680.

Degroot LJ, Jameson JL, eds. *Endocrinology*, 4th ed: WB Saunders, 2001.

Ginsburg-Fellner F. Insulin-dependent diabetes. *Pediatr Rev* 1990;11:239.

Kaufman FR. Type I diabetes mellitus. *Pediatr Rev* 2003;24:291–300.

Orr DP. Contemporary management of adolescents with diabetes mellitus. Part 1. Type 1 Diabetes. American Academy of Pediatrics. *Adolesc Health Update* 2000;12(2):4.

Orr DP. Contemporary management of adolescents with diabetes mellitus. Part 1. Type 2 Diabetes American Academy of Pediatrics. *Adolesc Health Update* 2000;12(3):1–8.

Rowell HA, Evans BJ, Quarry-Horn JL, et al. Type 2 diabetes mellitus in adolescents. *Adolesc Med State Art Rev* 2002;13(N9. 1):1–12.

Trachtenbarg DE. Diabetic ketoacidosis. *Am Fam Physician* 2005;71:1705–1714.

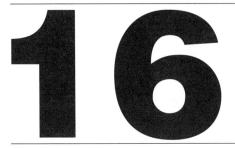

Thyroid Disease

I. **Description of the condition:** Thyroid disorders are common in adolescents. **Goiter (thyromegaly)** is the most common presenting physical abnormality. **Chronic autoimmune thyroiditis** is both the most prevalent clinical entity and the most common cause of goiter in the nonendemic goiter regions in the world. It causes at least 40% of the cases of goiter in adolescents. In many cases, the thyroid function studies of patients with goiter are normal and patients are clinically euthyroid. However, when there is an abnormality of thyroid function, **hypothyroidism is most commonly found. Hyperthyroidism, thyroid nodules, and thyroid cancer occur in adolescence but are much less prevalent.** Thyroid hormones are important because they affect growth, puberty, oxygen consumption, heat production, neurologic function, and the metabolism of lipids, carbohydrates, proteins, nucleic acids, vitamins, and organic ions. Thyroid disease can be easily missed since the presentation may be subtle.

A. **Epidemiology and classification:** One study of more than 4,800 11 to 18 year olds in the Southwestern United States found that 3.7% had a thyroid abnormality. The **most common abnormality in 19.3 of 1,000 individuals was euthyroid goiter.** Chronic lymphocytic thyroiditis was found in 12.7 of 1,000, and 4.6 of 1,000 had thyroid nodules, including two cases of papillary carcinoma. **Hypo- or hyperthyroidism was found in only 1.9 of 1,000 individuals.** Another study, of more than 7,700 9 to 16 year olds in four areas of the United States, found an overall prevalence of goiter of 6.8%. Most of these subjects had thyromegaly without clinical or biochemical evidence of a thyroid abnormality.

   Thyromegaly is defined as enlargement of the thyroid gland that can be diffuse, nodular, symmetrical, or asymmetrical. A nodule within the thyroid is a cystic or solid mass with a different consistency than the rest of the gland. According to the World Health Organization classification, a **goiter is an enlargement of the thyroid gland that is palpable and/or visible.** Thyromegaly is caused by stimulation [antithyroid drugs, iodine, goitregen agents, foods, and thyroid-stimulating hormone (TSH) secreting tumor], infiltration (neoplasia, cyst), or inflammation (bacterial, viral, noninfectious-autoimmune) of the thyroid gland. **In some cases of euthyroid goiter, thyroid autoantibodies can be found. They therefore may represent cases of mild autoimmune thyroid disease.** Although most patients with goiter are euthyroid, they may also have clinical signs and symptoms of hypo- or hyperthyroidism. Diffuse thyromegaly may regress spontaneously or progress to nodular goiter later in life (Table 16-1).

Table 16-1. Selected goitregenic agents

Environmental
  Pesticides
  Industrial chemicals (polychlorinated biphenyls, polybrominated biphenyls, dinitrophenols)
  Thiocyanate
  Iodine
Drugs
  Thioamides
  Anticonvulsants
  Lithium
  Amioderone

HYPOTHYROIDISM

I. **Description of the condition:**
   A. **Etiology:** Hypothyroidism can be congenital or acquired. **Congenital causes** of hypothyroidism that can present in adolescence are **thyroid dysgenesis,** in which an ectopic thyroid gland enlarges, and **thyroid dyshormonogenesis,** where there is a compensated defect in hormone synthesis. **Acquired hypothyroidism** is caused by either **primary hypothyroidism** from failure of the thyroid gland itself or **central hypothyroidism** from failure at the level of the pituitary/hypothalamic axis.

   The most common cause of acquired hypothyroidism is chronic autoimmune thyroiditis. Antithyroid antibodies directed against thyroglobulin, thyroid peroxidase enzyme, the sodium/iodide supporter protein, thyroid nuclei, and the TSH receptor are found in these patients. The **antiperoxidase and antithyroglobulin antibodies** are the most prevalent and diagnostically useful. Some investigators divide chronic autoimmune thyroiditis into **lymphocytic thyroiditis,** which only has lymphocytic infiltration, and **Hashimoto thyroiditis,** which also has findings of eosinophilic changes, atrophy, and fibrosis. Hashimoto thyroiditis is commonly referred to in the literature as **chronic lymphocytic thyroiditis** and presents with thyromegaly. **Atrophic thyroiditis** is a separate entity, which also has thyroid antibodies and is distinguished by the absence of a goiter. Unlike Hashimoto thyroiditis, atrophic thyroiditis is always associated with clinical and biochemical hypothyroidism. Approximately 20% of patients with chronic autoimmune thyroiditis revert to a euthyroid state. Chronic autoimmune thyroiditis can also present with transient hyperthyroidism because of release of hormone from damaged cells.
   B. **Other causes of hypothyroidism include:** (See Table 16-2)
      1. **Drug induced: Amiodarone** contains iodine resulting in decreased thyroid hormone synthesis; **anticonvulsants** such as carbamazepine, valproate, and phenobarbital are associated with low levels of serum thyroid hormones; **lithium** affects thyroid hormone synthesis and secretion; and **iodine** inhibits biosynthesis and release of thyroid hormone.
      2. **Endemic: Iodine deficiency** is a rare cause of hypothyroidism (<1%) in the United States because of the addition of iodine to salt and other foods. Iodine deficiency leads to increased TSH secretion, reduced iodination of thyroglobulin, depletion of thyroid colloid, gland hypertrophy, and in severe cases an inability to compensate with resultant hypothyroidism.

         Environmental goitrogens such as pesticides, industrial chemicals, and excessive iodine contribute to hypothyroidism.
      3. **Thyroid damage or infiltration:** This category includes irradiation (therapeutic radioiodine, external irradiation for nonthyroid tumors); surgical removal; infiltration (cystinosis, Langerhans cell histiocytosis, hemochromatosis).
      4. **Subacute thyroiditis (De Quervain syndrome):** This is a self-limited inflammation of the thyroid following a viral illness, for example, upper respiratory tract infection (URI) or mumps. It usually presents as transient hyperthyroidism related to release of stored hormone followed by transient hypothyroidism with recovery of the damaged thyroid cells. It has a course of 2 to 9 months and is usually not associated with antithyroid antibodies. Recovery occurs without residual effect. This is distinguished from **acute suppurative thyroiditis,** which is a rare form of bacterial infection commonly caused by *Staphylococcus aureus, Streptococcus hemolyticus,* pnemococcus, and anaerobes. Suppurative thyroiditis can occur when there is an embryologic remnant or pyriform sinus tract.
      5. **Postpartum thyroiditis:** This is the most common complication of chronic autoimmune thyroiditis in pregnancy. It occurs 2 to 6 months postpartum and resolves spontaneously within a year. It can present as hypothyroidism, hyperthyroidism, or hypothyroidism following hyperthyroidism. Even after initial recovery, 25% can have hypothyroidism 4 or more years later.
      6. **Hypothalamic-pituitary disorders:** There are deficiencies of TSH, and thyrotropin-releasing hormone (TRH). They occur in malformations such as septo-optic dysplasia and midline facial anomalies. Damage can occur to the hypothalamus or pituitary from trauma, neoplasms (craniopharyngioma), infectious or inflammatory processes (meningitis), irradiation, and surgery.
   C. **Genetics and familial transmission—contributing factors:** Autoimmune thyroiditis is familial. Females are 5 to 7 times more likely to be affected than males and are more likely to have a goiter. **Thyroid antibodies are found in up to 50% of**

Table 16-2. Differential diagnosis of acquired hypothyroidism

- Chronic autoimmune thyroiditis
  - Lymphocytic thyroiditis
  - Hashimoto thyroiditis
  - Atrophic thyroiditis
- Drug-induced hypothyroidism
- Endemic goiter
  - Iodine deficiency
  - Environmental goitrogens
- Thyroid damage/infiltration
  - External radiation of the thyroid
  - Surgical excision
  - Nephropathic cystinosis
  - Radioactive iodine
  - Langerhans cell histiocytosis
  - Hemochromatosis
- Subacute thyroiditis (de Quervain disease)
- Postpartum thyroiditis
- Hypothalalmic-pituitary disorders

Adapted from Lifshitz F, ed. *Pediatric endocrinology,* 4th ed. New York: Marcel Dekker, Inc; 2003, page 362.

first-degree relatives of patients with chronic autoimmune thyroiditis. This association implies a possible dominant inheritance. Both the **sex chromosomes and chromosome 21** may play a role in autoimmune thyroid disease. There is a higher prevalence in patients with certain genetic syndromes including Down syndrome, Turner syndrome, and Klinefelter syndrome. An association also exists with **other autoimmune-mediated diseases.** Thirty percent of children with diabetes mellitus have thyroid autoantibodies, and 10% have laboratory evidence of hypothyroidism.

Since concordance in monozygotic twins is only 20% to 50%, **environmental factors** may also play a role. Some examples of agents that are associated with an increase in the prevalence of autoimmune thyroid disease are **excessive iodine** intake and certain medications such as **lithium and interferon-α. Viral infections may also play a role.**

II. **Making the diagnosis:**
  A. **Signs and symptoms:** The signs and symptoms of clinical hypothyroidism may **be nonspecific,** such as weakness, lethargy, cold intolerance, constipation, dry skin, brittle hair, and change in school performance. Others include **decrease in growth velocity, which** may be the only symptom initially and can lead to **short stature,** the most common manifestation in children; delay in puberty (rarely precocious puberty); and overweight but not obesity. **Increased weight usually represents excess fluid.** Additional signs and symptoms are myxedematous facies; swelling in neck, puffy facies; dull or placid expression; goiter; slow return of deep tendon reflexes; bradycardia; galactorrhea (hyperprolactinemia); muscle tenderness, or dysphagia.

  Enlargement of the sella turcica may occur due to failure of the thyroid gland which can lead to hypertrophy of the pituitary thyrotropin cells. This is usually found incidentally during radiologic imaging of the head/brain and is usually asymptomatic. However, symptoms may include headache and visual disturbance. This condition is reversible with thyroxine therapy.

  B. **Physical exam: The most common clinical presentation of chronic autoimmune thyroiditis is asymptomatic goiter.** The gland is usually **diffusely enlarged, with a firm rubbery consistency.** There may be an irregular surface because of accentuation of the normal lobular structure. If fibrosis is present, there may be hard areas that can be confused with malignancy. Usually there is no tenderness and, if it is present, it is mild. Sometimes patients complain about a feeling of tightness of the neck. Pubertal development may be delayed and usually is proportional to retardation in skeletal maturation. In some cases, there may be precocious puberty (van Wyk-Grumbach syndrome) with menarche, breast development, and galactorrhea in females, and excessive enlargement of penis and testes in males. In most of these cases there is a lack of sexual hair development.

Table 16-3. Interpretation of thyroid function tests

Normal hypothalamic-pituitary axis function

TSH	Free T4	T3	Interpretation
Normal	Normal	Normal	Euthyroid
High	Low	Normal/low	Primary hypothyroidism
High	Normal	Normal	Subclinical hypothyroidism
Low	High/normal	High	Hyperthyroidism
Low	Normal	Normal	Subclinical hyperthyroidism

Abnormal hypothalamic-pituitary axis function

TSH	Free T4	T3	Interpretation
Normal/high	High	High	TSH mediated hyperthyroidism
Normal/low	Low/low normal	Low/normal	Central hypothyroidism

C. **Laboratory evaluation and tests:** (see Table 16-3)

    Serial growth charts are useful for plotting growth velocity and deviation from the previous growth curve.

    Minimal evaluation:

- **TSH and plasma free T4.** High TSH and low free T4 establishes a diagnosis of hypothyroidism originating from the thyroid gland. High TSH with normal free T4 indicates subclinical hypothyroidism. Normal to low TSH and low free T4 indicates a problem at the hypothalamic-pituitary axis. If total T4 is measured it should be done with a binding protein such as T3 resin uptake.
- **Low serum T4, normal TSH, and elevated reverse T3 are found in nonthyroidal illness** in patients with severe acute illness and chronic illness including malnutrition as is seen in anorexia nervosa.
- Total T3 should not be measured since it is usually normal.

    If there is primary hypothyroidism or goiter:

    Thyroid autoantibodies should be measured to rule out autoimmune disease. The two tests commercially available are thyroperoxidase and thyroglobulin antibodies. High levels are usually seen in autoimmune thyroiditis. Low levels can be seen in other thyroid conditions. If the antibody tests are negative they should be repeated in 3 to 6 months. Patients with negative antibody tests and persistent goiter should have additional evaluation. In community surveys, 50% to 70% of subjects with positive thyroid antibodies are euthyroid, 25% to 50% have subclinical hypothyroidism, and 5% to 10% have overt hypothyroidism.

    If a hypothalamic-pituitary cause is suspected:

    Perform pituitary function testing including provocative tests of adrenocorticopic hormone and growth hormone secretion as well as TRH stimulation of TSH. Computed tomography (CT) or magnetic resonance (MRI) of brain with sella views can be used to detect a hypothalamic-pituitary tumor.

    If goiter is present and thyroid antibodies are negative:

    Perform **radioiodide uptake test** with perchlorate discharge to exclude thyroid dysgenesis and inborn errors of thyroid hormone synthesis. **Ultrasound** of the thyroid will demonstrate the size and density of the gland. A diffuse hypoechogenic pattern is seen in 95% of patients with autoimmune thyroiditis. Fine needle aspiration (FNA) is not needed unless there is concern about a specific thyroid nodule or cyst.

III. **Management:**

  A. **Goals: The goal of treatment is restoration of euthyroid state.** The goiter will decrease in size if the TSH was elevated prior to treatment.

  B. **Medications:**

- Treatment for hypothyroidism is L-**thyroxine.**
- Replacement dose for adolescents is **2 to 4 μg per kg of body weight per day.**
- Begin with the lower dosage because excessive dosing can result in premature closure of epiphyses.
- Patients with central hypothyroidism may require lower doses of L-thyroxine.

  C. **Follow-up:** For primary hypothyroidism measure TSH and free T4 levels 6 to 8 weeks after beginning treatment and then every 6 to 12 months. **Serum free T4** should be in the upper half of the normal range; TSH should be in the lower half of the normal range. For central hypothyroidism measure only free T4 since TSH is not useful. Continue therapy through the adolescent growth spurt and pubertal development. Once complete, those with chronic autoimmune thyroiditis can be tested for remission by stopping treatment and retesting in 4 to 6 weeks. Therapy should resume if there are abnormal TSH levels. Follow patients with chronic autoimmune thyroiditis clinically and with thyroid function tests because those who are initially euthyroid may become hypothyroid.

HYPERTHYROIDISM

I.   **Description of the condition:**
   A. **Etiology: Thyrotoxicosis is uncommon in children and adolescents and 95% of the time is caused by Graves disease,** which is diffuse goiter with hyperthyroidism and infiltrative ophthalmopathy. Graves disease is an autoimmune thyroid disease but is not part of the spectrum of autoimmune thyroiditis. In Graves disease, **thyrotropin receptor-stimulating antibodies** bind to the TSH receptor, leading to gland hyperplasia and overproduction of thyroid hormones. The disease may go into remission.
        There are other causes of thyrotoxicosis. An **autonomously functioning thyroid adenoma** is the most common diagnosis after Graves disease. Patients with chronic autoimmune thyroiditis and subacute thyroiditis can present with **transient hyperthyroidism** because of release of thyroid hormones during the destructive inflammatory process. **Familial nonautoimmune hyperthyroidism** is rare but can be confused with Graves disease. It is caused by a germline mutation in the TSH receptor gene causing growth and increased function of thyroid follicular cells. It affects males and females equally because of autosomal dominant transmission. These patients do not have ophthalmopathy or TSH receptor antibodies and, unlike Graves disease, remission does not occur.
   B. **Genetics, familial transmission, and other factors:** Graves disease **peaks at 10 to 15 years of age. It is more common in females and is associated with a positive family history of autoimmune thyroid disease.** Chronic lymphocytic thyroiditis and Graves disease can be seen in the same family. There is a **concordance rate of 20% to 60% for monozygotic twins. A Danish study found that 80% of the risk of developing Graves disease is from genetic factors.** There may be an **association with other autoimmune endocrine diseases** such as diabetes and Addison disease and **nonendocrine autoimmune diseases** such as systemic lupus erythematosus, rheumatoid arthritis, pernicious anemia, myasthenia gravis, and vitiligo. Graves disease may occur concurrently with chronic autoimmune thyroiditis, creating challenges in diagnosis and management.

Table 16-4. Differential diagnosis of hyperthyroidism

- Graves disease
- Autonomous functioning nodule
  - Thyroid adenoma
  - Papillary or follicular carcinoma
  - McCune-Albright syndrome
- Familial nonautoimmune hyperthyroidism
- TSH-induced hyperthyroidism
  - Pituitary adenoma
  - Pituitary resistance to thyroid hormone
- Thyroiditis
  - Subacute thyroiditis
  - Hashimoto disease
- Exogenous thyroid hormone
- Iodine
- Tumor stimulating the thyroid
  - Hydatidiform mole
  - Choriocarcinoma

Adapted from Lifshitz F, ed. *Pediatric endocrinology*, 4th ed. New York: Marcel Dekker, Inc., 2003, page 372.

II. **Making the diagnosis:**
  A. **Signs and symptoms:** Although patients with Graves disease can present with classic signs and symptoms, subtle changes can occur for months prior to diagnosis. These include changes in academic performance and problems with insomnia, fatigue, lethargy, nervousness, and weight loss despite an increase in appetite. These **behavioral symptoms can be confused with attention-deficit hyperactivity disorder and hypothyroidism.** The signs and symptoms are similar to those of a hyperactive sympathetic nervous system.
  Other symptoms can include:
  - **goiter: almost always present** and if absent the diagnosis should be questioned
  - **tachycardia: present more than 80% of the time**
  - wide pulse pressure
  - systolic hypertension
  - heart murmur
  - palpitations
  - decreased exercise tolerance
  - **exophthalmos: present in more than 50% of patients**
  Eyelid lag, photophobia, blurred vision, diplopia, and lacrimation may accompany eye changes. There is infiltration in the ocular muscles, lacrimal glands, and retroorbital fat with mucopolysaccharides, lymphocytes, and edema fluid. **Eye changes are less common in adolescents than adults.**
  There can also be tremor, thyroid bruit, heat intolerance, excessive sweating, headache, myopathy (fatigability to periodic paralysis), diarrhea, urinary frequency, pubertal delay, amenorrhea, and nocturia. **Acceleration of growth and increase in height percentiles on growth curve can occur.** This is accompanied by accelerated epiphyseal closure, and **adult height is usually normal.**
  Thyroid storm, which is a **life-threatening event** with fever, tachycardia, high output cardiac failure, gastrointestinal disturbance (vomiting, diarrhea), and neurologic disturbance (confusion, seizures, coma), is rare. Infection, trauma, surgery, treatment with radioactive iodine, and withdrawal from antithyroid drugs may precipitate this event.
  B. **Physical exam:** Physical findings include a **diffuse goiter that is symmetrical, smooth, soft, and nontender.** There may be a palpable or audible thrill. Other common findings include tachycardia, elevated systolic blood pressure, heart murmur, wide pulse pressure, fine tremor, and brisk reflexes. Mild exophthalmos and lid lag are seen in over 50% of patients. The skin changes seen in adults with accumulation of mucopolysaccharides and pretibial edema are uncommon.
  C. **Laboratory evaluation and tests:**
  Minimal Evaluation:
  - **Serum TSH, free T4;** serum TSH should be suppressed with elevated free T4. If **free T4 is normal then measure serum T3,** which may be elevated prior to T4 or free T4; if TSH is not suppressed and free T4 and T3 are elevated this suggests a TSH secreting adenoma or pituitary resistance to thyroid hormone.
  - **Serum TSH receptor autoantibodies should be obtained for confirmation: TSH receptor stimulating antibody (TSA) and TSH binding inhibiting immunoglobulin (TBII).** Antithyroid antibodies may be detectable but at lower levels than patients with chronic autoimmune thyroiditis and are not indicated for diagnosing Graves disease. Patients with familial nonautoimmune hyperthyroidism will have negative antibodies.
  If a thyroid nodule is palpated or the thyroid gland is firm, tender, or asymmetric:
  - thyroid scan (radioiodine uptake) can be performed to differentiate Graves from other entities including adenoma, subacute thyroiditis, or chronic autoimmune thyroiditis. In Graves disease, uptake is increased in a homogenous fashion and uptake is decreased in thyroiditis.
III. **Management:**
  A. **Goal:** Achieve euthyroid state.
  B. **Treatment regimens:** In patients with severe symptoms of palpitations and tremor use a **β-adrenergic blocking agent (propanolol)** to control symptoms. Overall, **treatment choice is controversial in adolescents.**
  Therapeutic choices include **antithyroid drugs, radioiodine ablation, and subtotal thyroidectomy.**
  1. **Antithyroid drugs:** Most endocrinologists choose these as a first choice. **Their mechanism of action is to inhibit biosynthesis of thyroid hormone.** They may also have immunosuppressive activity. Antithyroid drugs can keep the

patient euthyroid until the disease remits. Initially 87% to 100% respond to antithyroid drug therapy but only 60 to 70% will have a permanent remission with drug therapy alone. It can take weeks to several months to achieve a euthyroid state. Therapy may be prolonged for several years and close supervision is needed. **The medications used are:**

- **Propylthiouracil (PTU):** dose 5 to 10 mg/kg/d.
- **Methimazole (MMI):** 0.5 to 1.0 mg/kg/d. The advantage of this drug is single daily dosing.

Minor side effects include urticarial or papular skin rash, transient granulocytopenia, arthralgia, and abnormal taste. **One serious toxic affect** is a lupuslike syndrome. **Baseline CBC and liver function tests (LFTs)** should be done before starting these medications. **All side effects are usually reversible.** The drug should be discontinued for a major side effect and another therapy instituted.

Follow up after initial therapy:

Thyroid function tests should be followed. Once a euthyroid state is achieved, the antithyroid medication can be continued at lower doses or continued at the same dose while thyroxine is given to prevent hypothyroidism. After several years, antithyroid medication can be tapered to see if the patient remains euthyroid or, alternatively, a T3 suppression test can be performed.

2. **Radioiodine therapy:** Radioiodide therapy is becoming more accepted for adolescents. Radioiodine is controversial because of concern over an increase in other tumors, effects on fertility, and teratogenicity. However, **studies have not shown an increase in thyroid or other tumors or congenital anomalies.** There is an increase in benign thyroid adenomas. **Oral radioactive iodine is used to cause ablation of the thyroid gland.** Initially, there may be an increase in thyroid hormones, but **ablation is complete in 6 to 18 weeks.** Beta-adrenergic blocking agents can be used to treat temporarily worsening hyperthyroid symptoms. Radioiodine therapy is contraindicated in pregnancy. **Hypothyroidism is a consequence of therapy,** and thyroid function tests should be monitored to guide initiation of thyroid hormone replacement therapy.

3. **Surgery:** Surgery is not recommended as first line therapy, but it is effective. The goal of surgery is subtotal thyroidectomy leaving less than 4 g of thyroid tissue. **Surgery is the most rapidly effective therapy** and is considered when other modalities fail and for those with severe ophthalmopathy who do not respond to antithyroid drugs. **Risks of surgery** include death, hypoparathyroidism, hypothyroidism, and vocal cord paralysis. **Hyperthyroidism may recur. An experienced surgeon is crucial.**

C. **Follow up:** Life-long follow up is required because of the risk of hypothyroidism with radioiodine or subtotal thyroidectomy and recurrent thyrotoxicosis with antithyroid drug therapy or surgery.

THYROID NODULES AND CANCER

I. **Description of the condition:**

A. **Epidemiology, etiology, and classification:** Thyroid nodules and cancer are uncommon in adolescents. Most patients with thyroid nodules are euthyroid and if the nodules are functional they are associated with hyperthyroidism. **Most (70%–80%) solitary nodules are cystic or benign adenomas, with only 15% to 20% of solitary nodules representing cancer. Radiation exposure** to the neck is a risk factor for developing thyroid carcinoma and males have a higher rate of cancer in nodules than females. There is also an increased risk if there is a **family history of papillary carcinoma** or if the patient has **an autosomal dominant multiple endocrine neoplasia syndrome mutation** that increases the risk of medullary carcinoma.

Less than 1% of functioning nodules represent cancers and most solitary solid nodules that are "cold" on radionuclide scan are benign. **Concern about a neoplasm should occur when there is a solitary mass with a consistency different from the rest of the thyroid gland.** A rapidly enlarging, painless, firm, hard nodule should raise suspicion. Most (60%–90%) of the thyroid cancers in adolescents are well-differentiated carcinomas, with 80% being papillary and 20% papillary-follicular. In general, these cancer types have a good prognosis compared to medullary or undifferentiated carcinomas that are much less common but have a higher mortality rate. Physical examinations can be difficult since nodules judged to

Table 16-5. Differential diagnosis of solitary nodules

* Lymphoid follicle from autoimmune lymphocytic thyroiditis
* Developmental anomaly
* Simple cyst
* Benign neoplasm
  * Colloid nodule
  * Follicular adenoma
  * Toxic adenoma
* Malignant neoplasm
  * Papillary carcinoma
  * Follicular carcinoma
  * Mixed papillary-follicular
  * Undifferentiated
  * Medullary carcinoma
* Nonthyroid
  * Lymphoma
  * Teratoma
* Abscess

Adapted from Hanna CE, LaFranchi SH. Adolescent thyroid disorders. *Adolesc Med State Art Rev* 2002;13:13–35.

be solitary at these examinations may actually represent multiple nodules when evaluated by ultrasound or radionuclide scan. Most multinodular goiter is caused by chronic autoimmune thyroiditis. (Tables 16-5 and 16-6)

II. Making the diagnosis:
  A. Signs and symptoms and the physical exam: Most nodules are asymptomatic. Findings that raise suspicion for cancer are rapid growth, size greater than 4 cm, fixation of the nodule, hoarseness or dysphagia, and enlarged regional lymph nodes. Medullary carcinoma usually appears in the upper half of the thyroid lobes. The presence of fever and a painful fluctuant mass suggest suppurative thyroiditis or abscess while signs of hypo- or hyperthyroidism point to subacute or chronic autoimmune thyroiditis or a functioning follicular adenoma.
  B. Laboratory evaluation and tests: TSH, serum free T4, T3, and antithyroid antibodies will detect hypo- or hyperthyroidism and help in differentiating autoimmune thyroiditis. Serum T3 will be high in a toxic adenoma. Positive antithyroid antibodies suggest that the nodularity is due to Hashimoto thyroiditis. Calcitonin is measured in cases of medullary carcinoma.
    Radiologic evaluation includes:
    1. Ultrasound: This will detect developmental abnormalities, whether the nodule is solid or cystic, and demonstrate if the lesion is solitary or multiple.

Table 16-6. Differential diagnosis of multinodular goiter

* Thyroiditis
  * Chronic autoimmune thyroiditis
  * Subacute thyroiditis
  * Acute suppurative thyroiditis
* Graves disease
* Goitrogen exposure
* Inborn error of thyroid hormone synthesis
* Iodine deficiency
* Colloid goiter
* Neoplasm

Adapted from Hanna CE, LaFranchi. SH Adolescent thyroid disorders. *Adoles Med State Art Rev* 2002; 13:13–35.

   2. Radionuclide scanning: This study should be done with iodine, which is trapped and organified, rather than with technetium, which is only trapped. The radionuclide scan will demonstrate whether the nodule is functioning as in a toxic adenoma or whether it is nonfunctioning or "cold." An autonomously functioning nodule will be the only tissue that shows uptake on thyroid scan. However, a non-functioning nodule does not imply malignancy since most are benign. The scan may also reveal uptake in the lungs or skeleton indicating possible metastatic spread of tumor. **A chest x-ray** should be done in patients with a solitary nodule.
   a. Fine needle aspiration (FNA) is recommended when physical signs of malignancy are absent. Positive or suspicious results are followed up with surgical excision.
   b. Surgical excision: Surgical excision should be performed on all solitary nodules that lack function on radionuclide scan and do not have negative FNA results. It also is done on nodules with negative FNA results but which subsequently increase in size.
   c. Surgical evaluation
III. **Management:**
   A. For nonmalignant nodules:
   • Hyperfunctioning nodules can be surgically excised.
   • Autoimmune thyroiditis with hypothyroidism is treated with L-thyroxine.
   B. For malignant nodules:
   • After surgery for malignancy, patients are given **L-thyroxine** therapy to suppress TSH stimulation of the gland. Serum T4 is kept in the upper part of the range and TSH is suppressed.
   • Patients with evidence of metastases or lymph node involvement are also given **ablative iodine therapy** after surgery. Patients are then followed with **serum thyroglobulin levels** to monitor for recurrence. **Calcitonin levels** are followed for medullary carcinoma.
IV. **Clinical pearls and pitfalls:**
   • Goiter is the most common clinical finding of thyroid disease in adolescents.
   • Most adolescents with goiter are euthyroid.
   • Chronic autoimmune thyroiditis is the most common clinical entity causing thyroid disease in adolescents.
   • Hypothyroidism is the most common functional abnormality.
   • Thyroid cancer is uncommon in adolescents, even those with solitary thyroid nodules.

BIBLIOGRAPHY

For the clinician

Dayan CM, Daniels GH. Chronic autoimmune thyroiditis. *N Engl J Med* 1996;335:99–107.
Foley TP. Hypothyroidism. *Pediatr Rev* 2004;25:94–100.
Hanna CE, LaFranchi SH. Adolescent thyroid disorders. *Adolesc Med State Art Rev* 2002;13:13–35.
Lifshitz F, ed. *Pediatric endocrinology*, 4th ed. New York: Marcel Dekker Inc, 2003.
Rallison ML, Dobyns BM, Meikle AW, et al. Natural history of thyroid abnormalities: prevalence, incidence, and regression of thyroid disease in adolescents and young adults. *Am J Med* 1991;91:361–370.
Sperling MA, ed. *Pediatric endocrinology*, 2nd ed. Philadelphia, PA: WB Saunders, 2002.
Trowbridge FL, Matovinovic J, McLaren GD, et al. Iodine and goiter in children. *Pediatrics* 1975; 56:82–90.

WEB SITES

www.tsh.org   Web site of the Thyroid Foundation of America
www.thyroid.org   Web site of the American Thyroid Association
www.nlm.nih.gov/medlineplus/thyroiddiseases   National Institute of Health information on thyroid disease

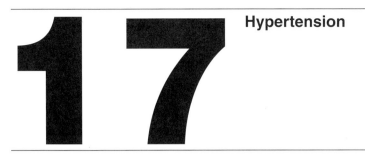

Hypertension

I. **Description of the condition:**
   A. **Definition:** For adolescents, **hypertension** is defined as systolic or diastolic blood pressure greater than the 95th percentile for the patient's age, height, and gender. Readings greater than 99th percentile are defined as **severe hypertension** whereas values between the 90th and 95th percentiles are defined as **prehypertensive.**

      The prevalence of hypertension in the pediatric population is 0.8% to 5%. On the basis of the 2001 United States census data, this equates to more than 350,000 children with significantly elevated blood pressure. Prevalence data have not been disaggregated for the adolescent age group.
   B. **Etiology:** Hypertension can be classified as **primary** or **secondary**. Although secondary hypertension is much more common in infants and children, primary hypertension becomes more prevalent as children enter adolescence. The incidence of primary hypertension in adolescents has further increased with the increasing prevalence of obesity in this age group.

      As a general rule, the more dramatic the increase in the blood pressure and the more difficult it is to control, the more likelihood there is of finding a secondary cause. Underlying kidney pathology is the most common cause of secondary hypertension in adolescents.

      Etiologies of secondary hypertension in adolescents are listed in Table 17-1.
II. **Making the diagnosis:** Most adolescents with hypertension are asymptomatic, and elevated blood pressure readings are noted during routine physicals or office visits. Several organizations, including the American Academy of Pediatrics (AAP), the American Heart Association (AHA), and the American Medical Association (AMA), recommend routine annual screening of children after the age of 3 years, including adolescents.

Table 17-1. Common etiologies of secondary hypertension in adolescents

Renal diseases	Glomerulonephritis
	Recurrent UTIs
	Polycystic kidney disease
Vascular diseases	Renal artery stenosis
	Coarctation of the aorta
Endocrine diseases	Cushing syndrome
	Hyperaldosteronism
	Pheochromocytoma
	Thyroid disease
Inheritable causes	Glucocorticoid remediable aldosteronism
	Apparent mineralocorticoid excess
Pharmacologic causes	Steroids
	Oral contraceptives
	Stimulant medications
	Decongestants
	Nicotine
	Caffeine
	Illicit drugs
Psychological stressors	

UTIs, urinary tract infections.
From Pappadis S, Somers M. Hypertension in adolescents: a review of diagnosis and management. *Curr Opin Pediatr* 2003;15:370–378, with permission.

Once an adolescent is found to have an elevated blood pressure, multiple readings (at least three) should be obtained on different occasions before hypertension is diagnosed (unless the blood pressure readings are in the severe category and the patient is symptomatic). Proper technique needs to be utilized to measure the blood pressure. The patient should have rested for at least 5 minutes. The right arm should be positioned at heart level and the inner cuff bladder width should be at least 40% of the mid-arm circumference. The cuff should cover 80% to 100% of the arm circumference. The first Korotkoff sound is used for systolic and the fifth Korotkoff sound is used to determine diastolic blood pressure in all ages. Tables 17-2 and 17-3 show the blood pressure levels for males and females depending on their age, height percentile, and gender.

Ambulatory blood pressure monitoring (ABPM) is fast emerging as a more useful tool for the evaluation of hypertension. As there are no standardized norms for the pediatric population, this caveat needs to be considered before using this modality for diagnosis. There are several studies in both pediatric and adult populations proving the utility of ABPM in the evaluation of borderline hypertension, white coat hypertension, and in the assessment of the efficacy of antihypertensive therapy.

Once the diagnosis of hypertension is confirmed, a complete history and physical examination is important to rule out secondary causes, to look for comorbid illnesses, for example, obesity, and also to assess end organ damage due to the elevated blood pressure. Laboratory tests and imaging studies are utilized as necessary to confirm diagnoses.

A. History:
- Important aspects of the **birth history** include history of prematurity, umbilical vein catheterization, or prolonged ventilation.
- **Past medical history** should focus on history of recurrent urinary tract infections or renal injury.
- **Family history** is important as children from hypertensive families have higher blood pressures than children of normotensive families. Also, patients with inherited forms of hypertension may have a history of early hypertension in family members.
- A **social history** with emphasis on use of medications, recreational drugs, tobacco, alcohol, and anabolic steroids by the adolescent is required, as all of these can contribute to elevated blood pressures.
- A thorough **review of systems** is necessary to confirm the presence or absence of symptoms of systemic illnesses that may have hypertension as a component, for example, endocrinopathies or systemic lupus erythematosis. Specific questions regarding headaches, visual changes, dyspnea, snoring, palpitations, chest pain, edema, pallor, and weight gain or loss should be asked.

B. Physical Examination:
- All patients require a complete physical examination.
- **Pulses** should be checked in all four extremities.
- **Blood pressure** should be measured in both an upper and a lower extremity to rule out vascular causes such as coarctation of the aorta.
- **Height** and **weight** should be measured and the **body mass index (BMI)** calculated.
- A **general exam** looking for specific body habitus features (e.g., buffalo hump) and skin changes should be performed.
- A **fundoscopic exam** is important to rule out arteriolar narrowing or arteriovenous nicking.
- A complete **cardiovascular exam** for tachycardia, arrhythmias, cardiomegaly, murmurs, and signs of early heart failure is important. Examination for carotid and abdominal bruits should be done.
- A thorough **neurologic exam** should be performed and a **musculoskeletal exam** to check for muscle weakness is important.

C. Laboratory Evaluations: A few basic screening tests should be ordered on all patients diagnosed with hypertension. Baseline complete blood count (CBC), electrolytes, fasting glucose, blood urea nitrogen (BUN), creatinine, and lipid profile along with a urinalysis, urine culture, and a renal ultrasound to rule out silent renal parenchymal scarring should be obtained. Electrocardiograms (EKGs) are not helpful in adolescents for the diagnosis of left ventricular hypertrophy (LVH). Echocardiography is a more sensitive test in the adolescent to rule out LVH.

Other tests to be considered, depending on clinical suspicion, include: thyroid function tests, renal Doppler study, and/or arteriography, computed tomography (CT) scan of the abdomen and pelvis, and levels of urinary catecholamines, aldosterone, and electrolytes. A pregnancy test should always be considered for the adolescent female.

Table 17-2. Blood pressure levels for males by age and height percentile

Age (yr)	BP (percentile)	Systolic blood pressure (mm Hg) height percentile							Diastolic blood pressure (mm Hg) height percentile						
		5th	10th	25th	50th	75th	90th	95th	5th	10th	25th	50th	75th	90th	95th
12	50	101	102	104	106	108	109	110	59	60	61	62	63	63	64
	90	115	116	118	120	121	123	123	74	75	75	76	77	78	79
	95	119	120	122	123	125	127	127	78	79	80	81	82	82	83
	99	126	127	129	131	133	134	135	86	87	88	89	90	90	91
13	50	104	105	106	108	110	111	112	60	60	61	62	63	64	64
	90	117	118	120	122	124	125	126	75	75	76	77	78	79	79
	95	121	122	124	126	128	129	130	79	79	80	81	82	83	83
	99	128	130	131	133	135	136	137	87	87	88	89	90	91	91
14	50	106	107	109	111	113	114	115	60	61	62	63	64	65	65
	90	120	121	123	125	126	128	128	75	76	77	78	79	79	80
	95	124	125	127	128	130	132	132	80	80	81	82	83	84	84
	99	131	132	134	136	138	139	140	87	88	89	90	91	92	92
15	50	109	110	112	113	115	117	117	61	62	63	64	65	66	66
	90	122	124	125	127	129	130	131	76	77	78	79	80	80	81
	95	126	127	129	131	133	134	135	81	81	82	83	84	85	85
	99	134	135	136	138	140	142	142	88	89	90	91	92	93	93
16	50	111	112	114	116	118	119	120	63	63	64	65	66	67	67
	90	125	126	128	130	131	133	134	78	78	79	80	81	82	82
	95	129	130	132	134	135	137	137	82	83	83	84	85	86	87
	99	136	137	139	141	143	144	145	90	90	91	92	93	94	94
17	50	114	115	116	118	120	121	122	65	66	66	67	68	69	70
	90	127	128	130	132	134	135	136	80	80	81	82	83	84	84
	95	131	132	134	136	138	139	140	84	85	86	87	88	88	89
	99	139	140	141	143	145	146	147	92	93	93	94	95	96	97

BP, blood pressure.
Adapted from National Heart, Lung, and Blood Institute. The fourth report on the diagnosis, evaluation, and treatment of high blood pressure in children and adolescents. *Pediatrics* 2004;114(2):555–576.

Table 17-3. Blood pressure levels for females by age and height percentile

Age (yr)	BP (percentile)	Systolic blood pressure (mm Hg) height percentile							Diastolic blood pressure (mm Hg) height percentile						
		5th	10th	25th	50th	75th	90th	95th	5th	10th	25th	50th	75th	90th	95th
12	50	102	103	104	105	107	108	109	61	61	61	62	63	64	64
	90	116	116	117	119	120	121	122	76	76	76	76	77	78	78
	95	119	120	121	123	124	125	126	79	79	79	80	81	82	82
	99	127	127	128	130	131	132	133	86	86	87	88	88	89	90
13	50	104	105	106	107	109	110	110	62	62	62	63	64	65	65
	90	117	118	119	121	122	123	124	76	76	76	77	78	79	79
	95	121	122	123	124	126	127	128	80	80	80	81	82	83	83
	99	128	129	130	132	133	134	135	87	87	88	89	89	90	91
14	50	106	106	107	109	110	111	112	63	63	63	64	65	66	66
	90	119	120	121	122	124	125	125	77	77	77	78	79	80	80
	95	123	123	125	126	127	129	129	81	81	81	82	83	84	84
	99	130	131	132	133	135	136	136	88	88	89	90	90	91	92
15	50	107	108	109	110	111	113	113	64	64	64	65	66	67	67
	90	120	121	122	123	125	126	127	78	78	78	79	80	81	81
	95	124	125	126	127	129	130	131	82	82	82	83	84	85	85
	99	131	132	133	134	136	137	138	89	89	90	91	91	92	93
16	50	108	108	110	111	112	114	114	64	64	65	66	66	67	68
	90	121	122	123	124	126	127	128	78	78	79	80	81	81	82
	95	125	126	127	128	130	131	132	82	82	83	84	85	85	86
	99	132	133	134	135	137	138	139	90	90	90	91	92	93	93
17	50	108	109	110	111	113	114	115	64	65	65	66	67	67	68
	90	122	122	123	125	126	127	128	78	79	79	80	81	81	82
	95	125	126	127	129	130	131	132	82	83	83	84	85	85	87
	99	133	133	134	136	137	138	139	90	90	91	91	92	93	93

BP, blood pressure.
Adapted from National Heart, Lung, and Blood Institute. The fourth report on the diagnosis, evaluation, and treatment of high blood pressure in children and adolescents. *Pediatrics* 2004;114(2):555–576.

Table 17-4. Common medications for treatment of hypertension in adolescents

Drug	Dosage	Common side effects
ACE inhibitors (ACEIs)		
Enalapril	0.08–0.6 mg/kg/d to 40 mg/d	• Dry cough, angioedema • Check for azotemia in renal insufficiency
Lisinopril	0.07–0.6 mg/kg/d to 40 mg/d	• Contraindicated in pregnancy and renal artery stenosis
Angiotensin receptor blockers (ARBs)		
Irbesartan	150–300 mg/d	• Contraindicated in pregnancy
Losartan	0.7–1.4 mg/kg/d to 100 mg/d	• Cough and angioedema less frequent than ACE inhibitors
Beta-blockers		
Atenolol	0.5–2.0 mg/kg/d to 100 mg/d	• Contraindicated in asthma and overt heart failure • May impair athletic performance
Propanolol	1–4 mg/kg/d to 640 mg/d	• Bradycardia, dizziness
Calcium channel blockers		
Amlodipine	2.5–5 mg/d	• May cause reflex tachycardia
Felodipine	2.5–10 mg/d	
Central alpha agonists		
Clonidine	0.2–2.4 mg/d	• Dry mouth, sedation • Rebound hypertension with sudden cessation
Diuretics		
Hydrochlorothiazide	1–3 mg/kg/d to 50 mg/d	• Caution in severe renal insufficiency
Furosemide	0.5–6 mg/kg/d	• Check for electrolyte imbalances
Vasodilators		
Minoxidil	5–100 mg/d	• Hypertrichosis with long-term use
Alpha antagonists		
Prazosin	0.05–0.5 mg/kg/d	• Hypotension, syncope

Adapted from the National Heart, Lung, and Blood Institute. The fourth report on the diagnosis, evaluation, and treatment of high blood pressure in children and adolescents. *Pediatrics* 2004;114(2):555–576.

III.   **Management:**
   A. Goals of treatment: The primary goal is to keep the systolic and diastolic blood pressure less than the 95th percentile for patient's age, height, and gender to ensure prevention of long-term cardiovascular, renal, and neurologic sequelae. More aggressive goals are set for patients with chronic renal disease and diabetes as blood pressures below the 90th percentile have proven to provide renal protective benefit in these clinical situations.

     For secondary hypertension, the underlying cause will also need to be addressed and treated.
   B. Treatment:
    1. Life style modifications: Regardless of the cause of hypertension, life style modifications have proven to be effective in controlling blood pressure. Emphasis is placed on dietary interventions, weight reduction, and exercise. **Reduced salt diets** help to decrease both the systolic and diastolic blood pressure. Potassium supplementation has not proven to be effective.

     Incorporating **regular exercise** into the adolescent's daily routine is beneficial. A 30 to 45 minute period of brisk walking daily can decrease blood pressure by up to 10 mm Hg. In obese adolescents, **weight loss** of only 5% has been shown to decrease blood pressure.

Discontinuing tobacco use, decreasing alcohol intake, and adopting a diet low in saturated fat and cholesterol are all important adjuncts in reducing blood pressure.

2. **Pharmacologic therapy:** Adolescents with hypertension are usually treated with the same broad range of medications as adults. Commonly used categories include diuretics, angiotensin converting enzyme inhibitors (ACE inhibitors), angiotensin receptor blockers (ARBs), and calcium channel blockers. Choice of a specific drug is dependent on the presumed underlying pathophysiology of hypertension, associated comorbid illnesses, the patient's ability to follow a prescribed regimen, and the clinician's experience with the selected medication.

   Diuretics, although commonly used in adults, have not been studied in the adolescent population. The only randomized controlled trial on hydrochlorothiazide found no improvement in the systolic or diastolic blood pressure compared to placebo. As diuretics can cause dehydration and hypokalemia, care should be taken if using this class of drug, particularly in the athletic adolescent. Also, compliance is an issue as many adolescents may skip doses to prevent frequent urination.

   ACE inhibitors are the most commonly prescribed antihypertensives in the adolescent population. Studies in children taking enalapril show an improvement in blood pressures similar to that seen in the adult population. Side effects, although uncommon, include cough and angioedema. ACE inhibitors should be used with extreme caution in patients suspected of having renal artery stenosis, as the decrease in the efferent artery pressure may cause renal hypoperfusion and exacerbate renal insufficiency. Also, because of their potential teratogenicity, ACE inhibitors should be avoided in sexually active adolescent females who are not using effective contraception.

   ARBs are similar to ACE inhibitors as far as efficacy and safety profile is concerned. The incidence of bradykinin mediated cough and angioedema is lower as these drugs work directly on the angiotensin receptor. ARBs also are contraindicated in pregnancy and should be used with caution in females who are sexually active.

   Beta-blockers are not used as often in adolescents as adults. They are contraindicated in patients with reactive airway disease and diabetes. Also, they can decrease exercise performance in athletic adolescents. Selective beta-blockers are of benefit in patients with migraine headaches or reflex tachycardia.

   Calcium channel blockers have been widely used in the pediatric population. Studies have shown good efficacy of these agents in this population. Amlodipine has been studied in the pediatric population and has been shown to decrease both systolic and diastolic blood pressure. Side effects include flushing, headache, lower extremity edema, and hypotension.

C. **Follow up:** Adolescents with hypertension should be evaluated every 2 months and more frequently if the blood pressure is severe or not under good control. Life style modifications should be restressed and adherence to the medication regimen assessed.

IV. **Special Circumstances:**
   A. **Participation in sports:** There are no restrictions to physical activity in a patient with mild to moderate hypertension. Patients are encouraged to exercise regularly as part of their treatment plan.

      In patients with severe hypertension, competitive sports and isometric exercises, for example, weight training, are restricted. Patients should be allowed to participate in aerobic physical activities, as it may help in reducing blood pressure.

V. **Clinical pearls and pitfalls:**
   - It is important to confirm the diagnosis of hypertension by repeated measurements on multiple occasions with use of an appropriate technique.
   - Primary hypertension is much more common in the adolescent population than in children.
   - Life style modifications including dietary intervention, weight reduction, and exercise are the first line of treatment.
   - Medications used in adolescents are similar to those used in the adult population. The choice of medications depends on the hypothesized pathophysiology of hypertension, the comorbid illnesses, the side effect profile, and the ease of following a regimen, and the providers' comfort with a specific medication.
   - There is no contraindication to sports and physical activity in patients with hypertension.
   - Patients should be followed every 2 months and more frequently if they have severe or uncontrolled hypertension.

BIBLIOGRAPHY

For the clinician

American Academy of Pediatrics. Committee on Sports Medicine and Fitness. Athletic participation by children and adolescents who have systemic hypertension. *Pediatrics* 1997;99(4):637–638.

Daniels S. Cardiovascular sequelae of childhood hypertension. *Am J Hypertens* 2002;15:61S–63S.

Flynn JT. Hypertension in adolescents. *Adolesc Med Clin* 2005;16:11–29.

Joint National Committee JNC VII. *Hypertension* 2003;42(6):1206–1252.

Morgenstern B. Blood pressure, hypertension, and ambulatory blood pressure monitoring in children and adolescents. *Am J Hypertens* 2002;15:64S–66S.

National High Blood Pressure Education Program's Updated Task Force on Blood Pressure in Children and Adolescents. NIH, 1996.

Pappadis S, Somers M. Hypertension in adolescents: a review of diagnosis and management. *Curr Opin Pediatr* 2003;15:370–378.

Sponsored by the National Heart, Lung, and Blood Institute. The fourth report on the diagnosis, evaluation, and treatment of high blood pressure in children and adolescents. *Pediatrics* 2004; 114(2):555–576.

WEB SITES

www.americanheart.org   Official Web site for the American Heart Association

www.familydoctor.org   Official Web site for the American Academy of Family Practice

www.noah-health.org   A patient-friendly Web site which gives answers to simple queries of patients and parents

www.lifeclinic.com   Industry-supported Web site with good information on hypertension, diabetes and cholesterol.

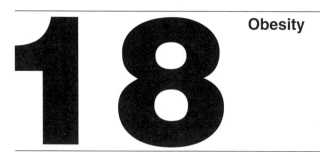

Obesity

I. **Description of the problem:** Obesity is rapidly becoming an epidemic among children and teenagers in the United States.

For the first time in American history, there are now more overweight and obese adults than there are normal-weight adults living in the United States. An overweight child has a 40% chance of becoming an overweight adult, but an overweight teenager is virtually guaranteed to become one (80% chance). Obesity is rapidly overtaking cigarette smoking as the number one most preventable cause of adult mortality and morbidity. Hospital costs for obesity-related illnesses have skyrocketed from $15 million in 1979 to $127 million in 1999.

A. **Definition:** Overweight and obesity are not single, well-defined diseases. Their causes are multifactorial (biologic, psychological, social), but they share the final common denominator that caloric intake exceeds energy expenditure. Body mass index (BMI) is now used to identify at-risk teenagers. Although BMI does not always correspond directly to body fat (e.g., certain athletes may be overweight but not have too much adipose tissue), it is easily available using weight and height measurements:

$$BMI = Weight\ (kg) \div Height\ (m^2)$$

Although adolescents sometimes get caught in the middle between childhood and adult definitions, the most common formulation uses BMI to define:

Overweight/At Risk of Overweight = BMI 85–95th percentiles (generally 25–30)

Obese = greater than 95th percentile (generally >30)

BMI charts are readily identifiable for teens to help clinicians identify at-risk patients (Figure 18-1). If charts are not immediately available, the 95th percentile BMI for male teens is approximately their age in years + 14, while the 95th percentile BMI for female teens is approximately their age in years + 13.

Obesity is also an excess of total body fat, which can be difficult to measure. However, by the end of the pubertal growth spurt, adolescent males should have 10% to 20% total body fat and adolescent females should have 17% to 27%.

B. **Epidemiology:** A series of National Health and Nutrition Examination Surveys (NHANES) examined nearly 1,500 teenagers in the most recent study (NHANES III, conducted between 1999 and 2000). Compared with the 1976–1980 survey, the prevalence of overweight has doubled among children 6 to 11 years of age and tripled among those 12 to 17 years of age. Nearly 16% of 12 to 19 year olds are at or above the 95th percentile for BMI. Currently, 35% of adults are overweight and 27% are obese, meaning that normal-weight adults are currently in the minority in the United States.

Certain subpopulations have even higher rates. A recent study using data from the National Longitudinal Survey of Youth found that men, African Americans, Hispanic Americans, and those living in southern states have the highest rates of overweight or obesity. More than one-fourth of Hispanic male teens and African-American female teens are obese. Between 1986 and 1998, the prevalence increased by 120% in African American youth and Hispanic youth, compared with 50% for white non-Hispanic youth. The recent National Heart, Lung, and Blood Institute Growth and Health Study (NGHS) studied 1,213 African-American and 1,166 white females, beginning at ages 9 or 10, for 9 years. By age 19, more than half of the African American females and a third of the white females were overweight. The prevalence of obesity was twice as high for African American teens (18%) as for white teens (8%).

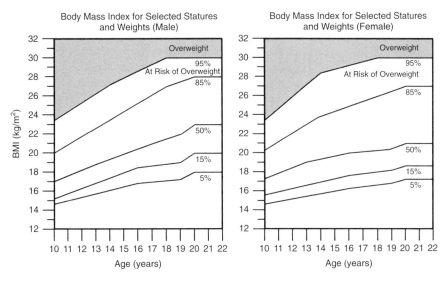

Figure 18-1. Body mass index for teenagers. BMI, body mass index. (From Green M, ed. *Bright futures: Guidelines for health supervision of infants, children and adolescents.* Arlington, VA: National Center for Education in Maternal and Child Health; 1994:266, Appendix G: Body Mass Index, with permission.)

Poorer adults tend to be more obese, but the relationship has not been settled for children or teens. In NHANES III, only poor white adolescents were 2.6 times more likely to be overweight.

C. **Etiology:** Adolescence appears to be a crucial period when overweight and obesity can occur. In males, abdominal fat is deposited; in females, the percentage of body fat increases. Puberty is also a time of relative insulin resistance. In addition, early menarche carries a two-fold increased risk of overweight. Ultimately, overweight and obese teenagers have an 80% likelihood of becoming overweight and obese adults.

1. **Nature versus nurture:** Perhaps nowhere in modern medicine is there more controversy than surrounding the causes of obesity. Is it nature or nurture, or both? Twin studies and studies of adopted children seem to demonstrate that 70% to 80% of the variance in obesity can be attributed to heredity. On the other hand, genetics cannot explain the significant association of fatness in spouses (nor the resemblance between overweight owners and their pets). Of course, the distinction becomes blurred when looking at the biologic family. A child with two obese parents has an 80% chance of becoming obese (odds ratio 10:1), a 40% chance if only one parent is obese, and only a 14% chance if both parents are of normal weight. At the moment, an educated scientific guess would put the genetic contribution at about 25%, and the environmental contribution at about 75%.

2. **Basic science:** Theories abound concerning the cause of obesity. One current theory holds that there are three critical periods during childhood for the development of obesity: infancy, adiposity rebound (age 5), and puberty. A competing theory states that humans are born with a finite number of adipocytes, which can undergo hyperplasia only in the first year or two of life. After that, fat cells can only undergo hypertrophy. Consequently, obesity is frequently determined during infancy.

Overweight and obesity represent a disturbance in basic energy balance: what goes in exceeds what is expended. Yet typically, weight gain is caused by a very small imbalance occurring over a long period of time. For example, 50 calories a day over a period of a year will result in a 5-pound weight gain. That can be negated by switching to skim milk, for example, or foregoing one pat of butter each day. Many hormones are involved in this process. One of the newest and most important is leptin, which correlates positively with BMI. It is secreted by adipose tissue and acts on the hypothalamus to increase satiety and lower food intake. Leptin levels in humans correlate with total body fat, and mice that lack leptin are extremely obese and have type 2 diabetes. Glucocorticoids inhibit leptin. Other important hormones include insulin, glucagon, tumor necrosis factor, neuropeptide Y, ghrelin, and adiponectin. Current research in this area could have a profound impact on the assessment and treatment of obesity in children and adolescents in the very near future.

3. **Physical activity:** National surveys document that children and adolescents are less physically active now than ever before. One in five young people ages 8 to 16 report two or fewer periods of vigorous exercise per week. In the NGHS study, levels of habitual activity decreased by 83% over 9 years. In the Youth Risk Behavior Survey of 2003, half of teens were not enrolled in physical education classes at school, and three-fourths had not participated in moderate physical activity for 5 of the previous 7 days. Other studies have found that American children average only 12 minutes of vigorous activity per day and that this figure declines with puberty.

Most energy expenditure (70%) comes from supplying the basal metabolic rate. Food intake and physical activity account for only 15% of the total energy equation. This helps to explain why losing weight is so difficult and why simply increasing the amount of exercise may not guarantee weight loss. Basal metabolic rates vary from individual to individual, but rates do tend to be similar among family members. Interestingly, basal metabolic rate (BMR) *increases* as body weight increases. Therefore, although obese people may expend less energy (e.g., riding an elevator instead of walking up stairs), they also use more energy per given activity. BMR also differs among different ethnic groups. For example, African-American women have lower BMRs than white women, which may help to explain why black women tend to be more obese.

4. **Nutrition:** The fast food industry has revolutionized the way Americans eat and contributed significantly to the current problem of obesity. In the year 2000, Americans spent $110 billion on fast food—more than on higher education, computers, or cars. Nearly half of every food dollar that Americans spend is on food eaten outside the home. Young people today get 10% of their total energy intake from fast foods, compared with 2% in the late 1970s. Between 1972 and 1995, the number of fast-food restaurants more than doubled. Every day, an estimated 30% of young people aged 4 to 19 years eat fast food, and 7% of the entire US population eats at McDonald's each day. Recent studies show that all adolescents eat too much fast food and that, in particular, overweight adolescents fail to compensate for their fast food intake by adjusting their energy intake for the rest of the day (*JAMA* 2004;291:2828–2833).

Fast food has infiltrated school cafeterias as well. Currently, there are more than 4,500 Pizza Huts and 3,000 Taco Bells in school cafeterias around the country. In a Harvard study of 6,212 children on 2 nonconsecutive days, children who ate fast food obtained 29% to 38% of their total energy intake from that source, with more fat, more sugar, and less healthful food. The researchers estimated that fast food contributes an additional 57 calories to the daily diet of young people in the US, which adds up to an additional 6 pounds of body weight per year.

Adolescents' intake of soda is also problematic. By age 14, 32% of females and 52% of males are consuming three or more sodas per day (Table 18-1). Contracts with soda manufacturers have generated $200 million for schools nationwide. A single can of soda has 140 calories in it; consumed daily, this amounts to

Table 18-1. Soft drink consumption

Children consuming 3 or more soft drinks per day

Age	Females	Males
6–8 yr	3%	7%
9–13 yr	21%	21%
14–18 yr	32%	52%

From US Department of Agriculture. www.healthinschools.org. Childhood obesity: What the research tells us. 2001.

51,110 calories per year. Since a pound gained is a net intake of 3,500 calories, this represents 14.6 pounds gained in a year. The single serving size for soda has changed dramatically, from the standard 6.5- and 10-ounce bottles to 12 to 24 ounces. At 7-11 stores, a Double Gulp cup holds 64 ounces of soda. A 2004 study of nearly 100,000 nurses from 1991 to 1999 found that increased consumption of soft drinks and fruit juices led to weight gain and a significant risk of type 2 diabetes in adult women (*JAMA* 2004;292:927–934). Women who consumed one or more sweetened drinks a day were twice as likely to develop diabetes as those who drank fewer than one per month.

5. **Television:** Television has been eyed suspiciously for many years as a significant contributor to obesity. One public health expert asserts that TV is the **single best predictor** of obesity in childhood and adolescence, much the same as cigarette smoking causes the majority of lung cancer. There are several reasons why TV may be an important contributor to the problem:
   - Studies show that children actually burn fewer calories while watching TV than while sleeping or reading quietly. American children and teens spend more time watching TV than in any other activity except for sleeping. Furthermore, TV displaces other, more calorie burning-intensive activities.
   - Children and teenagers view an estimated 40,000 ads per year on TV, and half are for food, especially sugared cereals, high-caloric snacks, and fast food. Watching TV and exposure to food ads each increase snacking behavior (teens now consume an average of 610 calories per day by snacking). By contrast, TV viewing is inversely associated with teens' intake of fruit and vegetables.
   - Six national cross-sectional studies have found a strong association between TV viewing and obesity. Of course, the causal arrow could run in either direction: Television could be causing obesity, or obese children and teens could be more sedentary and watching more TV. Several studies have found that young people who watch 4 or more hours of TV per day have higher BMIs than those who watch less than 2 hours. In addition, a recent study found that a child's risk for obesity increases 6% for every hour of TV viewed per day and that this risk increases an additional 31% for every hour viewed per day if he or she has a TV set in the bedroom.
   - The most powerful study showed that a simple 6-month curriculum to reduce total TV time in an elementary school could significantly increase all measures of adiposity including BMI, decrease high-fat food intake, and increase physical activity.

6. **Medical causes of obesity:** True medical causes of obesity are extremely rare (Table 18-2). In fact, probably 99% or more of adolescent obesity is primary in origin and *is not associated with any identifiable endocrine abnormality*. Knowledge

Table 18-2. Medical causes of obesity

Dysmorphic syndromes
Prader-Willi
Laurence-Moon-Biedl
Turner syndrome
Central nervous system disorders
Trauma
Tumor
Postinfectious
Endocrine
Hypothyroidism
Insulinoma
Cushing syndrome
Exogenous steroids
Polycystic ovary syndrome
Growth hormone deficiency
Pseudohypoparathyroidism (type 1)

Adapted from Dietz WH, Robinson TN. Assessment and treatment of childhood obesity. *Pediatr Rev* 1993;14:337.

of the normal growth dynamics during adolescence may help avoid unnecessary testing:

- Obese female preteens tend to enter puberty earlier than their leaner peers, whereas most endocrine causes of obesity are associated with poor growth, especially in height. Patients with hypothyroidism, Cushing disease, or growth hormone deficiency all present with short stature as well as obesity.
- Probably the most sensitive indicator of thyroid dysfunction is irregular menses. Females with regular menses are highly unlikely to have thyroid disorders. An obese teenager who is Tanner 4 or 5, in the 75th percentile for height, and has regular menses does not require thyroid function tests, despite the insistence of her mother that "it must be something glandular" or "we have thyroid disease running in our family."
- Use of Tanner staging, growth charts, and calculation of the BMI will enable the clinician to make an intelligent assessment about the need for endocrine testing.

7. **Toward a coherent theory of obesity:** The body seems to have a unique set point for body fat, sometimes called the "adipostat," located somewhere in the brain. This set point influences two types of largely voluntary behavior: eating and physical activity. The body seems to measure its own stores of body fat through leptin, which acts in a feedback loop that may affect the appetite and satiety centers of the brain. Like a thermostat, the adipostat can be reset by a variety of factors, including diet, activity, and drugs. It is also under heavy genetic influence. As people grow more sedentary with age, the adipostat veers upward. This combines with the decrease in basal metabolic rate that occurs around age 35 to produce increasingly overweight adults. Finally, weight loss is not simply a matter of cutting calories. The body seems to defend its own weight or set point by slowing the metabolic rate when energy input is curtailed. Thus, an adult who usually weighs 180 pounds has a metabolic rate that is 15% higher than someone does who used to weigh 205 pounds and recently lost 25 pounds.

D. **Complications:** Several studies have found that when obesity was present in adolescence, there is increased mortality among adult men, an increased risk of heart disease, and an increased incidence of diabetes in both men and women. The risk of early mortality over a 20-year period is 1.5 to 2.5 times increased if there is obesity at age 18.

Obesity has been known to be associated with many increased health risks, including:

- Type 2 diabetes: a three-fold increased risk. Adiposity in early adolescence is the single strongest predictor of the metabolic syndrome (hypertension, elevated fasting insulin or glucose levels, and type 2 diabetes). Remarkably, the estimated lifetime risk for an individual born in the year 2000 is now 32% for men and 38% for women.
- Hypertension: a five- to six-fold increased risk.
- Sleep apnea and Pickwickian syndrome. One study of 41 obese children found that one-third had symptoms of sleep apnea.
- Cardiovascular conditioning. A study of 48 males and females, ages 8 to 17, with BMIs greater than 40 kg per m^2 found significant cardiorespiratory morbidity, including severe lack of cardiovascular fitness (*J Pediatr* 2004; 144:766–769).
- Asthma, orthopedic problems, stroke, cancer, and a variety of other medical disorders.
- Mental health problems. Multiple studies show that obesity is associated with low self-esteem in some adolescents. Many overweight teens are also socially marginalized. Young children will choose a playmate with a major physical handicap over one who is obese. In one longitudinal study of more than 10,000 16 to 24 year olds, overweight women completed fewer years of school, were less likely to be married, and had greater rates of household poverty after 7 years.

E. **Metabolic syndrome:** Also known as Syndrome X, Metabolic syndrome is a recent clinical entity among adolescents. Previously, it was considered to be a problem only of middle age to older adults. The "classic" presentation of insulin resistance involves hyperglycemia, but Metabolic syndrome may present with one or more clinical features of insulin resistance instead:

- Acanthosis nigricans (pigmented skin over the neck and upper chest area, resembling someone who has not washed his or her neck recently)
- Accelerated or impaired linear growth
- Polycycstic Ovarian Disease (PCOS)
- Lipodystrophy
- Muscle cramps

Table 18-3. Diagnosis of Metabolic syndrome

National Cholesterol Education Program	World Health Organization
Any 3 of the following:	**Hyperinsulinemia or fasting BS >110 mg/dL** *plus* **at least 2 of the following:**
Abdominal obesity	Abdominal obesity
Waist >102 cm in males and >88 cm in females	Waist-to-hip ratio >0.9 BMI or waist >94 cm
Triglycerides >150 mg/dL	Dyslipidemia
HDL <40 mg/dL in males, or <50 mg/dL in females	Triglycerides >150 mg/dL or HDL <35 mg/dL
BP >135/85 mm Hg	BP >140/90
Fasting BS >110 mg/dL	

BS, blood sugar; BMI, body mass index; BP, blood pressure.

Metabolic syndrome puts teens at risk for the development of type 2 diabetes, PCOS, and early-onset cardiac, renal, and vascular disease. It has also been associated with liver pathology (fibrosis, cirrhosis, fatty liver).

A recent NHLB longitudinal study in Minneapolis found that adiposity in early or late adolescence, as measured by the BMI, is a strong predictor of who will have the Metabolic syndrome at age 26.

Diagnosis of Metabolic syndrome should be considered in any teenager who is obese. Criteria vary slightly (Table 18-3).

II. **Making the diagnosis:** Currently, the standard adult definitions of overweight (BMI ≥25) and obesity (BMI ≥30) are usually applicable to adolescents as well. Alternatively, teens' BMI can be plotted on a growth chart, with overweight in the 85th percentile or higher, and obese in the 95th percentile or higher.

Laboratory screening is rarely needed, but lipid levels may be useful. In addition, if type 2 diabetes is a consideration, then fasting insulin and glucose levels and a 2-hour postprandial glucose measurement will be needed.

III. **Management:** (Tables 18-4, 18-5, and 18-6).

A. **Clinical practice:** Clearly, the primary goal in clinical practice is to **prevent** overweight and obesity before it can appear. Early recognition of excessive weight gain should become routine in pediatric practices, as should the use of BMI. Because the treatment options are so fallible, prevention of overweight is critical and must begin in infancy.

Ideally, clinicians need a program in the community or at a tertiary care hospital to which to refer teens. The most successful programs employ a multidisciplinary approach, addressing:
- Changes in diet
- Increased activity
- Behavior modification
- Psychology and support
- Parental involvement
- Follow-up

Without access to such intensive programs, the average clinician can *still* make a significant difference, especially if they are in a general pediatric practice (Table 18-4). Obviously, since preventing obesity before it begins is the most important factor, the mothers of babies need to be instructed that, by far, *breastfeeding* offers the single best protection against obesity. Parents of children should be counseled to limit total media time, encourage physical activity, and avoid fast food. Most families should be switching to skim or 1% milk when their children reach age 2 and severely restricting intake of soda and sweetened juice during the childhood years. For teens, a few simple principles can make a major difference:
- **Setting appropriate goals.** A Tanner 5 adolescent may have an initial goal of a 10% reduction in weight. A Tanner 2 female or a Tanner 3 or 4 male may only need to *stabilize* their weights and let their height spurts kick in.
- **Making simple dietary adjustments.** Overweight patients consistently underreport their caloric intake. Tanner 5 teens can decrease their intake by up to 500 calories per day with a low-fat, high-fiber diet. Younger teens can simply switch from regular soda to diet soda, from full-fat ice cream to frozen yogurt, from

Table 18-4. Approach to managing overweight patients

- Establish diagnosis of overweight
- Exclude genetic causes by history and physical
- Assess comorbidity by history, physical, and labs
- Assess readiness for change
- Counsel on health consequences
- Establish dietary, activity, behavioral plan
- Ongoing monitoring
- Refer as appropriate

From Schwimmer JB. Managing overweight in older children and adolescents. *Pediatr Ann* 2004;33:39–44, with permission.

regular milk to skim milk, and from full-fat potato chips to baked chips or pretzels. Drinking just one can of soda a day increases a child's risk of obesity by 60%. Keeping a dietary journal may be useful. A nutritional assessment by a dietician can also be helpful. Patients need to be educated about the caloric density of different foods and be taught how to read food labels and gauge portion size.

For older adolescents, a reduced-glycemic load diet may be an alternative to a conventional low fat diet (*Arch Pediatr Adolesc Med* 2003;157:773–779). Glycemic load is determined by carbohydrates' immediate effect on blood glucose levels. Carbohydrates that break down quickly during digestion have the highest glycemic indexes. This may have implications in the causation of Metabolic syndrome.

In general, patients should be cautioned against low calorie diets (Table 18-5). The body defends itself against changes in weight by establishing a set point that it attempts to maintain by regulating the BMR. When intake is restricted, the body simply slows its BMR.

- **Increasing physical activity and decreasing sedentary activity.** Simply cutting TV and computer time in half will often result in a significant weight loss. At 1-year follow-up, young people who decreased their media time had significantly lower BMIs, regardless of their physical activity, than those who persisted in their viewing habits. On the other hand, increasing exercise alone will not result in weight loss.
- **Identifying behaviors that lead to increased eating (e.g., snacking while watching TV, eating at fast food restaurants after school).** Skipping breakfast is not an option. Having a TV set in the bedroom is a strong predictor of overweight.
- **Initiating a program of behavior modification that involves the entire family** (Table 18-6). Ultimately, the goal is to change the way the entire family eats, exercises, and plans their daily activities. Overweight or obesity is not just the teenager's problem; it is the family's problem.

B. **Drug therapy:** While research on pharmacotherapy to combat obesity is booming, there are very few options currently available that are risk-free, well tested, and clinically proven. On the horizon is a new drug called Acomplia (Sanofi-Aventis), which has recently been tested on more than 3,000 people throughout the United States,

Table 18-5. Does dieting work?

Diet	Design	Evidence supports use in primary care
Moderately low fat	20%–30% of calories	Yes
Low fat	<20% of calories	No
Low carbohydrate	<30% of calories	No
Very low calorie	<800 calories/d	No
Low glycemic index	Meals selected by influence on blood sugar	Yes/No
Meal replacement	Substitution for 1–3 meals/d	Yes/No

From Schwimmer JB. Managing overweight in older children and adolescents. *Pediatr Ann* 2004;33:39–44, with permission.

Table 18-6. Behavioral therapy for weight management

Strategy	Example
Goal setting	Lose 4 lb over 2 months
Self-monitoring	Record food intake and activity
Stimulus control	Keep high-calorie foods out of the home
Positive reinforcement	Family outing for completing food and activity log
Problem solving	Plan ahead for parties and holidays
Cognitive restructuring	Change self-defeating thoughts
Social support	Parents, peers

From Schwimmer JB. Managing overweight in older children and adolescents. *Pediatr Ann* 2004;33:39–44, with permission.

with 5% to 10% weight losses achieved that lasted up to 2 years (Associated Press, November 9, 2004). But for the time being, clinicians would be wise to refer morbidly obese patients to tertiary care programs that have specific research protocols in progress. The experience with "fen-fen" (i.e., fenfluramine and dexfenfluramine) and pulmonary hypertension and cardiac valve abnormalities should have taught everyone *to be extremely conservative in prescribing or asking for drugs to treat obesity.* Clinicians also need to be aware that using thyroid hormone supplementation in euthyroid patients is not only ineffective in producing weight loss but may lead to negative nitrogen balance and loss of lean body mass. However, there are a few drugs that have shown some promise in small research studies and appear to be relatively safe:

1. **Metformin:** Metformin is one of the mainstays of treatment for type 2 diabetes, but can it be used to treat obesity as well? A few studies involving teens have found that metformin decreases fasting glucose and insulin levels and can decrease BMI and weight, in conjunction with a low calorie diet. In one 8-week trial with 24 teens, an average weight loss of 6.5 kg was achieved. Early treatment with metformin has been shown to prevent the progression from precocious puberty to polycystic ovary syndrome in a group of 24 low birthweight females. The usual dosage is 500 mg twice a day.

2. **Sibutramine (Meridia):** Sibutramine is an appetite suppressant that inhibits the reuptake of norepinephrine, serotonin, and dopamine. In one trial with severely obese teens, two-thirds achieved 5% or more reductions in their BMIs after 6 months of treatment, in conjunction with behavioral therapy. Approximately a dozen adult studies have documented its effectiveness. Side effects include hypertension and tachycardia. It is not labeled for use in patients under 16 years of age.

3. **Orlistat (Xenical):** Orlistat is a drug that blocks gastric and pancreatic lipases in the stomach and small intestine, thus decreasing the absorption of triglycerides. Seven long-term studies of adults involving 2,400 patients have shown that an average of 12 pounds can be lost within 6 months. A few trials have involved adolescents as well. Side effects include effects on stools, including diarrhea, greasy stools, flatulence, leakage, and urgency. Use requires supplementation with fat-soluble vitamins and beta-carotene. It is not labeled for use in patients under the age of 18.

C. **Surgery:** Gastric stapling and bypass procedures should only be considered as a last resort—in teenagers who are morbidly obese and have access to tertiary care centers with considerable experience in these techniques. A recent report of ten teenagers, ages 17 and younger, undergoing gastric bypass surgery found an average weight loss of 30 kg, without any mortality (*J Pediatr* 2001;138:499–504). But this may also be the time of peak bone mineralization, and adult studies have shown significant morbidity and even mortality.

IV. **Clinical pearls and pitfalls:**
- Overweight and obesity pose one of the largest public health threats to adolescents in the United States. Both are increasing dramatically.
- As physical activity diminishes, media consumption increases, fast food intake soars, and soda intake climbs, American children and teenagers are getting fatter and fatter.
- Clinicians can make a difference, but only if they monitor growth curves closely, use BMI calculations, and are aggressive in providing counseling to patients and their families.
- From a societal viewpoint, increasing the number of breastfeeding mothers, decreasing portion sizes in restaurants, decreasing soda intake among children and teens in schools, and decreasing total media time would go far to heading off the current epidemic.

BIBLIOGRAPHY

American Academy of Pediatrics. Prevention of pediatric overweight and obesity. *Pediatrics* 2003;112:424–430.

Cuttler L, Whittaker JL, Kodish ED. The overweight adolescent: clinical and ethical issues in intensive treatments for pediatric obesity. *J Pediatr* 2005;146:559–564.

Dietz WH. Overweight in childhood and adolescence. *N Engl J Med* 2004;350:855–857.

Dietz WH, Robinson TN. Overweight children and adolescents. *New Engl J Med* 2005;352: 2100–2109.

Fowler-Brown A, Kahwati LC. Prevention and treatment of overweight in children and adolescents. *Am Fam Physician* 2004;69:2591–2598.

Kim SYS, Obarzanek E. Childhood obesity: a new pandemic of the new millennium. *Pediatrics* 2002; 110:1003–1007.

Neumark-Sztainer D. Addressing obesity and other weight-related problems in youth. *Arch Pediatr Adolesc Med* 2005;159:290–291.

Robinson TN. Television viewing and childhood obesity. *Pediatr Clin North Am* 2001;48:1017–1025.

Schneider MB, Brill SR. Obesity in children and adolescents. *Pediatr Rev* 2005;26:155–162.

Schwimmer JB. Managing overweight in older children and adolescents. *Pediatr Ann* 2004;33:39–44.

Sondike SB, Copperman NM, Jacobson MS. Bringing a formidable opponent down to size. *Contemp Pediatr* 2000;17:133–157.

WEB SITES

www.cdc.gov/growthcharts   Body mass index growth charts for gender and age

www.healthinschools.org   Center for Health and Health Care in Schools, at George Washington University

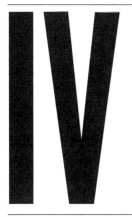

Common Behavioral Problems

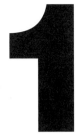
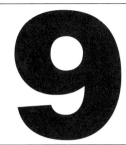

Attention-Deficit/ Hyperactivity Disorder

I. **Description of the condition:**
   A. **Diagnostic criteria:** Attention-Deficit/Hyperactivity Disorder (ADHD) is the most common neurobehavioral disorder of childhood and adolescence. The essential feature of the disorder, according to the *Diagnostic and Statistical Manual IV—TR*, is a persistent pattern of inattention and/or hyperactivity-impulsivity that is more frequently displayed and more severe than is typically observed in people at a comparable level of development. For the diagnosis to be made, some hyperactive-impulsive or inattentive symptoms must have been present before the age of 7 years. Table 19-1 lists the diagnostic criteria for ADHD.
   B. **Cause of ADHD:** The cause of ADHD is considered to be primarily genetic and neurologic. Several neuroimaging studies have shown that patients with ADHD, when compared with controls, have regions of the brain with reduced volume, specifically in the cerebellum, caudate nucleus, globus pallidus, and corpus callosum. These differences have been shown to be static and unrelated to stimulant therapy. Functional neuroimaging studies (position emission tomography) of children and adolescents with ADHD have shown hypoactivity of the frontal cortex and subcortical structures, usually on the right side.

   The frontal lobe of the brain represents the top level of circuitry in cognition, best described as "executive function" or "cognitive control." The impact of ADHD upon educationally relevant executive functions such as working memory, planning, reading comprehension, written composition, and general study skills continues to be an active area of research.

   Family and twin genetic studies have shown that ADHD is one of the most heritable conditions known, with a heritability factor between 0.80 and 0.88. Molecular genetic studies to date have shown associations between abnormalities in the dopamine D4 and the dopamine transporter genes and ADHD.
   C. **Prevalence of ADHD in children and adolescents:** ADHD affects 8% to 10% of children and persists into adolescence in approximately 80% of cases diagnosed during childhood. Certain subgroups of children with ADHD have less marked symptoms in childhood, and the diagnosis of ADHD is easily missed. These include the following subgroups:
   - Children (mainly females) who tend to exhibit fewer hyperactive symptoms, that is, the more obvious symptoms for teachers and parents to pick up on.
   - Individuals who exhibit mental rather than physical restlessness.
   - Children with a higher than average IQ.
   D. **Prevalence of ADHD in adolescents:** Recent prevalence data have shown that between 7.5% and 9.4% of adolescents have ADHD. Approximately 13.3% of males have ADHD by the age of 19. Approximately 50% of those identified with ADHD by age 19 were diagnosed after age 11.

   These data reveal that ADHD is one of the most common disorders among adolescents, particularly male adolescents.
II. **Making the diagnosis of ADHD in adolescents:** The diagnosis of ADHD in adolescents, especially in those adolescents in whom the diagnosis was not made in childhood, may be difficult and elusive. Complicating factors can influence the diagnosis:
   1. The classic diagnostic criteria have been based on experience with childhood ADHD and do not take into account symptoms first presenting in adolescence such as:
      a. physical hyperactivity can be transformed into much less obvious mental restlessness
      b. mental restlessness may make adolescents appear easily bored or impatient
      c. quieter individuals may be considered lazy or unmotivated
      d. the adolescent may become moody or uncommunicative

Table 19-1. Diagnostic criteria for Attention-Deficit/Hyperactivity Disorder

A. Either (1) or (2):
   (1) Six (or more) of the following symptoms of **inattention** have persisted for at least
       6 months to a degree that is maladaptive and inconsistent with developmental level:

   Inattention:
   (a) Often fails to give close attention to details or makes careless mistakes in schoolwork,
       work, or other activities.
   (b) Often has difficulty sustaining attention in tasks or play activities.
   (c) Often does not seem to listen when spoken to directly.
   (d) Often does not follow through on instructions and fails to finish schoolwork, chores,
       or duties in the workplace (not due to oppositional behavior or failure to understand
       directions).
   (e) Often has difficulty organizing tasks and activities.
   (f) Often avoids, dislikes, or is reluctant to engage in tasks that require sustained men-
       tal effort (such as schoolwork or homework).
   (g) Often loses things necessary for tasks or activities (e.g., toys, school assignments,
       pencils, books, or tools).
   (h) Is often easily distracted by extraneous stimuli.
   (i) Is often forgetful in daily activities.
   (2) Six (or more) of the following symptoms of hyperactivity–impulsivity have persisted for
       at least 6 months to a degree that is maladaptive and inconsistent with developmental
       level:

   Hyperactivity:
   (a) Often fidgets with hands or feet or squirms in seat.
   (b) Often leaves seat in classroom or in other situations in which remaining seated
       is expected.
   (c) Often runs about or climbs excessively in situations in which it is inappropriate (in
       adolescents or adults, may be limited to subjective feelings of restlessness).
   (d) Often has difficulty playing or engaging in leisure activities quietly.
   (e) Is often "on the go" or acts as if "driven by a motor."

   Impulsivity:
   (a) Often blurts out answers before questions have been completed.
   (b) Often has difficulty awaiting turn.
   (c) Often interrupts or intrudes on others (e.g., butts into conversations or games).
B. Some hyperactive-impulsive or inattentive symptoms that caused impairment were present
   before age 7.
C. Some impairment from the symptoms is present in two or more settings [e.g., a school (or
   work) and at home].
D. There must be clear evidence of clinically significant impairment in social, academic, or occupational functioning.
E. The symptoms do not occur exclusively during the course of a pervasive developmental disorders, or other psychotic disorder and are not better accounted for by another mental disorder
   (e.g., mood disorder, anxiety disorder, dissociative disorder, or a personality disorder).

Code based on type:

314.01 Attention-Deficit/Hyperactivity Disorder, Combined Type: if both Criteria A1 and
A2 are not met for the past 6 months.

314.00 Attention-Deficit/Hyperactivity Disorder, Predominantly Inattentive Type: If
Criterion A1 is met but Criterion A2 is not met for the past 6 months.

**314.01 Attention-Deficit/Hyperactivity Disorder, Predominantly Hyperactive-
Impulsive Type:** If Criterion A2 is met but Criterion A1 is not met for the past 6 months.

Coding Note: For individuals (especially adolescents and adults) who currently have symptoms
that no longer meet full criteria, "In Partial Remission" should be specified.

The characteristics of ADHD in adolescents are less well captured in the *DSM-IV-TR* ADHD criteria (which have been referred to as having a "child-based bias"). Compared with the characteristics defined in children, the above symptoms may be "typical" of adolescents who become distracted or bored when tasks do not interest them. Assessment of ADHD symptoms is further complicated by the presence of psychiatric comorbidities in as many as two-thirds of adolescents with ADHD.

Many of the teacher rating scales do not have adequate normative databases for children older than 12 years of age.

2. **Rating scales for schoolteachers, parents, and adolescents.** Schoolteachers are an important source of information for adolescents suspected of having ADHD. However, adolescents typically have five to eight teachers who see the student for only one or two periods per day and therefore may not have sufficient contact to provide meaningful information on ADHD-related behavior. Nevertheless, teacher information concerning a student's grade point average, standardized tests of achievement and IQ, and objective measures of rule breaking may be valuable in the total assessment of the adolescent. Because rating scales from teachers are an important component in the assessment of the adolescent suspected of having ADHD, a short questionnaire is preferable to some of the longer rating scales available. The 20-item Attention Problems Scale—Teacher Report Form and 28-item Conners Teacher Rating Scale—Revised (short form) are realistic alternatives to the longer rating scales. Information should be obtained from most of the adolescent's teachers, whenever this is practical.

Conners' abbreviated Parent Questionnaires (revised) come in both an 80-item long and a 27-item short form. The patterning of scores on the 80-item long form may help to distinguish between the ADHD inattentive versus ADHD combined subtypes. (Available from Multi-Health Systems, 908 Niagara Falls Blvd., North Tonawanda, NY 14120; 800-456-3003.) The Conners/Wells Adolescent Self-report of Systems (CASS) is a set of questions answered by the adolescent that screens for: (a) family problems, (b) emotional problems, (c) conduct problems, (d) cognitive problems, (e) anger control problems, and (f) hyperactivity. (Available from Multi-Health Systems, 908 Niagara Falls Blvd., North Tonawanda, NY 14120; 800-456-3003.) Rating scales should be a significant part of the assessment of the adolescent with possible ADHD. The assessment of the adolescent also should include a complete history and physical exam.

III. **Management:**

A. **Stimulant medication:**

1. **Basic principles:** The basic goal of stimulant medication is to help the adolescent improve the quality of daily life while not expecting a "cure" for this disorder. A positive response to stimulant medication does not confirm the diagnosis of ADHD because adolescents without ADHD can note a beneficial effect on attention with stimulant medication and also a rebound effect when off this medication.

The adolescent should be a willing participant in the management of ADHD with medication and should never be "forced" to take medication against his or her will.

Clear and realistic goals for the adolescent with ADHD who will be taking stimulant medication need to be set, such as the medication helping increase attention and limited task persistence and decreasing impulsivity. In general, the clinician begins a medication at a low dose and increases the dose until target symptoms improve to a level acceptable to the adolescent, parents, and teachers.

2. **Individual drugs, dosages, and dose schedules:** Although Ritalin and amphetamines are the stimulant medications of choice for adolescents with ADHD, many different preparations may be used. Available stimulant medications are listed in Table 19-2. Recent conclusions from the large, meticulously designed Multimodal Treatment Study of ADHD clearly indicate that aggressive titration of stimulants often results in substantially better treatment outcomes. Any clinician who attempts to manage adolescents with ADHD must be familiar with dosages, dose schedules, and side effects of these drugs. Several excellent references can be found at the end of this section.

B. **Other therapies used for adolescents with ADHD:** Although psychostimulant medication may be the cornerstone of therapy of adolescents with ADHD, other interventions have proven useful. These therapies include:

1. **Psychotherapy:** This intervention is designed to help those with ADHD learn to like and accept themselves, to understand their strengths and weaknesses, and to develop strategies to minimize the negative impact of their disorder.

2. **Behavior therapy:** The focus of this treatment method is to teach authority figures and parents how to increase appropriate behavior and decrease inappropriate behavior in the affected child.

Table 19-2. Available stimulant medications

Ritalin (Methylphenidate—short duration. Novartis)

Ritalin SR (20 mg methylphenidate tablet—long duration. Novartis)

Generic MPH (both short duration and long duration. Geneva)

Ritalin LA (Ritalin developed for 8-hour duration. Novartis)

Metadate ER [long-acting (8 hours) MPH, Celltech]

Methylin ER [long-acting (8 hours) MPH, Mallinckrodt]

Concerta (methylphenidate HCL, extended release tabs; 18 mg, 36 mg, 54 mg; up to 12 hour duration of MPH; McNeil)

Metadate CD methylphenidate HCL, extended-release 20 mg Capsules; 8–9 hours of MPH duration. Celltech)

Focalin (Dexmethylphenidate [purified D-methylphenidate to last 4–6 hours at half the usual dose] Novartis)

Dexedrine (dextroamphetamine tablets, GlaxoSmithKline)

Dexedrine Spansules (long-acting dextroamphetamine, GlaxoSmithKline)

Dextroamphetamine generic (Barr)

Dextrostat (dextroamphetamine, Shire US)

Adderall (combination of 4 amphetamine and dextroamphetamine salts, Shire US)

From Greydanus DE, Sloan MA, Rappley MD. Psychopharmacology of ADHD in adolescent. In *Neurologic and neurodevelopmental dilemmas in the adolescent. Adoles Med: State Art Rev* 2002;13(3):599–624, with permission.

3. **Cognitive-behavior therapy (CBT):** CBT is designed to help youth work on immediate issues and employs interventions that are intended to change behavior directly. CBT combines components of psychotherapy and behavior therapy to help adolescents rethink and restructure their thoughts and feelings about initiating behavior change.
4. **Biofeedback:** This treatment method combines physiological, cognitive, and behavioral techniques. It teaches a person how to control physiologic responses to stressors and to control and relax muscles that increase or decrease tension, anxiety, and stress.
5. **Psychosocial treatments:** These treatments address social, emotional, and behavioral functioning and include social skills training, support groups, parent training, teacher training, and peer mediation.

IV. **Comorbid conditions associated with ADHD:** Comorbid conditions (emotional/behavioral/psychiatric problems) are common in adolescents with ADHD. Other features commonly associated with ADHD can disrupt the life of the adolescent with ADHD and affect his or her family. According to one study, 87% of children and adolescents with ADHD had one comorbid condition. The presence of two or more comorbid conditions was seen in 67% of children and adolescents with ADHD.

These conditions include:

A. **Oppositional defiant disorder:** A pattern of negativistic, hostile, and defiant behavior lasting at least 6 months, involving loss of temper, frequent arguments with adults, refusing to comply with requests, deliberately annoying others, being angry and vindictive, and blaming others for one's mistakes. Fifty-nine percent of teens with ADHD have oppositional defiant disorder.
B. **Conduct disorder:** A repetitive pattern of antisocial behavior violating others' basic rights or societal norms, involving physical aggression, threats, use of weapons, cruelty to people or animals, destruction of property, deceitfulness, theft, repeated running away from home, frequent truancy, or sexual assault. Forty-three percent of teens with ADHD have a conduct disorder. There is sometimes a progression from oppositional defiant disorder to conduct disorder, and persistent conduct disorder is termed antisocial personality disorder in adulthood.
C. **Mood and anxiety disorders:** Many adolescents with ADHD are somewhat depressed because of their school and home problems. As a result, their self-esteem suffers. Twenty-five percent to 75% of referred adolescents with ADHD and 15% to 19% of community samples have one or more of the following types of mood disorders: major depressive disorder, dysthymic disorder, or bipolar disorder. Adolescents with ADHD and bipolar disorder are particularly challenging to treat. Twenty-seven percent to 30% of referred adolescents with ADHD and 7% to 26% of community samples have one or more of the following anxiety disorders: generalized anxiety disorder,

panic disorder, obsessive-compulsive disorder, social phobia, or posttraumatic stress disorder.

D. **Learning disabilities or academic achievement problems:** A significant discrepancy between average to above average intellectual ability and below-average academic achievement in reading, math, spelling, handwriting, or language are thought to reflect a processing deficit and result in academic underachievement. Between 19% and 26% of children with ADHD have learning disabilities in at least one area. Even though most adolescents with ADHD do not have learning disabilities, they do consistently show academic achievement problems, with scores on Standardized Achievement Tests lower than those of matched controls, and a greater likelihood of grade retentions, school dropout, or expulsions.

E. **Substance abuse:** Adolescents with ADHD show more cigarette and alcohol use than do matched controls. These conditions occur most commonly in the subgroup with conduct disorder. Marijuana is emerging as the most commonly used illicit drug among adolescents with ADHD.

F. **Driving behavior:** Adolescents with ADHD show less sound driving skills or habits than matched control groups, with greater likelihood of accidents, more bodily injuries associated with crashes, and more traffic citations, particularly for speeding. The subgroups with comorbid oppositional defiant disorder or conduct disorder are at the highest risk for such deficient driving skills or habits.

G. **Family relations:** Adolescents with ADHD and their parents display more negative, controlling interactions, fewer positive facilitative interactions, and more conflicts than matched controls. Mothers of adolescents with ADHD report more personal psychological distress than mothers of matched controls. The adolescents themselves underestimate the degree of family conflict, compared with their mothers.

H. **High-risk sexual behaviors:** A recent follow-up study found that adolescents with ADHD have an earlier age at first sexual intercourse, more sexual partners, less use of birth control, more sexually transmitted diseases, a greater frequency of testing for human immunodeficiency virus, and more teen pregnancies than their non-ADHD peers.

IV. **Clinical pearls and pitfalls:**
   - The treatment of ADHD requires expertise in many different treatment methods, no single one of which can address all of the difficulties likely to be experienced by people with this disorder.
   - Among the available treatments, education of parents, family members, and teachers about this disorder, psychopharmacology (chiefly stimulant medications), parent training in effective behavior management methods, classroom behavior modification methods, academic interventions, and special education placement appear to have the greatest efficacy or promise for dealing with children and adolescents with ADHD.
   - *Atomoxetine (Strattera)*
     - Atomoxetine is a nonstimulant drug promoted as an equally efficacious form of ADHD therapy as conventional agents (e.g., methylphenidate, dextroamphetamine, pemoline, buproxiprion, tugchic antidepressants). Controlled studies essential for evaluation of this agent have shown evidence of efficacy. Atomoxetine is also promoted as treatment for nocturnal enuresis and adult depression.
     - At present, Atomoxetine has been assessed only in short-term trials (8–9 weeks). Furthermore, direct comparative studies with other conventional ADHD treatments are lacking.
     - Atomoxetine cannot be recommended for treatment of ADHD over 9 weeks because of the lack of long-term studies.
     - Atomoxetine cannot be recommended over stimulant medication for the treatment of ADHD because it has not been shown to be more effective than conventional stimulant medications.

BIBLIOGRAPHY

For the clinician

AACHP. Practice parameter for the use of stimulant mediations in the treatment of children, adolescents and adults. *J Am Acad Child Adolesc Psychiatry* 2002;41:265–495.

American Academy of Pediatrics. Clinical practice guideline: diagnosis and evaluation of the child with attention-deficit/hyperactivity disorder. *Pediatrics* 2000;105:1158–1170.

American Psychiatric Association. *Diagnostic and statistical manual of mental disorder–TR*, 4th ed. Washington, DC: American Psychiatric Association. 2000.

Barkley RA. Adolescents with attention-deficit/hyperactivity disorder: an overview of empirically based treatments. *J Psych Practices* 2004;10(1):39–56.

Biederman J, Newcorn J, Sprich S. Comorbidity of attention-deficit/hyperactivity disorder with conduct, depressive, anxiety, and other disorders. *Am Psychiatry* 1991;148:564–577.

Biederman J, Wilen T, Mick E, et al. Pharmaco therapy of attention-deficit/hyperactivity disorder reduces risk for substance abuse disorder. *Pediatrics* 1999;104(2):e20.

Conners CK. *Conners parent rating scale—revised.* North Tonowanda, NY: Multi-Health Systems, 1997.

Conners CK, Wells K. *Conners/wells adolescent self-report scale.* North Tonowanda, NY: Multi-Health Systems, 1997.

Green M, Sullivan P, Eichberg C. Helping academic underachievers become achievers in their own right. *Contemp Pediatr* 2005;22(6):29–36.

Greydanus DE, Pratt HD, Sloane MA, et al. Attention-deficit/hyperactivity disorder in children and adolescents: inventions for a complex costly clinical conundrum. *Ped Clin N Am* 2003;50(5): 1049–1092.

Jensen PS, Hinshaw SP, Swanson JM, et al. Findings from the NIMH Multimodal Treatment Study of ADHD: implications and applications for primary care providers. *Dev Behav Pediatr* 2001;22:60–73.

Nahlik J. Issues in diagnosis of attention-deficit/hyperactivity disorder in adolescents. *Clin Pediat* 2004;43:1–8.

Schubiner H, Robin AL, Neinstein LS. *School problems and ADHD. Adolescent health care—a practical guide.* Philadelphia, PA: Lippincott Williams & Wilkins, 2002:1454–1475.

Wolraich ML, Wibbelsman CJ, Brown TE, et al. Attention-deficit/hyperactivity disorder among adolescents: a review of the diagnosis, treatment, and clinical implications. *Pediatr* 2005;115: 1734–1746.

For patients and parents

Levine M. *A mind at a time.* New York: Simon & Schuster, 2003.

Levine M. *The myth of laziness.* New York: Simon & Schuster, 2004.

Levine M. *Ready or not: Here life comes.* New York: Simon & Schuster, 2005.

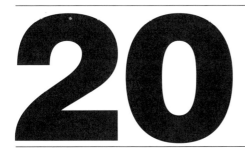

Substance Abuse

I. **Description of the problem:**
   A. **Epidemiology:** Substance abuse is the number one public health problem among adolescents.

   No other health problem among teenagers approaches the tragic effects of substance abuse in terms of adolescent mortality and morbidity and the devastating effects on the adolescent's family.

   Although this area of adolescent medicine is replete with statistics in terms of what drugs, including alcohol, adolescents are using, when they start using, and how often they use specific drugs, it is clear that adolescents who regularly abuse alcohol and drugs are putting their lives at risk and are, if they continue to abuse alcohol and drugs, not giving themselves a fair chance at life. These adolescents are limiting their futures in terms of what they can accomplish.

   Table 20-1 is a comprehensive list of risk factors and denotes which of these have the greatest effect at specific developmental stages.

   The current trends of individual drugs that are being used by teenagers are included in the "Comment" columns in Table 20-2.
   B. **Risk factors:** Not all adolescents are at equal risk for developing a substance abuse disorder. There are risk factors that make some adolescents more at risk, and some of these risk factors continue to emerge throughout adolescence.

   These risk factors are divided into four different domains: cultural/societal, interpersonal, psychobehavioral, and biogenetic. The greater the number of risk factors, the greater the risk of a substance use disorder (SUD). However, the strength and nature of risk factors can also influence the magnitude of risk.

   Psychiatric disorders make up interpersonal risk factors that can influence the development of an SUD throughout adolescence. Common psychiatric disorders influencing the development of substance abuse disorders in adolescents are:
   - Mood Disorders such as major depression, dysthymia, and bipolar disorder.
   - Anxiety Disorders such as generalized anxiety disorder, social anxiety disorder, and posttraumatic stress disorder.
   - Attention-deficit/Hyperactivity Disorder (ADHD), ADHD with conduct disorders, and ADHD untreated (treated ADHD reduces the risk for an SUD by 85%).
   - Conduct disorder.
   - Eating disorder: Bulimic patients have been found to have a greater risk for substance abuse than restrictive anorexics.
   - Suicidality: seventy percent of adolescents who complete suicide were drug and alcohol users.
   - Schizophrenia: Patients with schizophrenia are at increased risk of abusing marijuana.
   C. **Protective factors:** Protective factors can cushion the effect of risk factors and decrease overall negative outcomes. Protective factors include:
   1. Stable family and home environment.
   2. High degree of motivation for achievement.
   3. Strong parent–child bond.
   4. Consistent parental supervision and discipline.
   5. Boding to prosocial institutions (e.g., church-related youth groups).
   6. Association with peers who hold conventional attitudes.
   7. Exposure to community-wide antidrug messages.
   D. **Parental knowledge of their adolescent drug and alcohol use:** Several studies have shown that parents are remarkably unaware of their adolescent's drug and alcohol use. Teenagers' ability to deceive their parents about their use of mood-altering chemicals (including deceiving with half-truths) helps feed into the parents' denial about their children's use. When it comes to their drug and alcohol use, teenagers have deception down to a fine art.

Table 20-1. Domains of factors associated with drug use

I. Cultural/societal
  Laws favorable to drug use
  Social norms favorable to drug use
  Availability of drugs
  Extreme economic deprivations
  Neighborhood disorganization
II. Interpersonal
  a. Childhood interpersonal factors
    Family alcohol and drug behavioral and attitudes
    Poor and inconsistent family management practices
    Parent personality and other characteristics
    Family conflicts
    Physical or sexual abuse
  b. Adolescent interpersonal factors
    General stressful life events (i.e., relocation)
    Peer rejection in school and other contexts
    Association with drug using peers
III. Psychobehavioral
  a. Child and adolescent psychobehavioral influences
    Age
    Early and persistent behavior problem (including drug use)
    Academic failure
    Low degree of commitment to school
  b. Postadolescent psychobehavioral factors
    Occupational satisfaction and success
    Child rearing demands
    Multiple role obligations
    Achievement of sexual intercourse role expectations
    Intimate relationship functioning
    Educational/financial attainment and security
  c. Psychobehavioral antecedents and consequences throughout life
    Alienation, rebelliousness, or antisocial personality
    Sensation seeking
    Psychopathology (depression, anxiety)
    Attitudes favorable to drug use
    Cognitive motivations or expectancies for drug use
    Inability to delay gratification
IV. Biogenetic
  Inherited susceptibility to drug use
  Psychophysiologic vulnerability to drug use effects

From Newcomb MD. Psychosocial predictors and consequences of drug use: a development perspective within a prospective study. *J Addict Dis* 1997;16:57–89, with permission.

    E. Substances of abuse: Table 20-2 includes the most common drugs of abuse used by teenagers and includes pharmacology, intoxicating effects, intoxication treatment, withdrawal effects, and withdrawal treatment. The current use patterns of these substances by adolescents are also included. This table was first presented in 1994 in *Pediatrics in Review*. It has been updated by the author to include more recent trends and newer drugs of abuse have been added.

    It cannot be overstated that alcohol is the drug that has the most serious adverse consequences for adolescents in terms of morbidity and mortality, especially with binge drinking.

    An estimated 4.6 million adolescents aged 14 to 17 years have alcohol problems. Motor vehicle accidents as a result of driving under the influence of alcohol are the leading cause of death among the 15- to 24-year-old age group. Alcohol-related motor vehicle accidents result in approximately 8,000 adolescent deaths and 45,000 injuries each year. Alcohol use is also involved in approximately 40% of the 10,000 annual nonautomotive accidental deaths of adolescents and in a significant number of the 5,500 suicides and 5,000 homicides each year.

Table 20-2. Common drugs abused by adolescents

Pharmacology	Intoxication effects	Intoxication treatment	Withdrawal effects	Withdrawal treatment	Comments
Alcohol (Ethanol)					
Mechanism of action: central nervous system depression; increases fluidity of neuronal cell membranes	Mild (blood level <0.1 g/dL): disinhibition, euphoria, mild impaired coordination, mild sedation.	Mild intoxication: Observation (can be at home for adolescents who have stable home environment)	Mild hangover: headache, mild tremulousness, nausea/vomiting	Mild withdrawal: bed rest and hydration	Most commonly abused drug
Dose: approximately 10 g per drink (1 drink = 12 oz. beer, 4 oz. wine, 1.5 oz. 80 proof liquor); each drink increases blood concentration about 0.025 (varies by weight)	Moderate (0.1–0.2 g/dL): increased sedation, impaired mentation and judgment, mood swings, slurred speech, ataxia	Overdose (stupor, coma): • Airway protection, respiratory support • Gastric lavage and charcoal (avoid ipecac due to aspiration risk) • Thiamine 100 mg IV • Follow fingerstick glucose; administer IV fluid with glucose as necessary	Severe: • Prevalence: extremely rare in adolescents; only seen with chronic use • Onset: several hours after last drink • Eyes: dilated pupils • Neurologic: tremulousness, hyperactive reflexes, seizures • Cardiovascular: tachycardia, hypertension • GI: nausea/vomiting • Psychiatric: anxiety, agitation, insomnia, confusion, hallucinations.	Severe withdrawal: Benzodiazepine taper: • Chlordiazepoxide 25–50 mg q 4–6 h or diazepam 10 mg q 4–6 h • Decrease by 20% q.d. × 3–5 d • Consider antipsychotics for psychosis (but will lower seizure threshold)	Use in high school seniors 77% ever, 70% past year, 40% past month, 3% daily
Onset: 10 min (rapidly absorbed)	Severe (>0.3 g/dL): confusion, stupor; (>0.4 g/dL): coma, respiratory depression.				Major health risk: motor vehicle accidents, violence, other injuries secondary to intoxication
Peak: 40–60 min	Other effects: • Skin flushed				Significantly increased risk of toxicity when used with other sedatives
Elimination rate: 7–10 g/h	• Eyes: pupils normal size and sluggish, nystagmus • Neurologic: decreased reflexes				Diagnostic test: blood alcohol level; breath test used in law enforcement
Legal intoxication level: 0.05–0.10 g/dL (varies by state)	• GI: nausea/vomiting • Metabolism: hypoglycemia				Tolerance develops with prolonged use
					Acute complications (occur with large, single doses): • Gastritis • Pancreatitis

(continued)

Table 20-2. (Continued)

Pharmacology	Intoxication effects	Intoxication treatment	Withdrawal effects	Withdrawal treatment	Comments
	Blackouts: anterograde amnesia while intoxicated (with heavy use) Idiosyncratic intoxication: sudden onset, marked behavior change for example, impulsive, aggressive, depressed, with consumption of a small amount; lasts a few hours; most common in young men		Delirium tremens (DTs): · Chronic users only extremely rare in adolescents · Mortality: 20% in adults · Onset: 3–5 d after last drink · Autonomic hyperactivity, disorientation/clouding of consciousness, perceptual disturbances/hallucinations · Fluids and electrolytes important to manage		Chronic complications (extremely rare in adolescents): · Liver disease · Cardiomyopathy, hypertension, hyperlipidemia · Wernicke encephalopathy: delirium, eye muscle ataxia · Korsakoff syndrome: dementia with marked anterograde amnesia.
Ecstasy					
Active ingredient: 3,4 methylenedioxymethamphetamine (MDMA). An hallucinogenic methamphetamine. Onset: Approximately 1 min. after ingestion on empty stomach, a "rush"	General: A happy sociability. Cardiovascular: Hypertension and tachycardia are common. More severe: dysrhythmias, hypotension and shock	Activated charcoal—give as slurry (240 mL H₂O/30 g charcoal) Agitation/hallucinations: Diazepam 10 mg. PO or 5 mg IV Hypertension: Usually responds to benzodiazepines. If	No evidence of physically prominent or distinctive withdrawal syndrome If withdrawal, may resemble a mild form of stimulant withdrawal with	Symptoms of withdrawal usually resolve without treatment	Use of Ecstasy in high school seniors: 8.3% ever, 4.5% past year, 1.3% in past month May be long-term memory defects that are reversible with abstinence Neurotoxicity of MDMA is controversial

(continued)

Table 20-2. (Continued)

			anxiety, fatigue, depression and difficulty concentrating	MDMA may be found in the blood within 2 h after use and in the urine by GC/MS for 24 h
occurs lasting 30 min up to 3 h after ingestion. Extremely pleasurable feelings with trance-like movements.	Respiratory: Increased respiratory rate.	not, nitroprusside is drug of choice		
Usual dose: Approximately 120–180 mg of MDMA in one dose.	Pupils: Mydriasis	Hyponatremia: Free water restriction. Judicious use of 0.09% saline or 3% NaCl if life threatening		
	Neurologic: Excitement, agitation, ±nystagmus			
Candy shopping: Intermittent use of MDMA with ecstasy	Fluid-electrolyte: Hyponatremia associated with water loading before use. Syndrome of Inappropriate Secretion of Antidiuretic Hormone (SIADH) has been reported with MDMA use	Hyperthermia: Aggressive cooling measures, may need IV dantrolene		
Stacking: 3 or more MDMA tablets taken at once		Rhabdomyolysis: 0.9% NaCl IV to maintain urine output. Monitor urine output, serum electrolytes, CK, and renal function		
Mixing: MDMA taken with marijuana, alcohol, or ketamine to modulate the high	Musculoskeletal: Jaw clenching, tremors, muscle spasms, rhabdomyolysis	Overdose: Morbidity and mortality associated with hyponatremia, dehydration, hyperthermia, hypertensive crisis, cardiac dysrhythmias		
	Temperature: Hyperthermia			

(continued)

Table 20-2. *(Continued)*

Pharmacology	Intoxication effects	Intoxication treatment	Withdrawal effects	Withdrawal treatment	Comments
Marijuana					
Active agent: THC (Δ-9-Tetrahydro-cannibinol) Derived from leaves and stems of Cannabis sativa. Hashish is a high-potency resin derived from flower of female plant	Low dose: euphoria, laughter, relaxation, time distortion, auditory and visual enhancement; impaired concentration, thinking, memory	For severe anxiety or agitation: • Benzodiazepine • Calm environment Otherwise, no specific treatment	Relatively mild and occur with chronic use only • Psychiatric: irritability, sleep disturbances • Neurologic: tremor, nystagmus • GI: anorexia, nausea/vomiting, diarrhea	No specific treatment	Most commonly used illicit drug
Potency: 4%–5% THC typical; 20%–30% for hashish	High dose: mood fluctuations, depersonalization, hallucinations				Use in high school seniors—47% ever, 35% in past year, 21% in past month, 6% daily
Routes of administration: smoking (greater bioavailability), ingestions	Toxic reaction: anxiety, panic, delusions, hallucinations, paranoia, psychosis				Potentiates other drugs of abuse
Onset: 5–10 min smoked	Other effects: • GI: increased appetite, dry mouth, decreased nausea • Eyes: injected conjunctiva, normal to dilated pupils • Cardiovascular: increased heart rate, orthostatic hypotension (sometimes elevated blood pressure) • Neurologic: normal to increased reflexes,				May be adulterated by other drugs (e.g., PCP) without user's knowledge
Peak: 20 min smoked; 3–4 h ingested					Virtually no lethal potential other than from accident or injury secondary to intoxication
Duration: 3 h smoked; 6–8 h ingested					Detectability in urine: 5 d for single dose, 10 d for casual use, 14–30 d for daily use
Common street names: pot, weed, grass, reefer, joints (cigarettes), blunts (cigars)					Complications of chronic use: • Pulmonary (cough, bronchitis, decreased

(continued)

152

Table 20-2. (Continued)

	Signs and symptoms	Treatment	Withdrawal syndrome	Treatment of withdrawal	Comments
	drowsiness; impaired coordination, tracing, reaction times • Respiratory: bronchodilation (acutely) May precipitate seizures, psychosis, or emotional disorder in persons who have those underlying disorders				diffusion capacity and FEV$_1$) • Gynecomastia • Decreased sperm count and motility • "Amotivational Syndrome" (controversial); apathy, loss of ambition, withdrawal from work and recreational activities

PCP (Phencyclidine)

	Signs and symptoms	Treatment	Withdrawal syndrome	Treatment of withdrawal	Comments
Mechanism of action: dissociative anesthetic with analgesic, stimulant, depressant, and hallucinogenic properties Routes of administration: PO, IV, 1 M, snorting, smoking Available forms: liquid, powder, tablet, rock crystal, mixed with leaves (e.g., marijuana)	Low dose (<5 mg): • Psychiatric: illusions, hallucinations, disordered thought, distortion of body image, amnesia, euphoria, dysphoria, anxiety, psychosis, catatonia, paranoia, agitation, combative/violent behavior • Eyes: vertical and horizontal nystagmus, miosis, blank stare • Neurologic: analgesia, ataxia, dysarthria, hyper-reflexia, reduced	Reduce stimulation Do not try to "talk down" as for other hallucinogens Benzodiazepine for sedation, if necessary Respiratory and cardiovascular support Treat seizures Cooling blanket for hyperthermia	No specific syndrome	No specific treatment	Use in high school seniors: 2.5% ever, 1.3% past year, 0.6% past month, 0.2% daily Fat-soluble and may remain in body for prolonged periods Flashbacks occur; more common than with LSD Recovery usually within 24 h, but coma can last 5 d with high dose

(continued)

Table 20-2. (Continued)

Pharmacology	Intoxication effects	Intoxication treatment	Withdrawal effects	Withdrawal treatment	Comments
Dose: 3 mg smoked, 5 mg PO and snorted, 10 mg IV, on average	proprioception and sensation, impaired coordination • Cardiovascular: tachycardia, elevated blood pressure • Skin: diaphoresis, flushing	Treat hypertension with nitroprusside, labetalol, or phentolamine Restraints for violent behavior Haloperidol if needed for psychosis/very severe agitation (avoid phenothiazines)			Use caution in treating patients; behavior can be violent and unpredictable Detectability in urine: 1–2 wk
Onset: IV, sec; smoked and snorted, 2–5 min; PO, 30 min					
Peak: smoked and snorted, 15–30 min; PO, 2–5 h	Moderate dose (5–10 mg): see above plus hyperthermia, hypersalivation, myoclonus	Gastric lavage and charcoal; continuous nasogastric suction hastens removal			
Duration: up to 12 h					
Common street names: angel dust, dust, hog	High dose (>10 mg): see above plus unresponsiveness, muscle rigidity, eyes-open coma, hypoventilation, extensor posturing, seizures, arrhythmias, death, rhabdomyolysis, and renal failure	Acidifying urine increases excretion, but not recommended Diuresis is controversial			
Ketamine (common street name: "Special K") is a short-acting anesthetic that has psychoactive properties similar to PCP					

(continued)

Table 20-2. (Continued)

LSD and other hallucinogens

Active agent: LSD (D-lysergic acid diethylamide tartrate)	General: perceptual alterations, illusions, synesthesias (one sense is perceived as another), loss of time sense, body image changes, euphoria, depersonalization, derealization, hallucinations	Peaceful, calm environment	No specific syndrome	Use in high school seniors: 9% ever, 3.4% past year, 2.1% past month, 0.3% daily
Derived from an alkaloid in rye fungus		Help restore contact with reality-talk about familiar things and reassure patient ("talking down")		Detectability: not detected in standard urine screens
Mechanism of action: inhibits release of serotonin	Psychiatric: labile affect, anxiety, restlessness, paranoia, sleep disturbances	Benzodiazepine, if needed for sedation		No deaths have been reported from *direct* effect of drug
Route of administration: PO		Avoid phenothiazines because of possible synergistic anticholinergic and CNS depressant effects		Flashback: occurrence of effects after drug has worn off; selective serotonin reuptake inhibitor may induce or worsen
Available as tablets, gelatin squares, or applied to pieces of paper ("blotters")	Eyes: dilated pupils, conjunctival injection, lacrimation	Treat hypertension, hyperthermia, seizures as necessary	No treatment necessary	
Dose: usually 25–100 ~ g; >250 ~ g especially dangerous	Neurologic: dizziness, paresthesias, hyperreflexia, tremor, ataxia			
Onset: 30 min				
Peak: 2–4 h	GI: dry mouth, anorexia, nausea			
Duration: 6–12 h				
Tolerance: rapid and short lived	Temperature: elevated; flushing, piloerection			

(continued)

Table 20-2. (Continued)

Pharmacology	Intoxication effects	Intoxication treatment	Withdrawal effects	Withdrawal treatment	Comments
Common street name: acid	Cardiovascular: elevated blood pressure, tachycardia				
	Overdose: coma				
	Bad Trip: extremely negative response causing terror, panic, "feeling of going crazy"				
Cocaine					
Derived from leaves of cocoa bush, *Erythroxylon coca*	General: hyper-alertness, increased energy, confidence, restlessness, stimulation and enhancement of mood, elation, euphoria	Benzodiazepine for agitation, anxiety, seizures; helpful for hypertension	**Crash:** the immediate appearance of unpleasant effects; also a withdrawal syndrome that appears later	Consider antidepressant for depression	Use in high school seniors: 8% ever, 5% past year, 2% past month, 0.2% daily. (under-estimates actual use by adolescents due to higher use in high school dropouts)
Mechanism of action: Increased release and decreased reuptake of biogenic amines, causing:		For severe hypertension: nitroprusside, labetalol, or phentolamine	Craving for cocaine		
1. CNS and peripheral nervous system stimulation 2. Local anesthesia 3. Vasoconstriction	Psychiatric: insomnia, labile affect, agitation, anxiety, paranoia, delirium, hallucinations, psychosis	Cardiac monitor; treat arrhythmias (avoid lidocaine—can cause seizures)	Depression, dysphoria, anhedonia, irritability		Detectability in urine: 2–3 d (also detectable in blood)
Routes of administration: snorting, smoking (free base form, "crack"), intravenous	Eyes: dilated pupils		Lethargy, fatigue, weakness		Addicts use in binges with escalating doses and frequency
			Tremor		

(continued)

Table 20-2. (Continued)

Onset: very rapid	Neurologic: dizziness, paresthesias, hyperreflexia, tremor, local anesthesia, seizures	Treat ischemic chest pain with nitrates, heparin, aspirin, calcium channel blockers (beta-blocker use is controversial due to possible unopposed alpha agonist activity) Haloperidol for psychosis	Nausea, hunger	Crack has higher addiction potential due to more intense, shorter high and lower cost per dose
Peak: smoked, <1 min; snorted, 2–30 min; IV, 0.5–2 min	Cardiovascular: hypertension, tachycardia, arrhythmia			With concomitant ethanol use: prolonged effects due to formation of ethyl cocaine
Duration: smoked, 4–15 min; snorted, 30–60 min; IV, 12–30 min	GI: nausea, dry mouth, anorexia	Cooling blanket for hyperthermia		**Speedball:** cocaine and heroin used together IV
Common street names: coke, nose candy, snow; crack, rock (freebase)	Temperature: elevated; sweating			Sometimes smuggled in ingested packets
	Overdose: coma, toxic psychosis, chest pain/angina, myocardial infarction, hyperthermia, rhabdomyolysis, stroke, seizures			Complications of administration: • Nasal septum ulceration, epistaxis with snorting • Same IV complications as with IV heroin • Lung damage from smoking

(continued)

Table 20-2. (Continued)

Pharmacology	Intoxication effects	Intoxication treatment	Withdrawal effects	Withdrawal treatment	Comments
Heroin and other opiates					
Derived from opium poppy, *Papaver somniferum*, or synthesized	General: euphoria followed by sedation ("nod"), somnolence, analgesia	Overdose: · Respiratory and circulatory support · Treat any arrhythmias · Gastric lavage and charcoal may be useful if drugs taken PO	Seen with >3 wk of regular use; not seen with intermittent use	Primarily supportive (almost never fatal)	Heroin is the most widely abused of the opiates
Examples: heroin, morphine, meperidine, oxycodone, opium, codeine, methadone, hydromorphone, propoxyphene, fentanyl	Neurologic: slowed comprehension, impaired mentation, decreased reflexes Eyes: constricted/ pinpoint pupils	· Naloxone 2.0 mg (0.1 mg/kg in children) IV q 3 min until response or maximum of 10 mg; may need to re-administer in 2–3 h	Onset (varies by drug): 6–8 h after last dose of heroin; 24–48 h after methadone Duration: 7–10 d	Severe withdrawal: detoxification with methadone (20–40 mg qd tapered by 5 mg/d) and/or clonidine (0.2 mg tid-qid for 7–10 d, then tapered over 2–3 d)	Use of heroin in high school seniors: 1.8% ever, 1.1% past year, 0.4% past month, 0.1% daily; for other opiates: 13.2% ever, 9.3% past year, 4.1% past month, 0.2 % daily under-
Mechanism of action: binds to opioid receptors in central nervous system (CNS), causing CNS depression	Cardiovascular: decreased blood pressure, arrhythmias Temperature: decreased	or use IV drip (3$1$, of total initial dose/hour) because half-life is shorter than that of many opiates · Monitor for 24 h (72 h	General: drug craving, rhinorrhea, lacrimation, muscle aches, yawning Temperature: elevated; chills, hot and cold flashes, sweating, piloerection		(estimates actual use by adolescents due to higher use in high school dropouts) Potentially fatal interaction between meperidine and monamine oxidase inhibitors
Heroin: · Dose: 1–25 mg; concentration usually about 5%, but varies consider- ably (1%–20%) · Routes of administration: snorting (most common in adolescents), intra- venous ("shooting up," "mainlining"),	Respiratory: respiratory depression, cough suppression. GI: nausea/vomiting, constipation Urologic: urinary retention	for methadone and long-acting agents)	Respiratory: increased respiration rate GI: nausea/vomiting, abdominal cramps, diarrhea		Detectability in urine: 24 h for methadone, 3 d for heroin, 3 d for methadone; synthetic opiates such as fentanyl will not be detected

(continued)

Table 20-2. (Continued)

subcutaneous ("skin popping"), ingestion, smoking · Onset: IV, immediate; snorted, 30 min; SQ, 15 min · Duration: 3–6 h (IV) · Common street names: junk, smack, dope Methadone: · Onset: 30 min PO · Duration: more than 24 h	Overdose: · Hypotension, bradycardia, circulatory collapse · Severe respiratory depression, pulmonary edema · Stupor, coma, death. Seizures (especially with meperidine and propoxyphene)		Psychiatric: restlessness, anxiety, sleep disturbance Cardiovascular: hypertension, tachycardia Eyes: dilated pupils Neurologic: tremor	Complications of IV administration: "track marks," endocarditis, cellulitis, phlebitis; pulmonary emboli (septic and talc); hepatitis and human immunodeficiency virus (HIV) infection (with shared needles)
Inhalants Active agents: volatile solvents-toluene, benzene, other hydrocarbons, fluorocarbons Examples: model airplane glue, rubber cement, correction fluid, paint thinner, spray paint, shoe polish, gasoline, propane, butane, aerosol propellants Mechanism of action: CNS stimulation and excitement, progressing to depression	General: euphoria, giddiness, drowsiness, impaired judgment Psychiatric: hallucinations, psychosis Eyes: nystagmus, lacrimation Neurologic: dizziness, headache, ataxia, slurred speech, diplopia, diminished reflexes Respiratory: rhinorrhea, mucosal irritation	Respiratory and circulatory support Treat arrhythmias Avoid use of epinephrine or other proarrhythmic drugs, if possible Check CBC, PT/PTT, liver tests, and renal function tests	No withdrawal syndrome No withdrawal treatment	Use highest among young male adolescents, often as a group activity Use in eighth graders: 16% ever, 8.8% past year, 4% past month, 0.4% daily Use in high school seniors: 17% ever, 8% past year, 3% past month, 0, 1% daily May have rash on face, odor on breath, or irritation of eyes

(continued)

Table 20-2. (Continued)

Pharmacology	Intoxication effects	Intoxication treatment	Withdrawal effects	Withdrawal treatment	Comments
Route of administration: inhaled from a bag or cloth ("huffing") saturated with substance Onset: immediate Duration: 5–15 min	GI: anorexia, nausea, vomiting, salivation Overdose: respiratory depression, arrhythmia, cardiac arrest, seizure, delirium, stupor, coma Sudden sniffing death syndrome: sudden death, probably due to cardiac arrhythmias				Can cause permanent hepatic, renal, cardiac, CNS, and peripheral nerve damage Not detectable in blood

Other important hallucinogens:

- Peyote: cactus in southwest US and Mexico; tops contain hallucinogenic alkaloids, including mescaline.
- Mescaline (3,4,5-trimethoxyphenethylamine): effects similar to LSD but much less potent; fewer "bad trips"; dose: usually 100–500 ~ g; onset: 30–120 min; duration: 6–12 h; frequently accompanied by nausea/vomiting; drugs sold as mescaline are often LSD and/or PCP.
- Psychedelic mushrooms (psilocybin, psilocin): effects similar to LSD but much less potent; dose: 4–10 mg psilocybin; route: PO; onset: 15 min; peak: 90 min; duration: 5–6 h; common street names: mushrooms, shrooms.
- Morning glory seeds (*Rivea corymbosa* and *Ipomoea* sp): effects similar to LSD but less potent; often causes nausea, dizziness, and diarrhea.
- DMT (dimethyltryptamine): found in seeds from several plants in West Indies and South America; tobacco, marijuana, or parsley is soaked in the liquid and smoked; duration: 1–3 h.
- Nutmeg: contains lysergide and other hallucinatory alkaloids.
- Jimsonweed (*Daura stramonium*): grows wild in the southwest US; contains atropine and scopolamine; hallucinogenic and anticholinergic properties; may have anticholinergic syndrome (delirium, flushing, dry mucous membranes, dilated pupils); gastric lavage recommended; consider physostigmine in severe cases.

Other important inhalants:

- Nitrites [amyl nitrite ("poppers"), butyl nitrite, isobutyl nitrite]: cause vasodilatation and smooth muscle relaxation; common effects: lightheadedness ("rush"), giddiness, headache, dizziness, orthostatic hypotension, tachycardia, flushing; often abused for purpose of enhancing sexual pleasure; use can cause methemoglobinemia.
- Nitrous oxide ("laughing gas"): available as whipped cream propellant; usually inhaled from balloon; deaths have occurred with 100% N$_2$O.

From Johnston LD, O'Malley PM, Bachman JG, Schulenberg JE. *National results on adolescent drug use: Overview of key findings*, 2004. Bethesda, MD: National Institute on Drug Abuse, 2005; Ann Arbor, MI: News and Information Services of the University of Michigan, with permission.

Table 20-3. Criteria for substance dependence

A maladaptive pattern of substance use, leading to clinically significant impairment or distress, as manifested by three (or more) of the following, occurring at any time in the same 12-month period:

1. Tolerance, as defined by either of the following:
   a. a need for markedly increased amounts of the substance to achieve intoxication or desire effect.
   b. markedly diminished effect with continued use of the same amount of the substance.
2. Withdrawal, as manifested by either of the following:
   a. the characteristic withdrawal syndrome for the substance (refer to Criteria A and B of the criteria sets for withdrawal from the specific substances).
   b. the same (or a closely related) substance is taken to relieve or avoid withdrawal symptoms.
3. The substance is often taken in larger amounts or over a longer period than was intended.
4. There is a persistent desire or unsuccessful efforts to cut down or control substance use.
5. A great deal of time is spent in activities necessary to obtain the substance (e.g., visiting multiple doctors or driving long distances), use the substance (e.g., chain-smoking), or recover from its effects.
6. Important social, occupational, or recreational activities are given up or reduced because of substance use.
7. The substance use is continued despite knowledge of having a persistent or recurrent physical or psychological problem that is likely to have been caused or exacerbated by the substance (e.g., current cocaine use despite recognition of cocaine-induced depression, or continued drinking despite recognition that an ulcer was made worse by alcohol consumption). Specify if:

   With physiologic dependence: evidence of tolerance or withdrawal (i.e., either item 1 or 2 is present).

   Without physiologic dependence: no evidence of tolerance or withdrawal (i.e., neither item 1 nor 2 is present).

From *Diagnostic and statistical manual of mental disorders*, 4th ed. Washington, DC: American Psychiatric Association, 2000, with permission.

   The alcohol industry, with impunity and without restraint, advertises in magazines and TV programs that have a primarily young audience. The effect of this advertising is not inconsequential. Health care professionals should take the time to explain to parents and to their young patients the critical dangers of underage alcohol use.

II.   **Diagnosis:** If an adolescent is suspected of having a substance abuse disorder, he or she must meet the criteria for either substance dependence or substance abuse (see Tables 20-3 and 20-4). The hallmark for diagnosing either dependence or abuse is

Table 20-4. Criteria for substance abuse

A. A maladaptive pattern of substance use leading to clinically significant impairment or distress, as manifested by one (or more) of the following, occurring within a 12-month period:
   1. recurrent substance use resulting in a failure to fulfill major role obligations at work, school, or home (e.g., repeated absences or poor work performance related to substance use; substance-related absences, suspensions, or expulsions from school; neglect of children or household)
   2. recurrent substance use in situations in which it is physically hazardous (e.g., driving an automobile or operating a machine when impaired by substance use)
   3. recurrent substance-related legal problems (e.g., arrests for substance-related disorderly conduct) continued substance use despite having persistent or recurrent social or interpersonal problems caused or exacerbated by the effects of the substance (e.g., arguments with spouse about consequences of intoxication, physical fights)
   4. continued substance use despite having persistent or recurrent social or interpersonal problems caused or exacerbated by the effects of the substance (e.g., arguments with spouse about consequences of intoxication, physical fights)
B. The symptoms have never met the criteria for Substance Dependence for this class of substance.

From *Diagnostic and statistical manual of mental disorders*, 4th ed. Washington, DC: American Psychiatric Association, 2000, with permission.

continued use of the drug (including alcohol) despite harmful consequences. For example, if an adolescent continues to use marijuana despite failing grades, lack of motivation, disruption of family life, and/or previous legal problems because of marijuana use, this adolescent must be evaluated for a substance abuse disorder.

If the primary care clinician is not familiar with making the diagnosis of a substance abuse disorder and assessing its severity, referral of the adolescent and his or her family to someone who specializes in the area of addiction medicine is appropriate.

III. **Management:** If an adolescent is thought to have a substance abuse disorder, he or she should be properly assessed for the severity of the disorder by someone specializing in addiction medicine. The severity of the disorder will dictate the level of treatment the adolescent needs. The levels of treatment include outpatient treatment, intensive outpatient treatment, residential treatment, or inpatient treatment. If the adolescent needs only counseling, this should be done with someone knowledgeable in adolescent substance abuse.

Most primary care clinicians will not be involved in the treatment of the substance-abusing adolescent except to provide support and encouragement to the patient and family.

Urine drug screens are often indicated when an adolescent is in outpatient counseling, and these should be performed weekly and be done randomly with monitoring of the collection of the specimen.

IV. **Clinical pearls and pitfalls:**
- Most adolescents, by the age of 18 years, will have been offered tobacco, alcohol, and/or marijuana.
- Preventative counseling for older children and adolescents should include the risk of underage drinking and drug use.
- Marijuana is not a "safe" drug. The use of marijuana is illegal, and marijuana is an addictive drug.
- If an adolescent is thought to have a substance abuse disorder, he or she should have a substance abuse assessment by someone specializing in addiction medicine.
- If an adolescent has a substance abuse disorder, the adolescent should receive treatment for this disorder at the appropriate level of care.
- There is a difference between counseling and treatment for a substance-abusing adolescent. "Counseling" for this disorder is often unrewarding.
- Marijuana is the common "illicit" drug of abuse by teenagers. Twenty-five percent of high school seniors admit to having used marijuana in the past month.
- Approximately 30% of high school seniors admit to binge drinking in the previous 2 weeks.
- Adolescents who regularly abuse drugs and/or alcohol often need a major intervention in their lives to stop this behavior.
- Alcohol, marijuana, and tobacco are "universally" available to adolescents.

BIBLIOGRAPHY

Cole JC, Sumnall HR. Altered states: The clinical effects of ecstasy. *Pharmacol Ther* 2003;98:35–58.

Graham AW, Schultz TK, eds. *Principles of addiction medicine*, 3rd ed. Chery Chase, MD: American Society of Addiction Medicine, 2003.

Green AR, Mechan AO, et al. The pharmacology and clinical pharmacology of 3,4-Methylenedioxymethamphetamine. *Pharmacol Rev* 2003;55:463–508.

Grube JW, Waiters E. Alcohol in the media: content and effects on drinking beliefs and behaviors among youth. *Adolesc Med Clin* 2005;16.

Hallucinogenic amphetamines. Poisondex Managements. Micromedex. Healthcare series. Vol. 122.

Johnston LD, O'Malley PM, Bachman JG, et al. *National results on adolescent drug use: Overview of key findings*, 2004. Bethesda, MD: National Institute on Drug Abuse, 2005.

Kulig JW, the Committee on Substance Abuse. Tobacco, alcohol and other drugs: the role of the pediatrician in prevention, identification, and management of substance abuse. *Pediatr* 2005;115: 816–821.

Mandl KD, Lovejoy FH. Peripheral brain: common poisonings. *Pediatr Rev* 1994;15:151–152.

Neinstein LS. *Adolescent health care: A practical guide*. Baltimore, MD: Williams and Wilkins, 1996:985–1017, 1032–1087.

Rogers PD, Heyman RB. Addiction medicine. Adolescent substance abuse. *Pediatric Clinics of North America* 2002;49(2):245–246.

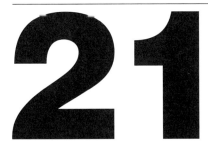

Adolescent Tobacco Use

I. **Description of the condition:** Tobacco use is the most preventable cause of disease and death in the United States. Despite major efforts to prevent and reduce smoking, initiation of tobacco use among children and adolescents remains high. Tobacco is the only legal substance that, when used as intended, causes death and disease.

   A. **Epidemiology:** Each day in the United States approximately 4,400 youths aged 12 to 17 years try their first cigarette. An estimated one-third of these young smokers are expected to die from a smoking-related disease.

   The National Youth Tobacco Survey (NYTS) conducted in 2002 provides estimates of usage among US middle and high school students for various tobacco products [i.e., cigarettes, cigars, smokeless tobacco, pipes, bidis (leaf wrapped, flavored cigarettes from India), and kreteks (clove cigarettes)] (Table 21-1).

   B. **Smoking initiation in adolescents:** Few people initiate smoking or become regular smokers after adolescence. Moreover, the younger a person is when initiating smoking the more likely that person is to be a current smoker in adulthood.

   Smoking onset has been considered a time-dependent developmental process that includes:
   - Preparation—never smoked
   - Initiation—trying the first cigarette
   - Experimentation—repeatedly trying cigarettes
   - Nicotine dependence

   Progress through these stages is presumed to take at least 2 years, and quitting becomes more difficult as a smoker progresses through the continuum. Because a young person may become a regular smoker in only 2 to 3 years, the adolescent period of development is a critical time for prevention efforts. Consequently, the stage model of smoking onset indicates that interventions targeting children at the preparation stage (i.e., those who have never smoked) are more effective than interventions targeting more advanced stages.

   C. **Factors influencing tobacco initiation and use:**
      1. **Gender:** Females are more likely than males to report social norms as a reason to initiate smoking, and females who start smoking are more likely to have parents or friends who smoke than females who do not smoke.

Table 21-1. Findings from youth tobacco surveillance. United States, 2002

- 28.4% of high school students reported current use of any tobacco product, down from 34.5% in year 2000.
- Cigarettes (23%) were the most commonly used tobacco product, with no difference by sex; however, white students were more likely to use cigarettes than were black, Hispanic, or Asian students.
- Cigars (11.6%) were the second most common tobacco product, followed by smokeless tobacco (6%), pipes (3%), kreteks (2.7%), and bidis (2.6%).
- High school and middle school males were more likely than females to use all tobacco products except for cigarettes.
- White high school and middle school students were more likely to use smokeless tobacco than were students in other racial/ethnic groups.
- During 2000–2002, cigarette use decreased from 28% to 23% among high school students.
- [a]Tobacco use among middle school students dropped from 15% in 2000 to 13.3% in 2002.

[a]Editorial Note: The lack of any statistically significant decline in tobacco usage among middle school students is cause for concern.
Adapted from youth tobacco surveillance—United States, 2002. *MMWR Morbidity Mortality Weekly Report* 2003;52(45):1096–1098.

Smoking has been associated with low self-esteem in females, but not in males. Females, when compared with males, were more likely to smoke to control weight. Females who diet more frequently were more likely to become smokers, suggesting that dieting among females exacerbates the risk of beginning smoking.

Females are more likely to smoke out of rebelliousness and risk-taking than are males.

2. **Ethnicity:** White high school students (24.9%) have higher rates of current cigarette smoking than black (15.1%), Hispanic (18.4%), and Asian (12.8%) students.

3. **Parental factors:** Among adolescents in the United States, about 40% are currently exposed to at least one parent who smokes, and parental smoking is associated with increased risk of smoking initiation. In particular, low parental monitoring of smoking, easy access to cigarettes, and absence of restrictions on smoking in the home are indicators for smoking initiation.

Intervening in parental behavior may be an important area for future prevention efforts.

D. **Preventive counseling:** The American Academy of Pediatrics recommends that tobacco use prevention counseling be part of routine preventive counseling for youth. To be most effective, physicians must address the use of tobacco products repeatedly and should target their patients' perception of cigarettes, the parents' possible motives to use tobacco products including family and peer behavior and media messages.

Cognitive developmental considerations among adolescents include challenging parents on their behavior and a belief in their own invulnerability, both of which make the risk of smoking high. The themes used in brand advertising not only sell cigarettes, they also sell the social acceptability of smoking.

The adolescent's learning and practicing resistance skills can help provide "social inoculation" and, thus, help youth to avoid these unhealthy behaviors.

The National Cancer Institute (NCI) has developed a variety of materials for primary care clinicians to use to help their patients not smoke.

NCI resource materials are available free by calling 1-800-4 Cancer.

II. **Making the diagnosis:**

A. **Approach to the adolescent who uses tobacco:** See Table 21-2 for summaries of recommendations of the panel from the U.S. Public Health Service. See Table 21-3 for counseling techniques for patients.

Table 21-4 lists some strategies to use for the patient who is willing to quit.

Table 21-2. Recommendations for clinicians for treating adolescents who use tobacco

Recommendation	Strength of evidence
Clinicians should screen pediatric and adolescent patients and their parents for tobacco use and provide a strong message regarding the importance of totally abstaining from tobacco use.	C
Counseling and behavioral interventions shown to be effective with adults should be considered for use with children and adolescents. The content of these interventions should be modified to be developmentally appropriate.	C
When treating adolescents, clinicians may consider prescriptions for bupropion SR or NRT when there is evidence of nicotine dependence and desire to quit tobacco use.	C
Clinicians in a pediatric office setting should offer smoking cessation advice and interventions to parents to limit children's exposure to second-hand smoke.	B

NRT, nicotine replacement therapy.

Strength of evidence criteria:

B = Some evidence from randomized clinical trials supports this recommendation, but the scientific support was not optimal (e.g., few trials exist, existing trials were somewhat inconsistent, or trials not directly relevant to the recommendation).

C = Reserved for important clinical situations where the panel achieved consensus on the recommendation in the absence of relevant controlled clinical trials.

Table 21-3. The "5 As" for brief intervention

A	Intervention
Ask about tobacco use.	Identify and document tobacco use status for every patient at every visit (see Brief Strategy A1).
Advise to quit.	In a clear, strong, and personalized manner, urge every tobacco user to quit (see Brief Strategy A2).
Assess willingness to make a quit attempt.	Is the tobacco user willing to make a quit attempt at this time? (see Brief Strategy A3).
Assist in quit attempt.	For the patient willing to make a quit attempt, use counseling and pharmacotherapy to help him or her quit (see Brief Strategy A4).
Arrange follow-up.	Schedule follow-up contact, preferably within the first week after the quit date (see Brief Strategy A5).

Table 21-4. Brief strategies for helping patients who are willing to quit

Action	Strategies for implementation
Brief Strategy A1. Ask: Systematically identify all tobacco users at every visit.	
Implement an office-wide system that ensures that, for *every* patient at *every* clinic visit, tobacco-use status is queried and documented.	Expand the vital signs to include tobacco use, or use an alternative universal identification system.[a] For example: Vital signs: Blood Pressure _____ Pulse: _____ Weight: _____ Temperature: _____ Respiratory rate: _____ Tobacco use: Current Former Never (circle one)
Brief Strategy A2. Advise: Strongly urge all tobacco users to quit.	
In a *clear, strong,* and *personalized* manner, urge every tobacco user to quit.	Advice should be: *Clear:* "I think it is important for you to quit smoking now, and I can help you." "Cutting down while you are ill is not enough." *Strong:* "As your clinician, I need you to know that quitting smoking is the most important thing you can do to protect your health now and in the future. The clinic staff and I will help you." *Personalized:* Tie tobacco use to current health or illness, its social and economic costs, patient's motivation level and readiness to quit, and/or the impact of tobacco use on children and others in the household.
Brief Strategy A3. Assess: Determine willingness to make a quit attempt.	
Ask every tobacco user if he or she is willing to make a quit attempt at this time (e.g., within the next 30 days).	Assess the patient's willingness to quit: If the patient is willing to make a quit attempt at this time, provide assistance (see Brief Strategy A4). If the patient will participate in an intensive treatment, deliver such a treatment or refer to an intensive intervention. If the patient clearly states he or she is unwilling to make a quit attempt at this time, provide a motivational intervention. If the patient is a member of a special population (e.g., adolescent, pregnant smoker, racial/ethnic minority), consider providing additional information.

(continued)

Table 21-4. *(Continued)*

Action	Strategies for implementation
Brief Strategy A4. Assist: Aid the patient in quitting.	
Help the patient quit with a plan.	In preparation for quitting, instruct the patient to: Set a quit date. Ideally the quit date would be within 2 weeks. Tell family, friends, and coworkers about quitting, and request understanding and support. Anticipate challenges to planned quit attempt, particularly during the critical first few weeks. These include nicotine withdrawal symptoms. Remove tobacco products from your environment. Prior to quitting, avoid smoking in places where you spend a lot of time (e.g., work, home, car).
Provide practical counseling (problem solving or skills training).	*Abstinence:* Total abstinence is necessary. "Not even a single puff after the quit date." Past quit experience: Identify what helped and what hurt in previous quit attempts. Anticipate triggers or challenges in upcoming attempt: Discuss challenges/triggers and how patient will successfully overcome them. *Alcohol:* Because alcohol can cause relapse, the patient should consider limiting or abstaining from alcohol while quitting.[b] Other smokers in the house: Quitting is more difficult when there is another smoker in the household. Patients should encourage housemates to quit with them or not smoke in their presence.
Provide intratreatment social support.	Provide a supportive clinical environment while encouraging the patient in his or her quit attempt. "My office staff and I are available to assist you."
Help patient obtain extratreatment social support.	Help patient develop social support for his or her quit attempt in his or her environments outside of treatment. "Ask your spouse [or partner], friends, and coworkers to support you in your quit attempt.
Recommend the use of approved pharmacotherapy, except in special circumstances.	Recommend the use of pharmacotherapies found to be effective in these guidelines (Table 21-5). Explain how these medications increase smoking cessation success and reduce withdrawal symptoms. The first-line pharmacotherapy medications include bupropion SR, nicotine gum, nicotine inhaler, nicotine nasal spray, and nicotine patch.
Provide supplementary materials.	*Sources:* Federal agencies, nonprofit agencies, or local/state health departments. *Type:* Culturally, racially, educationally, and age appropriate for the patient. *Location:* Readily available at every clinician's workstation.

(continued)

Table 21-4. (Continued)

Brief Strategy A5. Arrange: Schedule follow-up contact.

Schedule follow-up contact, either in person or over the telephone.

Timing: Follow-up contact should occur soon after the quit date, preferably during the first week. A second follow-up contact is recommended within the first month. Schedule further follow-up contacts as indicated.

Actions during follow-up contact: Congratulate success. If tobacco use has occurred, review circumstances and elicit recommitment to total abstinence. Remind patient that a lapse can be used as a learning experience. Identify problems already encountered, and anticipate challenges in the immediate future. Assess pharmacotherapy use and problems. Consider use or referral to more intensive treatment.

[a]Alternatives to expanding the vital signs are to place tobacco-use status stickers on all patient charts or to indicate tobacco use status using electronic medical records or computer reminder systems.
[b]Alcohol use is illegal for adolescents younger than 21 years.
Adapted from Fiore MC, Bailey WC, Cohen SJ, et al. *Treating tobacco use and dependence. Clinical practice guideline.* Rockville, MD: U.S. Department of Health and Human Services, Public Health Service;2000:23–35.

III. Treatment:

A. Pharmacotherapy: The role of pharmacotherapy has not been extensively studied with adolescent smokers, The Clinical Practice Guideline suggests that nicotine replacement therapy (NRT) and bupropion therapy should be considered when there is evidence of nicotine dependence and there is a genuine desire to quit. The nicotine patch may be effective for adolescents who desire to quit.

The nicotine patch is available under a number of brand names. Although specific instructions vary, one generally prescribes the highest strength patch for 4 to 8 weeks and then the lower strength patch for an additional 4 to 8 weeks.

Those who smoke fewer than 10 cigarettes per day may start directly on the lower dosage patch and should be treated for up to 8 weeks. Table 21-5 lists the drugs used for smoking cessation.

B. Counseling for the adolescent who is unwilling to quit: Tobacco dependency is a chronic disease. Thus, smoking cessation is a process, and clinicians are encouraged to use the "five R's" strategy in motivating to quit (Table 21-6).

C. Preventing relapse: Clinicians should provide brief, effective relapse prevention treatment. Most relapses occur within the first 3 months after quitting. Relapse prevention interventions should be part of every encounter with a patient who has recently quit.

Relapse prevention interventions can be divided into two categories: minimal practice and prescriptive interventions.

Prescriptive relapse prevention techniques deal directly with the problems in maintaining abstinence from tobacco.

Table 21-7 shows the two categories of relapse prevention.

IV. Clinical pearls and pitfalls:

- Each day more than 4,000 teenagers try their first cigarette.
- One-third of adolescents who smoke regularly will die of a tobacco-related illness.
- Few people initiate smoking after adolescence.
- Clinicians must address the use of tobacco products frequently and encourage their young patients not to start any use of tobacco products.
- Medications used to treat adolescent smokers are available. The use of bupropion and the nicotine patch may be the best pharmacotherapy for teenagers who smoke more than 10 cigarettes per day and who are motivated to quit.
- There are guidelines available for clinicians to briefly intervene with their patients who smoke.
- Most adolescents who relapse after quitting use of tobacco products relapse during the first 3 months after quitting.
- Relapse prevention strategies are very important, especially during the first 3 months after quitting.

Table 21-5. Drugs used for smoking cessation

Nicotine-replacement therapy

Product	Daily dose	Length of treatment	Common side effects	Advantages	Disadvantages
Transdermal patch[a]	7-, 14-, or 21-mg patch worn for 24 h[b]		Skin irritation, insomnia	Provides steady level of nicotine; easy to use; unobtrusive; available without prescription	User cannot adjust dose if craving occurs; nicotine released more slowly than in other products
24 h (e.g., Nicoderm CQ)		8 wk			
16 hr (e.g., Nicotrol)	15-mg patch worn for 16 h	8 wk			
Nicotine polacrilex gum (Nicorette)[a]	1 piece/h (<24 pieces/d)	8–12 wk	Mouth irritation, sore jaw, dyspepsia, hiccups	User controls dose; oral substitute for cigarettes; available without prescription	Proper chewing technique needed to avoid side effects and achieve efficacy[c]
2 mg <25 cigarettes/d					
4 mg (≥25 cigarettes/d)					
Vapor inhaler (Nicotrol Inhaler)[a]	6–16 cartridges/d (delivered dose, 4 mg/cartridge)	3–6 mo	Mouth and throat irritation, cough	User controls dose; hand-to-mouth substitute for cigarettes	Frequent puffing needed; device visible when used
Nasal spray (Nicotrol NS)[a]	1–2 doses/h (1 mg total; 0.5 mg in each nostril)	3–6 mo	Nasal irritation; sneezing, cough, teary eyes	User controls dose; offers most rapid delivery of nicotine and the highest nicotine levels of all nicotine-replacement products	Most irritating nicotine-replacement product to use[d]; device visible when used

(continued)

Table 21-5. (Continued)

Non-nicotine therapy

Drug	Dose	Duration	Side effects	Advantages	Comments
Sustained-release bupropion (Zyban or Wellbutrin SR)[a]	150 mg/d for 3 d, then 150 mg twice a d[e]	7–12 wk (up to 6 mo to maintain abstinence)	Insomnia, dry mouth, agitation	Easy to use (pill), no exposure to nicotine	Increases risk of seizure (≤0.1%)
Nortriptyline[f]	75–100 mg/d[g]	12 wk	Dry mouth, sedation, dizziness	Easy to use (pill), no exposure to nicotine	Side effects common; should be used cautiously in patients with coronary heart disease
Clonidine[f]	0.1–0.3 mg twice a d	3–10 wk	Dry mouth, sedation, dizziness	No exposure to nicotine	Side effects limit use

[a]This product has been approved by the Food and Drug Administration as a smoking-cessation aid. The Public Health Service clinical guidelines also recommend it as a first-line drug for smoking cessation.

[b]The starting dose is 21 mg/d unless the smoker weighs less than 45.5 kg (100 lb) or smokes fewer than 10 cigarettes per day, in which case the starting dose is 14 mg/d. The starting dose should be maintained for 4 weeks, after which the dose should be decreased every week until it is stopped.

[c]The user should chew the gum slowly until he or she experiences a distinct taste, indicating that nicotine is being released. The user should then place the gum between cheek and gum until the taste disappears to allow the nicotine to be absorbed through oral mucosa. The sequence should be repeated for 30 minutes before the gum is discarded. Acidic beverages (such as coffee and soft drinks) reduce the absorption of nicotine and should be avoided for 30 minutes before and during chewing.

[a]Tolerance develops to local side effects during the first week of use.

[c]Treatment should be started 1 week before the quitting date.

[f]This agent has not been approved by the Food and Drug Administration as a smoking-cessation aid. The Public Health Service clinical guidelines recommend it as a second-line drug for smoking cessation.

[g]Treatment should be started 10–28 days before the quitting date at a dose of 25 mg/d, and dose should be increased as tolerated.

From Rigotti NA. Treatment of tobacco use and dependence. *N Engl J Med* 2002;346:506–512, with permission.

Table 21-6. The "Five Rs" strategy

- Relevance

  Encourage the patient to quit for reasons that are personally relevant, such as chronic cough or problems with sports participation; young teens with children of their own or family members with health problems should be educated about the effects of environmental tobacco smoke.
- Risks

  Identify relevant ones, such as decreased stamina, shortness of breath, yellow teeth, and even sexual impotence—issues that are dear to the heart of all adolescents.
- Rewards

  Teens who quit tobacco use will save money and have improved health; they and their clothes will smell and look better; food will smell and taste better; and they will prove their ability to control a behavior and may, in fact, eliminate a major source of parental nagging.
- Roadblocks

  Teens recognize and identify the same problems as adults, including the cravings for tobacco, their loss of a powerful mood-altering agent, and the likelihood of weight gain. The clinician must be honest about these issues and offer ongoing support in addressing them.
- Repetition

  Practicing pediatricians are accustomed to achieving success with their clinical interventions, and the resistance with which the issue of smoking cessation frequently is received may be frustrating. The clinician must repeat the message at every opportunity, preferably identifying how health and wellness issues are affected by tobacco use.

From Fiore MC, Bailey WC, Cohen SJ, et al. *Treating tobacco use and dependence. Clinical practice guideline.* Rockville, MD: U.S. Department of Health and Human Services, Public Health Service; 2000:23–35, with permission.

Table 21-7. Smoking cessation relapse prevention

Brief Strategy C1. Components of minimal practice relapse prevention

These interventions should be part of every encounter with a patient who has quit recently.

Every ex-tobacco user undergoing relapse prevention should receive congratulations on any success and strong encouragement to remain abstinent.

When encountering a recent quitter, use open-ended questions designed to initiate patient problem solving (e.g., How has stopping tobacco use helped you?). The clinician should encourage the patient's active discussion of the following topics:

- The benefits, including potential health benefits, the patient may derive from cessation.
- Any success the patient has had in quitting (e.g., duration of abstinence, reduction in withdrawal).
- The problems encountered or anticipated threats to maintaining abstinence (e.g., depression, weight gain, alcohol, other tobacco users in the household).

Brief Strategy C2. Components of prescriptive relapse prevention

Problems	Responses
Lack of support for cessation	Schedule follow-up visits or telephone calls with the patient.
	Help the patient identify sources of support within his or her environment.
	Refer the patient to an appropriate organization that offers cessation counseling or support.
Negative mood or depression	If significant, provide counseling, prescribe appropriate medications, or refer the patient to a specialist.
Strong or prolonged withdrawal symptoms	If the patient reports prolonged craving or other withdrawal symptoms, consider extending the use of an approved pharmacotherapy or adding or combining pharmacologic medications to reduce strong withdrawal symptoms.

(continued)

Table 21-7. *(Continued)*

Weight gain	Recommend starting or increasing physical activity; discourage strict dieting.
	Reassure the patient that some weight gain after quitting is common and appears to be self-limiting.
	Emphasize the importance of a healthy diet.
	Maintain the patient on pharmacotherapy known to delay weight gain [e.g., bupropion SR, nicotine replacement therapies (NRTs), particularly nicotine gum].
	Refer the patient to a specialist or program.
Flagging motivation or feeling deprived	Reassure the patient that these feelings are common.
	Recommend rewarding activities.
	Probe to ensure that the patient is not engaged in periodic tobacco use.
	Emphasize that beginning to smoke (even a puff) will increase urges and make quitting more difficult.

From Fiore MC, Bailey WC, Cohen SJ, et al. *Treating tobacco use and dependence. Clinical practice guideline.* Rockville, MD: U.S. Department of Health and Human Services, Public Health Service; 2000:23–35, with permission.

BIBLIOGRAPHY

Camenga DR, Klein JD. Adolescent smoking cessation. *Curr Opin Pediatr* 2004;16:368–372.

Centers for Disease Control and Prevention. Prevalence of cigarette use among 13 racial/ethnic populations—United States, 1999–2003, *MMWR Morbidity and Mortality Weekly Report* 2004; 53:49–52.

Cigarette Use Among High School Students—United States, 1991–2003. *MMWR Morbidity and Mortality Weekly Report* 2004;53.

Fiore MC, Bailey WC, Cohen SJ, et al. Treating tobacco use and dependence. *Clinical Practice Guideline.* Rockville, MD: US Department of Health and Human Services. Public Health Service, June 2000.

Hanson K, Allen S, Jensen S, et al. Treatment of adolescent smokers with the nicotine patch. *Nicotine and Tobacco Research* 2003;5:515–526.

Klein JD, Camenga DR. Tobacco prevention and cessation in pediatric patients. *Pediatr Rev* 2004; 25:17–26.

Klesges LM, Johnson KC, Somes GW, et al. Use of nicotine replacement therapy on adolescent smokers and non smokers. *Arch Pediatrics Adol Med* 2003;157:517–522.

Myers MG, MacPherson L. Smoking cessation efforts among substance abusing adolescents. *Drug and Alcohol Dependence* 2004;73:209–213.

Sargent JD. Smoking in movies: impact on adolescent smoking. *Adolesc Med Clin* 2005;16: 345–370.

Vickers KS, Thomas JL, Patten CA, et al. Prevention of tobacco use in adolescents: review of current findings and implications for healthcare providers. *Curr Opin* 2002;14:708–712.

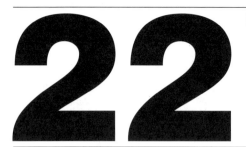

Eating Disorders

I. **Description of the condition:**
   A. **Epidemiology:** The prevalence of anorexia nervosa is estimated to be 0.5% of adolescent females in the United States. Bulimia nervosa is more common than anorexia, with a prevalence of 1% to 5% of adolescent females. Up to 5% to 10% of all cases of eating disorders occur in adolescent males. There are also many adolescents who do not meet all of the Diagnostic and Statistical Manual of Mental Disorders, Fourth Edition (DSM-IV), criteria for anorexia or bulimia nervosa but still suffer many of the physical and psychological consequences of having an eating disorder. Such adolescents may be diagnosed as eating disorder not otherwise specified (EDNOS).
   B. **Contributing factors:** Cultural, social, and environmental factors certainly play a role in the development of eating disorders, in addition to psychological factors in both the adolescent and the family. Genetically mediated biologic factors are under investigation. Biochemical changes in the brain also likely play a role in the onset and continuation of both anorexia and bulimia nervosa.

II. **Making the diagnosis:**
   A. **Signs and symptoms:**
      1. **Anorexia nervosa:**
         - The hallmark feature of the "restricting type" is persistent and severe caloric restriction, often in combination with compulsive exercise.
         - A relentless desire and drive to be thinner, leading to progressive weight loss.
         - 'Binge eating/purging type' anorexia nervosa patients intermittently engage in 'bulimic' behaviors.
         - The patient who is significantly malnourished can have various signs and symptoms, including constipation, dizziness, cold intolerance, hair loss, and psychological symptoms such as irritability or depression.
         - The presenting complaint may be secondary amenorrhea, abdominal pain, syncope, "Raynaud phenomenon" (cold, mottled, purple hands), as well as weight loss. Often the adolescent has no complaint and it is the parents who are concerned.
      2. **Bulimia nervosa:**
         - Frequently there are no signs or symptoms.
         - The patient can be of normal weight, overweight, or underweight.
         - Symptoms can include binge eating immediately followed by some compensatory behavior to rid the body of the ingested calories.
         - Purging is a compensatory mechanism used by most patients who have bulimia nervosa (e.g., self-induced vomiting, or laxative use). The key feature of bulimia nervosa is the binge eating, not the purging.
         - The nonpurging type involves fasting or exercise as ways to lose or maintain weight.
         - Most patients have menstrual irregularity (oligomenorrhea) but not secondary amenorrhea.
   B. **Clinical features:** (See Table 22-1.)
   C. **Differential diagnosis:**
      - Malignancy, brain tumor.
      - Gastrointestinal system: inflammatory bowel disease, malabsorption, celiac disease.
      - Endocrine: diabetes mellitus/insipidus, hyper- or hypothyroidism, hypopituitarism, Addison disease.
      - Psychiatric: depression, obsessive–compulsive disorder.
      - Other chronic disease or chronic infection, for example, human immunodeficiency virus (HIV).
      - Stimulant abuse, for example, cocaine or methamphetamine.

Table 22-1. DSM-IV diagnostic criteria for anorexia nervosa and bulimia nervosa, and description of eating disorder not otherwise specified

Anorexia nervosa

1. Refusal to maintain body weight at or above a minimally normal weight for age and height (e.g., weight loss leading to maintenance of body weight less than 85% of that expected; or failure to make expected weight gain during period of growth, leading to body weight less than 85% of that expected).
2. Intense fear of gaining weight or becoming fat, even though underweight.
3. Disturbance in the way in which one's body weight or shape is experienced, undue influence of body weight or shape on self-evaluation, or denial of the seriousness of the current low body weight.
4. In postmenarchal females, amenorrhea, that is, the absence of at least three consecutive menstrual cycles. (A woman is considered to have amenorrhea if her periods occur only following hormone, e.g., estrogen administration.)

Specify type:

Restricting type: during the current episode of anorexia nervosa, the person has not regularly engaged in binge-eating or purging behavior (i.e., self-induced vomiting or the misuse of laxatives, diuretics, or enemas).

Binge-eating/purging type: during the current episode of anorexia nervosa, the person has regularly engaged in binge-eating or purging behavior (i.e., self-induced vomiting or the misuse of laxatives, diuretics, or enemas).

Bulimia nervosa

1. Recurrent episodes of binge eating, characterized by both of the following:
   a. eating in a discrete period of time (e.g., within any 2-hour period), an amount of food that is definitely larger than most people would eat during a similar period of time and under similar circumstances.
   b. a sense of lack of control over eating during the episode (e.g., a feeling that one cannot stop eating or control what or how much one is eating).
2. Recurrent inappropriate compensatory behavior in order to prevent weight gain, such as self-induced vomiting; misuse of laxatives, diuretics, enemas, or other medications; fasting; or excessive exercise.
3. The binge eating and inappropriate compensatory behaviors both occur, on average, at least twice a week for 3 months.
4. Self-evaluation is unduly influenced by body shape and weight.
5. The disturbance does not occur exclusively during episodes of anorexia nervosa.

Specify type:

Purging type: during the current episode of bulimia nervosa, the person has regularly engaged in self-induced vomiting or the misuse of laxatives, diuretics, or enemas.

Nonpurging type: during the current episode of bulimia nervosa, the person has used other inappropriate compensatory behaviors, such as fasting or excessive exercise, but has not regularly engaged in self-induced vomiting or the misuse of laxative, diuretics, or enemas.

Eating disorder not otherwise specified (EDNOS)

The EDNOS category is for disorders of eating that do not meet the criteria for any specific rating disorder. Examples include

1. For female patients, all of the criteria for anorexia nervosa are met except that the individual has regular menses.
2. All of the criteria for anorexia nervosa are met except that, despite significant weight loss, the individual's current weight is in normal range.
3. All of the criteria for bulimia nervosa are met except that the binge eating and inappropriate compensatory mechanisms occur at a frequency of less than twice a week or for a duration of less than 3 months.
4. The regular use of inappropriate compensatory behavior by an individual of normal body weight after eating small amounts of food (e.g., self-induced vomiting after the consumption of two cookies).
5. Repeatedly chewing and spitting out, but not swallowing, large amounts of food.
6. Binge-eating disorder: recurrent episodes of binge eating in the absence of the regular use of inappropriate compensatory behaviors of bulimia nervosa.

From *Diagnostic and statistical manual of mental disorders,* 4th ed. Washington, DC: American Psychiatric Association, 1994, with permission.

D. Physical examination:
   1. Anorexia nervosa:
   - Height and weight to determine body mass index and percentage below ideal body weight for height.
   - Vital signs may reveal hypothermia, bradycardia, or orthostasis.
   - Hypotension in severe cases.
   - Cardiac murmur (one-third have mitral valve prolapse).
   - Hair loss, dry skin, and lanugo hair may be seen.
   - Peripheral edema, acrocyanosis, or decreased capillary refill also occur.
   - Signs of purging (e.g., eroded tooth enamel, scars on knuckles, or parotid enlargement).

   2. Bulimia nervosa:
   - Usually normal weight or overweight.
   - Cardiac arrhythmias (related to electrolyte imbalance).
   - Look for signs of purging activity as with anorexia patients.
   - Bilateral parotid enlargement is common.
   - Dental enamel erosions.
   - Calluses may be present on the back of knuckles (Russell sign) when patients use their fingers to induce emesis.

E. Laboratory evaluation and tests: The diagnosis of an eating disorder is a clinical one. The laboratory tests are not confirmatory or diagnostic but rather help to assess medical complications.
   - Initial screening tests done on all patients with eating disorders should include a complete blood count (malnutrition can cause neutropenia and, rarely, anemia or thrombocytopenia), electrolytes (hypo- or hypernatremia may be detected if patient is manipulating water intake; vomiting and laxative or diuretic use can cause a hypokalemic, hypochloremic metabolic alkalosis), and urinalysis (check specific gravity in patients with anorexia nervosa, who may consume large amounts of water before medical appointments to add extra weight).
   - Additional tests to consider include: total cholesterol (starved patients with anorexia nervosa often have high cholesterol levels); liver function tests (fatty liver seen with anorexia nervosa); and thyroid function tests (serum thyroxine and triiodothyronine may be low in anorexia nervosa).
   - Consider hormone studies in patients with amenorrhea (luteinizing hormone, follicle-stimulating hormone, prolactin, estradiol).
   - Adolescents with eating disorders are at risk for the development of osteopenia or osteoporosis. If the patient is amenorrheic for longer than 6 months, the physician should order a dual energy x-ray absorptiometry (DEXA) scan to determine bone density. For adolescents, DEXA results should be compared with those of age-matched standards (use Z-score, not T-score).
   - Electrocardiogram in patients with significant bradycardia or significant purging behaviors (prolonged QTc interval can result from severe hypokalemia).

III.   Management: The treatment for eating disorders requires a multidisciplinary approach. Medical and nutritional management is needed in coordination with mental health treatment. Most adolescents with eating disorders are treated in outpatient settings. Those with more severe disorders require inpatient hospitalization (Table 22-2).

   While most patients with anorexia nervosa are able to eat, some require assisted enteral or parenteral nutrition in order to receive sufficient calories to restore weight. Patients with bulimia nervosa need to relearn normal eating patterns that will decrease the likelihood of binge-and-purge behaviors.

A. Comprehensive treatment goals:
   - Identify and treat medical complications of starvation and/or bingeing and purging.
   - Encourage a balanced diet with adequate calories to restore a normal nutritional state.
   - Use behavioral techniques to reward weight gain or fewer bingeing and purging episodes.
   - Provide sound guidance about nutrition and exercise.
   - Change attitudes about eating and body image.
   - Optimize family support through counseling and education.
   - Psychotherapy [e.g., cognitive behavioral therapy (CBT)].

B. Pharmacotherapy:
   - Antidepressant medications, specifically selective serotonin reuptake inhibitors (SSRIs), have not been shown to help with weight gain in patients with anorexia

Table 22-2. Indications for hospitalization in an adolescent with an eating disorder

Anorexia nervosa
- <75% ideal body weight, or ongoing weight loss despite intensive management
- Refusal to eat
- Body fat <10%
- Heart rate <50 beats per minute daytime; <45 beats per minute nighttime
- Systolic pressure <90
- Orthostatic changes in pulse (>20 beats per minute) or blood pressure (>10 mm Hg)
- Temperature 35.6°C (96°F)
- Serum potassium concentration <3.2 mmol/L
- Serum chloride concentration <88 mmol/L
- Arrhythmia
- Severe infection in a starved patient (e.g., pneumonia)
- Acute medical complications (e.g., pancreatitis, syncope, seizures)
- Arrested growth and pubertal development in young adolescents
- Failure to respond to outpatient treatment
- Psychiatric emergencies (e.g., suicidal ideation or attempt, psychosis)

Bulimia nervosa
- Serum potassium concentration <3.2 mmol/L
- Serum chloride concentration <88 mmol/L
- Cardiac arrhythmias including prolonged QTc
- Intractable vomiting
- Acute medical complications (e.g., hematemesis, esophageal tears)
- Failure to respond to outpatient treatment
- Psychiatric emergencies (e.g., suicidal ideation or attempt)

From American Academy of Pediatrics Committee on Adolescence Policy Statement. Identifying and treating eating disorders. *Pediatrics* 2003;111:204–211, with permission.

nervosa, although they may be useful in treating the depression and/or the obsessive–compulsive disorder that can often be both the cause and effect of the eating disorder. Recent studies suggest that SSRIs may help recovering patients with anorexia nervosa to prevent relapse.
- SSRIs have been shown in multiple clinical studies to have an antibulimic effect independent of their antidepressant effect that results in a significant reduction in bingeing and purging episodes. The United States Food and Drug Administration has approved fluoxetine for the treatment of bulimia nervosa.

IV. **Prognosis:**
- On the basis of the outcome measures of sufficient weight gain, return of menstrual periods, and psychosocial functioning, about half of adolescents with anorexia nervosa fully recover, and 30% achieve partial recovery. In 20% there is no significant improvement.
- Reported mortality rates average at about 5%, usually from cardiac dysfunction and/or electrolyte imbalance.
- There is less data about the prognosis of adolescents with bulimia nervosa. Patients who have significant depression or a history of sexual abuse may be more difficult to treat.

V. **Clinical pearls and pitfalls:**
- Eating disorders are prevalent in the adolescent population and have serious medical and psychological consequences if left untreated.
- Early diagnosis and treatment of eating disorders leads to a better prognosis.
- Clinicians should identify variations of eating disorders that do not meet the full criteria for either anorexia or bulimia nervosa but still deserve medical and psychiatric attention.
- Patients with bulimia nervosa may be more difficult to identify because they usually do not have the extreme weight loss seen in those with anorexia nervosa.
- Growth stunting, failure to attain peak bone mineral mass, and structural brain changes are potentially irreversible complications of eating disorders in adolescents and provide the rationale for early diagnosis and aggressive treatment, especially in pre- and peripubertal children.

BIBLIOGRAPHY

For the clinician

American Academy of Pediatrics Committee on Adolescence Policy Statement. Identifying and treating eating disorders. *Pediatrics* 2003;111:204–211.

American Psychiatric Association. Eating disorders. In: *Diagnostic and statistical manual of mental disorders*, 4th ed. Washington, DC: American Psychiatric Association, 1994:539–550.

Eating Disorders in Adolescents. Position paper of the Society for Adolescent Medicine. *J Adolesc Health* 2003;33:496–503.

Fisher M. Eating disorders. In: Holland-Hall, C Brown RT, eds. *Adolescent medicine secrets*. Philadelphia, PA: Hanley & Belfus, 2002:255–263.

Fisher M, Golden NH, Jacobson MS, eds. The spectrum of disordered eating: anorexia nervosa, bulimia nervosa, and obesity. *Adolesc Med Clin* 2003;14:1–182.

Hillman JK. 'Just dieting' or an eating disorder? a practical guide for the clinician. *Adolesc Health Update* 2001;13:1–8.

Kreipe RE, Dukarm CP. Eating disorders in adolescents and older children. *Pediatr Rev* 1999;20: 410–421.

Misra M, Aggarwal A, Miller KK, Almazan C, et al. Effects of anorexia nervosa on clinical, hematologic, biochemical, and bone density parameters in community-dwelling adolescent girls. *Pediatr* 2004;114:1574–1583.

Phillips EL, Pratt HD. Eating disorders in college. *Psychiatr Clin North Am* 2005;52(1):85–96.

Rome ES, Ammerman S. Medical complications of eating disorders: an update. *J Adolesc Health* 2003;33:418–426.

For patients and parents

Pipher M. *Hunger pains: The modern woman's tragic quest for thinness*. New York: Random House, Rev ed. 1997.

Sacker IM, Zimmer MA. *Dying to be thin: Understanding and defeating anorexia nervosa and bulimia—a practical, lifesaving guide*. New York: Warner Books, 1987.

WEB SITES

www.anad.org   The National Association of Anorexia Nervosa and Associated Disorders
www.bulimia.com
www.edap.org   National Eating Disorders Association
www.kidshealth.org

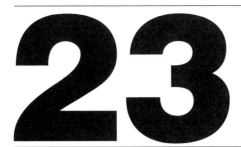

Mood and Anxiety Disorders

MOOD DISORDERS

I. **Description of the condition:** Adolescence certainly can be filled with experiences that may elicit dramatic emotional responses (e.g., romantic encounters and break-ups, arguments with friends and parents), but these responses are typically short-lived and ultimately have little impact on the adolescent's overall functioning. In fact, most adolescents report that they are happy most of the time. Occasionally an adolescent's mood becomes so abnormal that his or her functioning is impaired. This impairment may occur in the domains of family functioning, school performance, or peer activities and interactions. In these instances, a mood disorder may be to blame.

A. **Epidemiology:** Mood disorders have been diagnosed in adolescents with increasing frequency over the past decades. In addition to better recognition of these disorders in young people, it appears that the incidence of these disorders in adolescents is actually rising.

- The point prevalence of **major depressive disorder (MDD)** among adolescents is about 4% to 8%; by the end of adolescence, up to 20% of persons will experience a major depressive episode.
- Six to 10% of depressed youth go on to experience chronic, treatment-resistant depression.
- After puberty, the ratio of female adolescents to male adolescents with depression is greater than 2:1.
- Up to 8% of adolescents experience dysthymia.
- Mania is less common, with a lifetime prevalence of up to 2% during adolescence.
- Up to 25% of high school students state they have considered suicide during the past year.
- An estimated 70% to 80% of depressed adolescents do not receive treatment.

B. **Clinical features:** The criteria for a **major depressive episode** are described in the *American Psychiatric Association's Diagnostic and Statistical Manual of Mental Disorders, 4th edition (DSM-IV-TR)*. The primary criteria are presented in Table 23-1. Adolescents with depression may report the typical sadness characteristic of depressed adults; alternatively, they may experience chronic irritability, boredom, or apathy as the primary feature of their depression. This must cause the adolescent

Table 23-1. Criteria for major depressive episode

At least one of the following symptoms, nearly every day for a 2-week period, representing a change from the previous level of functioning:
- Depressed, bored, or irritable mood most of the day
- Diminished interest or pleasure in all or almost all activities

In addition, at least four of the following must be present:
- Significant weight loss, decreased appetite, weight gain, or failure to gain weight appropriately (in a child or young adolescent)
- Insomnia or hypersomnia
- Psychomotor agitation or retardation
- Fatigue or loss of energy
- Feelings of worthlessness or excessive or inappropriate guilt
- Diminished ability to think or concentrate, or indecisiveness
- Recurrent thoughts of death, suicidal ideation

Adapted from American Psychiatric Association. *Diagnostic and statistical manual of mental disorders,* 4th ed. Text Revision. Washington, DC: American Psychiatric Association; 2000.

Table 23-2. Criteria for a manic episode

Distinct period of elevated, expansive, or irritable mood for at least 1 week.
In addition, at least three of the following must be present:
• Inflated self-esteem or grandiosity
• Decreased need for sleep
• More talkative than usual
• Flight of ideas or racing thoughts
• Distractibility
• Increase in goal-directed activity
• Excessive involvement in pleasurable activities (potentially risky)

Adapted from American Psychiatric Association. *Diagnostic and statistical manual of mental disorders,* 4th ed.
text revision. Washington, DC: American Psychiatric Association; 2000.

significant distress and/or impaired functioning, and it must represent a change from the adolescent's previous level of functioning. The presence of this persistent negativity is a more reliable predictor of depression than mood lability. Adolescents typically manifest many of the cognitive and behavioral symptoms of depression; they are less likely to experience the neurovegatative symptoms common among adults. They may present with vague, chronic somatic symptoms and have limited insight into the role their mood plays in their symptoms.

Substantially less research exists on adolescents with mania and bipolar disorder, in which depressive and manic symptoms occur in a mixed or cyclic fashion. The symptoms of a **manic episode** are presented in Table 23-2. A manic episode must be associated with significant impairment of functioning or social interactions. The excessive involvement in pleasurable activities may include risky behaviors such as reckless driving, spending or giving away money inappropriately, or hypersexual behaviors. A **hypomanic episode** is characterized by a shorter duration (at least 4 days) and a lesser degree of impairment but still represents an unequivocal change from baseline functioning. It is believed that bipolar disorder has been underrecognized in children and adolescents, and its diagnosis has increased dramatically in the past decade. Both unipolar depression and bipolar disorder are likely to have a recurrent course, with symptoms persisting into or reemerging in adulthood.

Adolescents with mood disorders often have additional psychiatric diagnoses as well. Among adolescents with MDD, 40% to 70% have a comorbid psychiatric condition such as an anxiety disorder (present in 25% to 50% of depressed youths), dysthymic disorder, attention deficit hyperactivity disorder (ADHD) or another disruptive behavior disorder, or a substance abuse disorder. The comorbid condition typically precedes the first major depressive episode. The exception to this is substance abuse, which is often the result of "self-medicating" for depressive symptoms. The presence of a comorbid disorder is associated with longer duration of depressive symptoms, a worse response to treatment, and a higher rate of recurrence.

C. **Contributing factors:** The child of a parent with MDD has a 2- to 4-fold increased risk of developing MDD, corresponding with a lifetime risk of 15% to 60%. Conversely, 30% to 50% of first-degree relatives of adolescents with MDD have MDD themselves. Twin and adoption studies strongly support a genetic contribution to depressive disorders. Although the physiologic basis for mood disturbance is poorly understood, it appears to be associated with alterations in central serotonergic and noradrenergic neurotransmission.

Personal risk factors for the development of a mood disorder include the presence of an anxiety disorder or another psychiatric disorder, stressful life events such as the early death of a parent, parental conflict or divorce, history of abuse or neglect, presence of a chronic medical illness, minority race, and lower socioeconomic status. Certain medications such as corticosteroids may cause depressive symptoms. Limited evidence supports a link between the use of hormonal contraception and mood disturbances, and to date no causal association has been proven between the use of isotretinoin (Accutane) and depression or suicidality.

II. **Making the diagnosis:**
A. **Diagnostic/clinical features of specific disorders:** MDD is the most commonly diagnosed mood disorder. The mean duration of a major depressive episode (without treatment) is 7 to 9 months; 90% of affected persons experience remission within

1 to 2 years. Longer duration of symptoms is associated with comorbid psychiatric disorders, poor psychosocial functioning, and other environmental risk factors. Recurrence is the norm: 40% of patients experience another major depressive episode by 2 years and 72%, within 5 years. Young age of onset, greater severity of the initial presentation, and psychiatric comorbidity are predictors of recurrence.

Adolescents with **dysthymic disorder** experience depressive symptoms that are less intense but more chronic than those diagnostic of MDD. The adolescent must experience a depressed mood or irritability on most days, for most of each day, for at least 1 year. In addition, the adolescent must report at least two of the following symptoms: poor appetite, sleep disturbance, low self-esteem, impaired concentration or decision-making capacity, fatigue or low energy, and hopelessness. The mean duration of dysthymic disorder is 3 to 4 years, and it may be associated with extensive psychosocial impairment. Seventy percent of adolescents with this disorder develop MDD, typically 2 to 3 years after the onset of the dysthymia.

Up to 40% of adolescents with MDD develop **bipolar disorder,** experiencing both depressive and manic episodes, within 5 years of the first major depressive episode. Even more patients may exhibit subthreshold manic symptoms that do not meet criteria for a manic episode. Most adolescents experience a depressive episode as the first manifestation of bipolar disorder, but a small proportion may experience mania first. The risk of bipolar disorder is increased in patients with a family history of this disorder, patients with psychotic features to their depression, and those who have a manic or hypomanic response to antidepressant therapy. Adolescents with bipolar disorder are more likely than adults to experience **rapid cycling,** alternating between manic and depressive symptoms within a period of a few days or even hours. They are also more likely to have **mixed** episodes in which they experience symptoms of mania and depression simultaneously. Bipolar disorder typically persists and/or recurs in adulthood. It can be difficult to treat, and the associated morbidity may be great. Affected patients have a particularly high rate of suicide attempts and completions.

An adolescent may be diagnosed with **adjustment disorder with depressed mood** if he or she presents with mood symptoms within 3 months of the onset of an identifiable stressor other than the death of a loved one. The symptoms must be in excess of what would be expected in response to the stressor, or they must cause impaired functioning. The adolescent must not meet criteria for a major depressive episode. The symptoms are self-limited and must resolve within 6 months of the termination of the stressor.

Premenstrual dysphoric disorder occurs in up to 5% of menstruating adults; its prevalence among adolescents is unknown. Affected women have severe mood symptoms that may be similar to those of a major depressive episode. Symptoms are greatest during the last week of the leuteal phase, begin to remit with the onset of menses, and resolve completely by 1 week following menses.

Persons with mood disorders may exhibit **psychotic features,** such as delusions or hallucinations. Psychotic features are present in 30% of patients with MDD; their presence is associated with an increased risk of developing bipolar disorder.

B. **History:** A few simple questions may be asked to screen for depressive symptoms during routine health checks or when evaluating chronic somatic complaints:
- What do you do for fun?
- Tell me some things you are good at.
- Have there been any changes or problems with your eating or sleeping?
- Are you more often happy or sad? What kinds of things make you sad?
- Have you had any thoughts about hurting yourself or not wanting to be alive any more?

If the adolescent's responses raise the suspicion of a mood disorder, a more comprehensive assessment is necessary. The parents should be interviewed as well since they may provide a more objective report of observable symptoms such as behavioral problems, school problems, and abnormal sleeping or eating patterns. In addition to eliciting specific symptoms and diagnostic criteria of a mood disorder, the provider must assess the impact of the patient's symptoms on his or her own functioning and on the functioning of the family. Specific sources of stress at school and at home should be elicited.

The provider must inquire explicitly about suicidality. If an adolescent endorses any suicidal thinking, the provider must determine whether he or she has a specific plan for self-harm, and assess the lethality of that plan. The provider must determine

Table 23-3. Risk factors for suicide completion

Chronic depression
Substance abuse
Impulsivity
History of physical or sexual abuse
Same-sex attraction and sexual activity
Family history of a suicide attempt or completion
Access to effective means of suicide (e.g., firearms)

as well whether the adolescent has access to firearms, medications, or other lethal means of suicide. Risk factors for suicide completion are listed in Table 23-3.

  C. **Evaluation tools:** The **Beck Depression Inventory (BDI)** is the most commonly used screening tool for depression in adolescents. This self-administered questionnaire consists of 21 items, each scored 0 to 3. A total score greater than 12 may be considered significant. Research has demonstrated reasonable sensitivity and specificity of the BDI for detecting depression in community samples but not in clinical or referred populations of adolescents. The BDI has been criticized as a tool that measures general psychological distress more than depression severity *per se.* It should be considered a screening tool only and should not be relied upon for definitive diagnosis of a depressive disorder or to determine the severity of depression in an adolescent. It may be useful to monitor changes in symptoms over time and response to therapy. The Mood and Feelings Questionnaire (available at http://devepi.mc.duke.edu/mfq.html) is a more recently developed self-assessment tool. The short form consists of 13 items, and with further research it may prove to be a more sensitive and specific screening tool for depression in adolescents. It is reasonable to consider administering both depression and anxiety self-assessment tools together to assist in differentiating between these disorders. In any case, the clinician must follow up the use of a screening tool with a more comprehensive history and assessment of the diagnostic criteria for specific disorders.
  D. **Differential diagnosis:** In addition to distinguishing between the various mood disorders, the clinician must consider other psychiatric disorders in the differential diagnosis. Anxiety disorders, eating disorders, substance abuse disorders, ADHD and other disruptive behavior disorders all may mimic or coexist with a mood disorder. An adolescent with mild mental retardation or a learning disorder may develop depressive symptoms secondary to low self-esteem and frustration with poor academic performance.

  Medical conditions commonly associated with mood symptoms include anemia, mononucleosis, hyper- or hypothyroidism, collagen-vascular diseases such as systemic lupus erythematosus, and human immunodeficiency (HIV) infection. In addition, the presence of any chronic disease (e.g., diabetes, epilepsy, cystic fibrosis) may predispose adolescents to the development of a mood disorder. Medication-induced mood symptoms may develop in patients using corticosteroids, stimulants, neuroleptics, or hormonal contraceptives.
  E. **Physical examination:** A comprehensive physical examination must be performed but most likely will be normal in a patient with a mood disorder. Particular attention should be paid to the general appearance of the patient: Does he or she make eye contact with the interviewer? Is personal hygiene maintained? Is the affect flat or blunted? Stigmata of physical abuse or substance abuse should be noted. A complete neurologic examination should be performed. Any somatic complaints should be evaluated appropriately.
  F. **Ancillary studies:** Laboratory studies typically are not indicated or useful. They may be appropriate for the evaluation of a particular somatic symptom or physical examination finding. Urine drug screening may be indicated in specific situations (see Chapter 20, on substance abuse) but is not recommended as a routine practice. In rare instances in which the patient or family reports abrupt or bizarre personality changes, brain imaging may be indicated.
 III. **Management:**
  A. **Education of the patient and family:** The patient and family must understand that a mood disorder is a prevalent and well-recognized disease, rather than a "character flaw" in the affected individual. Realistic expectations should be set for a gradual

return to functioning with appropriate treatment. Many depressed adolescents feel a sense of disbelief and hopelessness that they will ever feel well again. The clinician must identify and attempt to mitigate these feelings. The primary care clinician, patient, and family must develop a crisis intervention plan at the outset of treatment, so that the family knows how to respond if the adolescent becomes suicidal, manic, or otherwise unmanageable by the parents while awaiting treatment or treatment effect. This plan may include utilization of local emergency departments, suicide hotlines, mental health facilities, and the "on call" coverage for the primary care provider. The family must do everything possible to ensure the patient's safety at home. This includes locking up medications and other toxic substances and removing firearms from the home. Unfortunately, families often are reluctant to adhere to the latter recommendation.

B. **Treatment:** Overriding goals of treatment include: (1) a return to family, academic, and peer-related functioning, and (2) the resumption of progression of normal adolescent psychosocial development, if this has been impaired or interrupted. Treatment may include psychotherapy, pharmacotherapy, or both. A recent study, funded by the National Institute of Mental Health, found that adolescents with MDD who were treated with both fluoxetine and cognitive-behavioral therapy (CBT) in combination showed greater improvement than those treated with either therapy alone. The same study found that adolescents who received only fluoxetine did better than subjects who received only CBT. Patients with severe or chronic depression are likely to need both. For less severely affected adolescents it is reasonable to begin with psychotherapy and add medication if no response is demonstrated in 6 to 8 weeks. Close follow-up with the primary care provider is essential, even in patients who are referred to mental health specialists, since adolescents with depression demonstrate high rates of nonadherence to both mental health counseling and antidepressant medication.

C. **Psychotherapy:** Among the psychotherapeutic techniques, the most evidence exists for the efficacy of CBT in the treatment of adolescent depression. CBT includes identifying and restructuring the adolescent's negative, self-critical thoughts and views and challenging these negative perceptions. The behavioral component includes increasing pleasurable activities, decreasing behaviors that reinforce the depression, and improving interpersonal skills. Other types of therapy may be employed as well, including general supportive therapy, interpersonal therapy, and family therapy. Group therapy may be useful for adolescents who experience isolation and need to improve their social skills. Typical psychotherapy continues for 6 to 16 sessions. In order to prevent relapse, ongoing visits with decreased frequency may be appropriate rather than abrupt cessation of therapy.

D. **Pharmacotherapy:** Medication may be used for the treatment of moderate-to-severe MDD in adolescents. It may be prescribed as first-line treatment or when there has been an inadequate response to psychotherapy. Medication may be considered to treat the depressive symptoms of a patient with dysthymic disorder, but no evidence exists for efficacy in this situation. Fluoxetine is the only antidepressant approved by the Food and Drug Administration (FDA) for the treatment of MDD in adolescents, although other medications are widely used as well.

Selective serotonin reuptake inhibitors (SSRIs) are the most commonly prescribed antidepressants for adolescents, due to their demonstrated efficacy and low side effect profile. Both fluoxetine and citalopram have been shown to be more effective than placebo in the treatment of adolescents with depression. Nonetheless, the response rate to SSRIs is a modest 60%. Paroxetine and venlafaxine, which inhibits both serotonergic and noradrenergic reuptake, have recently been shown to be ineffective and should not be used. Side effects of SSRIs include gastrointestinal upset, agitation, sexual dysfunction, sedation, and sleep disturbances including insomnia. They may cause behavioral activation including disinhibition, hypomania, or mania in susceptible patients. Although the therapeutic effect of an SSRI typically takes 4 to 6 weeks to become apparent, the side effects often are noted within the first few weeks of use. SSRIs inhibit the cytochrome P450 system to varying degrees, so drug interactions must be monitored.

When an SSRI is prescribed, the clinician should begin with half the usual dose (e.g., fluoxetine or citalopram 10 mg daily) for 1 week (Table 23-4). If this dose is tolerated without side effects, it should be increased to a therapeutic dose (e.g., 20 mg). Dosing can be further increased at intervals of at least 4 weeks, to a maximum daily dose equivalent to fluoxetine 60 mg. There is some evidence that adolescents metabolize SSRIs faster than adults, so high doses may be required to

Table 23-4. Guidelines for prescribing SSRIs

Dosing:
- Begin with half the usual dose (e.g., fluoxetine 10 mg daily) $\times$ 7 d
- Increase to therapeutic dose (e.g., fluoxetine 20 mg daily) if no side effects
- Titrate up to maximum dose (e.g., fluoxetine 60 mg daily) as needed, at 4-wk intervals

Patient and parent counseling: Call provider immediately for the following[a]
- Suicide attempt
- New or increasing suicidal thoughts
- Worsening depression or anxiety symptoms
- New or worsening panic attacks
- New or worsening agitation or impulsivity
- New or worsening mania or hypomania

FDA Recommended Follow-up[a]:
- Weekly for first 4 wk
- Every 2 weeks for next 4 wk
- End of 12th wk
- More often if any problems are encountered

SSRIs, Selective serotonin reuptake inhibitors.
[a]Recommended for all antidepressants.

achieve a therapeutic effect. The SSRI may be given in the morning or evening, depending on whether it causes sedation or insomnia in a given patient. Successful pharmacotherapy should be continued for at least 6 months following clinical improvement to reduce the risk of relapse. Lack of response to treatment with one SSRI does not imply that others will be ineffective; it is reasonable to switch to another SSRI if initial treatment fails or is terminated due to side effects. SSRIs, particularly those with short half-lives (e.g., sertraline), should be tapered before discontinuing.

Despite their frequent use, there is no evidence that **tricyclic antidepressants (TCAs)** are more effective than placebo in the treatment of adolescent depression. The narrow therapeutic window and high lethality in overdose also make TCAs an inappropriate first-line therapy for depressed adolescents, particularly if they are suicidal. If used, they should be dispensed in limited quantities.

Other antidepressants have been used in adolescents as well, although their safety and efficacy are not well studied in this age group. Trazodone is reasonably safe but quite sedating; it is most commonly prescribed to treat the insomnia caused by depression or SSRIs. Bupropion hydrochloride has demonstrated efficacy in an open-label trial for adolescents with both MDD and ADHD. Mirtazepine and nefazodone are being prescribed with increasing frequency by mental health specialists. There is evidence to support the use of St. John's Wort (*Hypericum perforatum*) in adults with mild-to-moderate depression, but no studies on adolescents have been published.

Recently, concerns have been raised and highly publicized regarding the risk of suicidality among children and adolescents using antidepressant medications, particularly SSRIs. A meta-analysis of 24 studies was performed, which included more than 4,400 children and adolescents using antidepressant medications for various psychiatric disorders. Of these subjects, 78 demonstrated suicidality. Among patients with MDD, the risk of suicidality in patients taking antidepressants was 4%, compared to 2% in the patients taking placebo. No suicides occurred in either group. There was no difference in suicidality between the two groups among patients being treated for anxiety disorders. Although this area remains controversial, the FDA now requires that all antidepressants contain a "black box" warning regarding their association with suicidality in children and adolescents. This information should be carefully explained to patients and their parents, and the potential risks and benefits of antidepressant use should be weighed on a case-by-case basis. Careful counseling and close follow-up are recommended, as described in Table 23-4.

Table 23-5. Indications for primary physician care and specialty care in adolescents with depression

Indications for primary physician care
 Initial episode of depression
 Recent onset of depression
 Absence of coexisting conditions
 Ability to make no-suicide contract
Indications for specialty physician care
 Chronic, recurrent depression
 Lack of response to initial course of treatment[a]
 Coexisting substance abuse[a]
 Recent suicide attempt, current suicidal ideation with plan, or both[a]
 Psychosis[a]
 Bipolar disorder[a]
 High level of family discord
 Inability of family to monitor patient's safety[a]

[a]The presence of this factor indicates the need for more urgent or more intensive care.
From Brent DA, Birmaher B. Adolescent depression. *N Engl J Med* 2002;347(9):667, with permission.

Antidepressants should not be prescribed to adolescents with bipolar disorder, and they should be used with caution in depressed adolescents with a family history of bipolar disorder. These patients are best treated by a mental health professional. Mood stabilizers such as lithium, divalproex, and carbamazepine have all been used in this age group. Primary care providers should be aware that divalproex, the most commonly used mood stabilizer in adolescents, may be teratogenic and in rare cases can cause agranulocytosis. Lithium may cause hypothyroidism.

E. Criteria for referral: Primary care providers are often able to initiate treatment of mild-to-moderate depression without the aid of a psychiatrist or mental health specialist, depending on the severity of symptoms, clarity of the diagnosis, and experience and comfort level of the provider. Brief counseling interventions may include identifying negative thinking patterns and encouraging "reality checks" with regard to such negative perceptions, and encouraging scheduled participation in enjoyable activities. Indications for specialty physician care are presented in Table 23-5. Inpatient treatment may be required for severely affected adolescents, including those who are acutely suicidal, who have substance dependence, or whose psychotic, manic, or severe depressive symptoms cause such great impairment that outpatient treatment is unlikely to be effective.

ANXIETY DISORDERS

I. Description of the condition:

A. Epidemiology: Anxiety disorders are, as a whole, among the most common psychiatric disorders experienced by adolescents. Although precise prevalence estimates vary among different studies, 8% to 14% of adolescents experience at least one anxiety disorder that causes significant dysfunction. Both male and female adolescents are affected; significant gender discrepancies are not seen for most disorders. Most never seek care for these conditions.
- In one study, 6% of adolescents experienced social phobia over a 12-month period.
- In community samples, 3.6% to 7.3% have general anxiety disorder (GAD).
- Up to 3% of adolescents have obsessive-compulsive disorder (OCD).
- Up to 44% of sexually abused children and adolescents develop posttraumatic stress disorder (PTSD).
- More than 50% of children and adolescents with anxiety meet diagnostic criteria for two anxiety disorders; 30% have three anxiety disorders.

B. Genetics/familial transmission: Adolescents whose parents have anxiety disorders are more likely to develop these disorders themselves. There is strong evidence for a genetic component predisposing to these disorders, especially panic disorder, OCD, and GAD.

C. Clinical features: Anxiety is the emotional disturbance associated with the perception or anticipation of danger. It may be accompanied by the physiologic changes that exist to ready an individual for "fight or flight" in a threatening situation. When anxiety is excessive and causes significant functional impairment, an anxiety disorder may be present. In general, the cycle of anxiety disorders begins with exposure to a **trigger** that causes the adolescent to feel anxious. The adolescent engages in an **escape behavior,** such as avoidance of the trigger or a compulsive behavior. This behavior reduces the adolescent's level of anxiety, thereby reinforcing the behavior until it becomes **habitual.** Although adults with anxiety disorders generally realize that their anxiety is excessive or unreasonable, young people who are affected are less likely to acknowledge this.

Adolescents with anxiety disorders may present with overt anxiety symptoms, but they often present with vague somatic complaints. Younger adolescents, in particular, may have minimal insight into the role anxiety plays in their symptoms. School avoidance, excessive school absence, and other avoidant behaviors are common. Although the symptoms and severity may vary over time, the condition often persists into adulthood and may cause lifelong impairment.

In addition to a high prevalence of coexistence of two or more anxiety disorders, there is high comorbidity between anxiety disorders and other mental health disorders. Comorbidities are more prevalent among older adolescents and those with more severe symptoms.

- Thirty to 60% of adolescents with an anxiety disorder also have a depressive disorder; in these individuals anxiety symptoms typically precede depression.
- Disruptive behavior disorders, particularly ADHD, are more common among affected adolescents.
- Substance abuse disorders are prevalent, often developing from an attempt to self-medicate for anxiety symptoms.
- The risk of suicide is increased.

II. **Making the diagnosis:**
A. **Recognizing anxiety symptoms:** The presence of an anxiety disorder should be suspected in patients who present with poorly defined somatic complaints and chronic complaints such as headache, chest pain, and abdominal or pelvic pain. They may have several visits for the same or varying symptoms. Anxiety disorders should also be considered in patients with other mental health diagnoses or a family history of anxiety.
B. **Signs and symptoms:** Patients with anxiety disorders may report psychological symptoms including:
  - Feeling excessively anxious or worried
  - Feeling scared or fearful
  - Feeling nervous, restless, fretful, or unsettled
  - Fearing death or impending doom or disaster
  - Hyperarousal or hypervigilance, easily startled
  In addition, patients may report several physiologic symptoms including:
  - Rapid heart rate or palpitations
  - Rapid breathing, shortness of breath, or chest pain
  - Skin changes, flushing, or excessive perspiration
  - Dizziness, light headedness, fainting
  - Tremulousness
  - Paresthesias or "numbness"
  - Gastrointestinal symptoms
  The severity of symptoms is disproportionate to the stressor, if any is identified, that precipitates them.
C. **Diagnostic/clinical features:** The above symptoms may be present in varying combinations, but in order for the diagnosis of an anxiety disorder to be made they must cause significant distress and/or impairment of functioning. Specific anxiety disorders are described below. Complete diagnostic criteria may be found in the DSM-IV-TR.
  1. **Specific phobias** are persistent, excessive, and unreasonable fears of specific objects or situations, causing avoidance of those triggers.
  2. **Social phobia,** the most prevalent anxiety disorder, is characterized by marked, persistent fear in one or more social or performance situations. An affected individual fears criticism or public humiliation in these situations, which may include speaking, eating, or writing in public, attending parties, or using a public restroom. Patients may experience physical symptoms such as choking, flushing, palpitations, or tremulousness in these situations. Adolescents must experience these symptoms not only in the presence of adults or authority figures, but in front of their peers as well. Refusing to go to school and avoiding extracurricular activities often ensues.

3. **Generalized anxiety disorder (GAD),** formerly classified as overanxious disorder of childhood, is diagnosed in the adolescent with excessive anxiety that is difficult to control and causes more than 6 months of functional impairment. There is no specific focus or environmental context for the anxiety, which often includes unrealistic worries about the future. Affected adolescents experience at least one additional symptom of restlessness, fatigue, poor concentration, sleep disturbance, irritability, or muscle tension. Chronic somatic complaints are common. This disorder exhibits substantial chronicity, with nearly half of affected patients reporting persistent symptoms 8 years after diagnosis.

4. Adolescents with **panic disorder** experience discrete episodes ("panic attacks") of severe psychological and physiologic anxiety symptoms. Symptoms commonly include shortness of breath, chest pain or tightness, palpitations, and fear of dying. Affected patients often fear they are having a heart attack. Episodes are recurrent and generally have an abrupt onset and a more gradual resolution. They often occur at night or in response to specific situations, but many adolescents cannot identify specific triggers. Agoraphobia may be present, and patients who are severely affected may report avoiding social situations out of fear that they will experience an attack in front of other people. Female adolescents are more likely to be affected than are male adolescents.

5. Adolescents with **obsessive-compulsive disorder (OCD)** experience obsessions and/or compulsions that are psychologically distressing and/or time consuming. Most (80%) experience both obsessions and compulsions. Common obsessions include thoughts of harm to self or others, issues of cleanliness and contamination, concerns with environmental exposures such as exhaust and electricity, and symmetry urges. Compulsions classically include washing, checking (e.g., locks, electrical outlets), counting, and arranging or ordering behaviors. OCD is likely to persist into adulthood, though symptoms may wax and wane over time.

6. **Posttraumatic stress disorder (PTSD)** may occur following an incident in which an adolescent experiences the actual or perceived threat of death or serious injury to himself or herself or others. Incidents commonly preceding PTSD include physical or sexual abuse or assault, natural disasters, acts of terrorism, and parental loss. The adolescent **reexperiences** the episode through dreams or flashbacks when exposed to environmental cues evoking memories of the experience. **Avoidance** of such stimuli occurs, and the adolescent may become detached, disinterested, and have a sense of a foreshortened future. Sleep disturbance, irritability, problems with concentration, and hypervigilance are manifestations of the **increased arousal** that is characteristic of PTSD. Symptoms must be present for more than 1 month. **Acute stress disorder** is characterized by similar symptoms lasting less than 1 month after the inciting incident.

7. Adolescents with marked anxiety symptoms that lead to impaired functioning in response to a specific, identifiable stressor may be diagnosed with **adjustment disorder with anxiety.**

D. **History:** A comprehensive history including a complete mental health and psychosocial history must be obtained, as well as a careful history of medication use and substance abuse. Specific physical and psychological symptoms should be elicited, as described above. Symptoms of mood and disruptive behavior disorders should be elicited, as described elsewhere. Parents should be interviewed as well, to assess the family's response to the patient's symptoms and the degree of impairment of family functioning. Key questions may include:
- Do you worry more than other people your age? More than other family members?
- On a scale of zero (never worry) to 10 (always worry), how much do you worry about things?
- Do symptoms occur only in certain settings, or when you are thinking about certain things?
- What impact do symptoms have on your functioning?
- Are you afraid you might die from your symptoms?
- How much school have you missed in the last year? How often are you late for school?
- Do you avoid certain places or activities?
- Do you participate in extracurricular activities and social activities with peers?
- Did you experience any very upsetting or traumatic events before the symptoms started?
- Are other people in your family worriers? Is there a family history of panic disorder, OCD, or other anxiety disorders?
- Do you have any behaviors or rituals that you think are unusual?

- How many minutes do you spend doing these behaviors every day?
- How often are you late to school or other places because you were engaging in these behaviors?
- Do you ever get so worried or bothered by your symptoms that you think about hurting yourself or killing yourself?

E. **Differential diagnosis:**
  - Other and/or comorbid anxiety disorders
  - Mood disorder
  - ADHD or other disruptive behavior disorder
  - Hyperthyroidism
  - Pheochromocytoma
  - Cardiac arrhythmia
  - Vocal cord dysfunction
  - Hypoglycemia
  - Prescription medication use: corticosteroids, sympathomimetics, asthma medications
  - Over the counter medication use: diet pills, ephedra derivatives, "cold" medications, caffeine
  - Illicit substance abuse: amphetamines, cocaine, phencyclidine (PCP), anabolic steroids, nicotine
  - Withdrawal from illicit substance use: alcohol, benzodiazepines, opioids, marijuana

F. **Physical examination:** A complete physical examination should include a thorough neurologic examination, examination of the heart and lungs, and palpation of the thyroid gland. Localizing somatic symptoms should be evaluated as indicated.

G. **Laboratory evaluation and ancillary studies:** Laboratory and ancillary studies usually are not necessary or helpful, but they may be indicated if the clinician suspects a thyroid disturbance, or to evaluate a specific somatic symptom or finding. Persistent tachycardia may suggest hyperthyroidism. Tachycardia or palpitations that have abrupt onset, abrupt discontinuation and are not accompanied by convincing evidence of an anxiety disorder may be evaluated with the use of a cardiac event monitor or Holter monitor and/or electrocardiography.

H. **Evaluation tools:** Several evaluation tools exist to assist the clinician with the diagnosis of an anxiety disorder. Some are designed as self-rating scales that may be used as screening tools by primary care providers; others are administered by an experienced clinician. These tools are generally useful for distinguishing adolescents with anxiety disorders from normal controls, and for monitoring changes in symptomatology over time and in response to treatment. Their utility is limited by their inability to reliably differentiate between specific anxiety disorders, and some do not discriminate well between anxiety and mood disorders. They should therefore be used in conjunction with other diagnostic modalities when assessing an adolescent for an anxiety disorder. The Multidimensional Anxiety Scale (MASC) and the Screen for Child Anxiety Related Emotional Disorders (SCARED) are self-report scales that aim to address some of these weaknesses, and they may be useful in the primary care setting.

III. **Management:**
A. **Goals of treatment:** Return to normal personal and psychosocial functioning should be the primary goal of treatment. Return to school and specific situations, places, or activities that have been avoided may be used as specific, more tangible goals.

B. **Treatment:** The treatment team may include the patient, parents, siblings, primary care provider, mental health provider, and psychopharmacologist. Other prominent people in the adolescent's life may be included as well, such as teachers, coaches, employers, etc., who may need to respond to the adolescent's symptoms.

Treatment should begin with educating the patient and family about the diagnosis and reassuring them that you have helped adolescents with these symptoms in the past. Explicit reassurance about the benign nature of specific physical symptoms (e.g., "I am certain that you are not having a heart attack") may be particularly comforting to the patient and family. Acknowledge that the symptoms the patient is experiencing are very real, not "all in his head," but that sometimes a primary problem in the brain or thought process can cause physical symptoms in the body. Specific, everyday illustrations of this concept may make it more acceptable to the adolescent (e.g., blushing when one is embarrassed; feeling one's heart pound while watching a scary movie). Patients who are only mildly affected may respond well to this simple reassurance and explanation of their symptoms.

Both psychotherapy and pharmacotherapy have been shown to be effective for the treatment of anxiety disorders, but evidence-based recommendations for adolescents are lacking. It is reasonable to start with psychotherapy and consider adding a medication if the former is not successful. Therapy should ideally be undertaken by a mental health professional skilled and experienced with the treatment of anxiety disorders in children and adolescents. Cognitive behavioral therapy may be effective. This may include gradual exposure to the anxiety-producing stimulus and elimination of the escape/avoidant behavior (**exposure plus response prevention**). General supportive "talk" therapy is less likely to be effective, particularly for adolescents with moderate-to-severe symptoms.

C. **Medications:** Medications have been shown to reduce many of the symptoms of anxiety disorders, but they may not necessarily lead to improvements in psychosocial functioning. The best data exist for the efficacy of medications in the treatment of OCD; findings are mixed for the treatment of other anxiety disorders. Most medications are not approved by the FDA for the treatment of anxiety disorders in adolescents; use is "off-label" for this indication.

1. **Selective serotonin reuptake inhibitors (SSRIs)** are considered first-line pharmacotherapy for anxiety disorders in all age groups. The low side effect profile and relative safety in overdose are attractive qualities of this class of medication. Several studies support their safety for use in adolescents, and efficacy studies are gradually accumulating. Sertraline and fluvoxamine have been approved by the FDA for the treatment of OCD in children and adolescents, and other SSRIs have been shown effective for this condition as well. Paroxetine has been shown effective for treatment of social phobia. Treatment with an SSRI should be initiated at low doses and titrated up on a weekly basis. Rapid increases may cause worsening of anxiety or panic symptoms. Patients should be informed that the medication may take several weeks to achieve maximal efficacy. Once the therapeutic dose is achieved, it should be continued for at least 1 month before it is considered ineffective. Further information on using SSRIs may be found earlier in this chapter (see also Table 23-4).

2. There are some small studies indicating that **tricyclic antidepressants (TCAs)** may be useful in the treatment of some adolescents with anxiety disorders, but the evidence is quite limited. Side effects (anticholinergic and antiadrenergic) and high lethality with overdose further limit their utility. If used, baseline electrocardiography should be obtained, and it should be repeated prior to each dose increase to monitor for conduction delays. Blood pressure and pulse, both supine and standing, should be monitored. TCAs should be started at low doses and titrated gradually. They should be tapered before discontinuing.

3. **Benzodiazepines** are commonly used for adults with anxiety, but they should be considered second-line treatment in adolescents due to their addictive potential and the limited data supporting their safety and efficacy in this population. They may be used intermittently for relief of acute, severe anxiety episodes such as panic attacks or debilitating OCD associated with the inability to sleep. Benzodiazepines may be used in conjunction with an SSRI, particularly during the early stages of treatment while the SSRI dose is being titrated upward and full efficacy has not yet been attained. Side effects include sedation and paradoxical agitation. For acute symptom relief, benzodiazepines with a short half-life, such as lorazepam or alprazolam, should be used. A test dose equivalent to 0.5 mg of lorazepam should be given to evaluate for behavioral activation or disinhibition; ultimately a higher dose may be needed for symptom relief. Clonazepam has a long half-life and may be used for short periods of time, divided into two doses daily. It should be tapered prior to discontinuation if used for more than a few days.

4. **Buspirone** is widely used in adults with GAD due to its demonstrated safety and efficacy in that population, and the low potential for addiction or tolerance. It is poorly studied in children and adolescents, and is therefore not recommended as first-line therapy for anxiety disorders in this population.

D. **Support for families:** Families should be educated regarding the adolescent's specific diagnosis. Family therapy may be useful, particularly for families in which the adolescent's symptoms have a significant impact on overall family functioning. Family members must learn to respond appropriately to the adolescent's symptoms and escape behaviors. They should understand that relapse is common, and that many anxiety disorders persist for years with waxing and waning symptoms. They should be referred to local or Internet-based support groups if interested.

E. **Criteria for referral:** Most adolescents with anxiety disorders are best served by a mental health professional experienced with the treatment of these disorders in young people. Patients with moderate to severe symptoms and all patients with OCD should be strongly encouraged to seek treatment. Patients with substance abuse disorders should have these addressed first, even if the substance use developed as an attempt to self-medicate for anxiety symptoms. Patients who do not respond to SSRI treatment in conjunction with counseling may be best served by a psychiatrist.

IV.   **Clinical pearls and pitfalls:**
   - High degrees of comorbidity exist between mood and anxiety disorders, substance use disorders, and ADHD; when one diagnosis is made, evaluate for others.
   - Psychotherapy, medications, or both may be used to treat these disorders; decisions should be made on a case-by-case basis.
   - SSRIs are first-line pharmacotherapy for depression and anxiety disorders in adolescents.
   - Careful counseling and close follow-up should be performed and documented when SSRIs are prescribed, due to concerns that they may increase the risk of suicidality in adolescents with MDD.
   - Follow-up visits with the primary care provider are important for patients with mental health disorders, in order to monitor symptoms and adherence to therapy.
   - Substance abuse disorders may lead to mood and anxiety symptoms, or they may develop from attempts to "self-medicate" for these symptoms. In either case, it is critical to treat the substance use disorder before, or concurrent with, the mood or anxiety disorder.
   - Suicidality should routinely be assessed with initial evaluation and during subsequent visits for adolescents with these disorders; asking about suicidality does not increase a patient's risk of suicidal behaviors.

BIBLIOGRAPHY

For the clinician

American Psychiatric Association. *Diagnostic and statistical manual of mental disorders*, 4th ed., text revision. Washington, DC: American Psychiatric Association, 2000.
Beasley PJ, Beardslee WR. Depression in the adolescent patient. *Adolesc Med* 1998;9(2):351–362.
Birmaher B, Yelovich AK, Renaud J. Pharmacologic treatment for children and adolescents with anxiety disorders. *Pediatr Clin North Am* 1998;45(5):1187–1204.
Bostic JQ, Martin A. Psychopharmacology. *Psychiatr Clin North Am* 2006 (in press).
Brent DA, Birmaher B. Adolescent depression. *N Engl J Med* 2002;347(9):667–671.
Kreipe R, Hodgman C. Adolescent Psychiatry. *Adolesc Med Clin* 2006 (in press).
Lewinsohn PM, Seeley JR, Buckley ME, Klein DN. Bipolar disorder in adolescence and young adulthood. *Child Adolesc Psychiatr Clin N Am* 2002;11:461–475.
March J, Silva S, Petrycki S, et al. Fluoxetine, cognitive-behavioral therapy, and their combination for adolescents with depression: Treatment for Adolescents with Depression Study (TADS) randomized controlled trial. *JAMA* 2004;292(7):861–863.
Varley CK, Smith CJ. Anxiety disorders in the child and teen. *Pediatr Clin N Am* 2003;50(5):1107–1138.

For patients and parents

Pruitt D, ed. *Your Adolescent. Emotional, behavioral and cognitive development from early adolescence through the teen years.* New York: HarperCollins, American Academy of Child and Adolescent Psychiatry, 2000.

WEB SITES

www.aacap.org   The American Academy of Child and Adolescent Psychiatry. Includes "Facts for Families," describing several mental health diagnoses affecting children
www.childanxiety.net   The Child Anxiety Network, run by Boston University
www.mentalhealth.samhsa.gov   The National Mental Health Information Center of the Substance Abuse and Mental Health Services Administration
www.fda.gov/cder/drug/antidepressants/   The Food and Drug Administration's page on adolescent depression, including information for providers and parents regarding the use of SSRIs and suicidality
www.nimh.nih.gov/healthinformation/childmenu.cfm   Information for patients, families, and providers from the National Institute of Mental Health
www.parentsmedguide.org   A joint project of the American Psychiatric Association and the American Academy of Child and Adolescent Psychiatry. An excellent resource for both patients/parents and professionals, discussing the management of depression in young people. In particular, it addresses the issue of antidepressants and the new black box warnings.

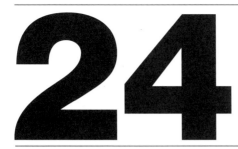

Psychosomatic Problems in Adolescence

It is more important to know what sort of person has a disease than to know what sort of disease a person has.

—Hippocrates

I. **Description of the problem:** Treating the adolescent who may have a psychosomatic problem is one of the most difficult dilemmas in adolescent medicine. No other set of disorders calls for the same diagnostic and management skills. Dealing successfully with psychosomatic illness represents the "art" of medicine. Unfortunately, at present, the science of psychosomatic medicine is still in its infancy. Making a correct diagnosis will benefit the teenager and his or her family greatly; making an inaccurate diagnosis will result in "doctor-shopping," repeated and expensive tests, and occasionally even unnecessary surgery.

A. **Basic principles:** There are three important principles involved in making the diagnosis of a psychosomatic disorder:
1. Organic disease needs to be ruled out.
2. Psychosocial dysfunction needs to be ruled in.
3. Ideally, as the psychosocial dysfunction improves, the symptoms of the illness should abate.

The term "psychosomatic" is often interpreted as if the mind and the body were separate. In fact, all illnesses have a physiologic and a psychological component to them. Expressions used in everyday life confirm that people believe in the connection even if science is sometimes skeptical:
- "pissed off"
- "all choked up"
- "gut reaction"
- "you're going to give me a heart attack"
- "you make me sick"
- "I'm so angry I can't see straight."

Every clinician in America is taught the first principle. Unfortunately, the teaching about psychosomatic illness frequently ends here. **Psychosomatic illness is not what the patient has when no organic illness can be discovered.** In other words, it is a diagnosis of inclusion as well as exclusion. In addition, the pains are real; they are not simply "all in your head," as many patients are led to believe.

The second principle may be even more difficult than the first. Patients are not typically aware of any psychosocial distress. **If patients could identify specific sources of their stress or anxiety, then they would not subconsciously have to resort to somatization.** For example, a 16-year-old male is anxious about his parents' divorce and feels that it is partially his fault. By developing acute chest pains, he does not have to deal consciously with his feelings. Instead, he can elicit sympathy from both parents while rechanneling his distress about their divorce into more acceptable channels. If he could verbalize his feelings of anxiety and guilt, it is unlikely that he would have developed chest pains in the first place. But **in contemporary society, physical illness is far more acceptable than emotional distress.**

B. **Epidemiology:** Arguably, today's teenagers are more stressed than in the history of American society (Tables 24-1 and 24-2). And teenagers frequently worry about their bodies and their health—more than half, in one study. Recurrent abdominal pain accounts for 5% of all pediatric office visits and at least 10% of teenagers report either frequent headaches, chest pain, nausea, or fatigue. In one survey of 12- to 16-year-olds, significant somatic symptoms were found in 11% of females and 4% of males. In another, 24% of 1,500 middle school students reported headaches and 13% reported

Table 24-1. What me worry? The top 10 worries of adolescents

Male adolescents
1. Terrorism
2. Feelings that I'm a bad person
3. Having sex or thoughts about having sex
4. Eating too little or too much
5. My parents' physical or mental health
6. Too much free time
7. Getting special recognition at school
8. Going out on a date
9. Popularity with friends and classmates
10. Trouble with the law

Female adolescents
1. Terrorism
2. My parents' physical or mental health
3. My periods
4. Feelings that I'm a bad person
5. Getting bad grades
6. Having sex or thoughts about having sex
7. Death or illness of a friend or family member
8. People being afraid of me
9. Going out on a date
10. Getting special recognition at school

From Kaufman KL, Brown RT, Graves K, et al. What, me worry? A survey of adolescents' concerns. *Clin Pediatr* 1993;32:8, with permission.

abdominal pains occurring either daily or several times a week. For actual psychosomatic illness, one researcher found an incidence of 8% to 10% in a seven-center study of outpatient clinics.

Apparently, psychosocial problems are on the rise. In a study of nearly 12,000 children aged 4 to 15 years of age, spanning 1979 to 1996, psychosocial problems identified by clinicians increased from 7% to 19% of all visits (using the same format and categories). This is striking, given that clinicians often fail to recognize psychosocial problems—83% went undetected in one study. In addition, some clinicians may underreport such problems because of concerns about insurability, reimbursement, or stigma.

Where is all of this stress, and all of these problems, coming from? A variety of sources, some new and some old:
- Psychosocial problems and stress are more common among single-parented teens and those from lower socioeconomic groups.

Table 24-2. Common adolescent stresses[a]

Stress	Reported incidence
Failing grades on report card	34%
Increased arguments between parents	28%
Serious family illness	28%
Broke up with boy/girlfriend	24%
Death in family	22%
Problem with siblings	21%
Teacher problems	14%
Parents divorced	13%
Death of a close friend	11%

[a]Survey of 172 11 to 19 year olds in a general adolescent clinic.
Adapted from Greene JW, Walker LS, Hickson G, et al. Stressful life events and somatic complaints in adolescents. *Pediatr* 1985;75:19.

- As many as 40% of all American children will experience the divorce of their parents by age 18, and nearly half will spend part of their childhood with only one parent.
- More than 2.5 million children and teens have lost at least one parent through death.
- Each year, nearly 18% of children move with their families to a new home.
- An estimated 27% of women and 16% of men report having been sexually abused as children or teenagers.
- In one British study of nearly 3,000 schoolchildren ages 8 and 9 who had physical complaints and were consulting their school nurse, those who had been bullied were 2.5 times more likely to be having abdominal pains or headaches.
- Because of high rates of early sexual intercourse and of drug use and the "super-peer" influence of the media, today's teenagers have to develop coping strategies earlier than ever before.
- Teenagers continue to be concerned about how the threat of nuclear war, terrorism, and pollution of the environment may cut short their future.

C. Pathophysiology: The relatively new field of psychoneuroimmunology has identified links between the central nervous system, the peripheral nervous system, hormones, and the immune system. For example, stress can alter the susceptibility of individuals to infection:

- A landmark study in 1962 found that the incidence of streptococcal illness increases according to levels of social stress.
- Other studies (Figure 24-1) of children have found correlations between amount of stress and:
  - Injuries
  - Duration of illness
  - Hospitalizations
  - Asthma and allergic rhinitis
  - Recurrent colds
  - Increased incidence of flu
- At the organ level, psychiatric "stress interviews" have been shown to induce motility disturbances in the sigmoid colon. In one infamous experiment, a group of medical student volunteers underwent sigmoidoscopy and were told that a bowel carcinoma was "accidentally discovered." When the hoax was explained, the readings from the sigmoid probes returned to normal (Figure 24-2).

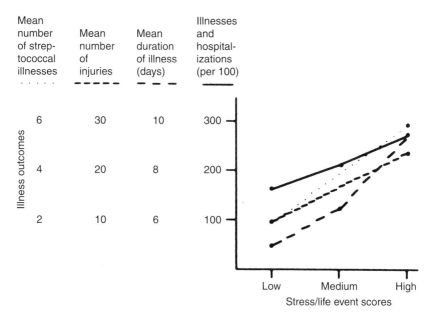

Figure 24-1. Results of four studies in which health outcome correlated with amount of stress. (From Boyce WT. Stress and child health: an overview. *Pediatr Ann* 1985;14:539. Copyright © Slack Inc. Reprinted with permission.)

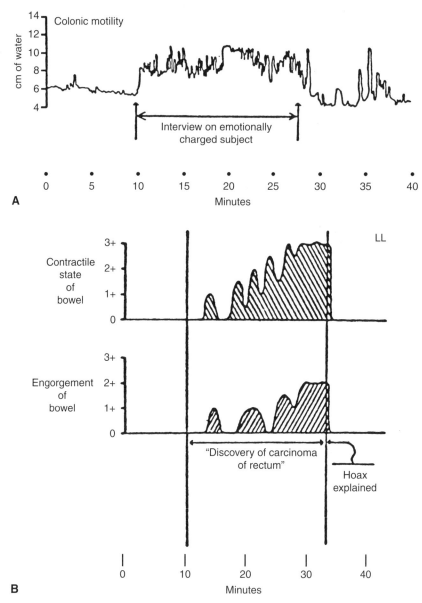

Figure 24-2. Gastrointestinal reactions to stress. **A:** Alterations in colonic motility during a stress interview. **B:** Sigmoidoscopic observations before, during, and after a normal medical student volunteer was informed—as a hoax—that he had a carcinoma of the rectum. (From Drossman DA, Powell DW, Sessions JT Jr. The irritable bowel syndrome. *Gastroenterology* 1977;73:811. Copyright 1997. Reprinted with permission from the American Gastroenterological Association.)

How these responses are mediated is a topic of active investigation. In the presence of stress or depression, certain immune responses are blunted, including lymphocyte proliferation, T-cell suppression, delayed hypersensitivity, and natural killer cell activity. For colds, the flu, and asthma, the important mediator may be salivary IgA, which is decreased in stressful circumstances.

Somatic symptoms are often a learned behavior. At a young age, children in certain families learn that somatic complaints are more acceptable than expressed feelings. Children or teens with somatic symptoms often have been exposed to a family member who has a chronic physical illness. Finally, adolescents with a history of physical or sexual abuse are far more likely to develop somatic complaints or a psychosomatic disorder.

II.   **Making the diagnosis:**

    A. Evaluation/assessment: The most frequent concern that clinicians have with making a psychosomatic diagnosis is, "How can I be sure I'm not missing a rare disease?" This often leads to just one more test or consultation. Because there is no one test for psychosomatic illness, there is no safety in making the diagnosis. It hinges on observing the three basic principles mentioned at the beginning of this discussion. In addition, there is no urgency in diagnosing rare medical disorders, and *they are rare!* Astute practitioners follow and reassess their patients frequently, rather than pursuing an immediate "shotgun" approach to testing.

    Many researchers have commented on the need to proceed with the organic and the psychological investigations simultaneously, giving the implicit message to the family and patient that each is as important as the other. In many cases, however, the medical workup is done first. When it is negative, the patient is shuttled off to see a psychiatrist. Understandably, most patients (and their families) resent this, and *it is antitherapeutic.* The underlying message is, "The pains are all in your head, and I'm sending you to a 'shrink' to take care of them."

    In assessing a patient who may have a psychosomatic disorder, the first step to take is to maintain a high index of suspicion, especially if the teen is complaining of chronic abdominal pain, chest pain, or headaches. On the other hand, *even very astute practitioners cannot expect to elicit the source of stress or anxiety at the first visit, no matter how thorough a history is taken.* Other factors that may alert the practitioner to a psychosomatic diagnosis are:

- A previous history of multiple somatic complaints.
- Dysfunction in key areas of normal adolescent development: family, peers, and school.
- A history of multiple visits to different physicians.
- Presence of a "role model" within the family who has chronic or recurring symptoms.
- Presence of an "enmeshed family," in which parents tend to avoid conflict and feelings and are overprotective.
- The patient's reaction to the symptoms, which may be curiously disproportionate to his or her actual disability.

    Despite this approach, patients and their families may still be reluctant to accept the diagnosis of a psychosomatic disorder. To counteract this reluctance, clinicians can:

- Refer to the problem as "stress-related" instead of using the term "psychosomatic" or "somatoform."
- Do the organic and psychological workups simultaneously.
- Use projective testing if patients or their families are reluctant to see a mental health professional.
- Explain that a stress-related disorder is usually quite preferable to having an organic disease (e.g., stress-related abdominal pains vs. ulcerative colitis; stress headaches vs. a brain tumor).
- Try to get parents to accept the notion of stress-related problems by using common analogies: "exam diarrhea," the tension headache at the end of a busy workday, etc.
- Reassure the patient and family that further testing can always be done in the future, as needed.

      1. Chronic abdominal pain: In a classic study of 1,000 British schoolchildren, aged 4 to 15 years, 10% fit the criteria for chronic abdominal pain—at least three episodes, severe enough to restrict activity, occurring over a period of at least 3 months. All 100 of these youngsters were hospitalized for an intensive diagnostic workup, and only 5% to 8% were found to have organic lesions. Therefore, the clinician confronted with a teenager who has chronic abdominal pains can say, with perhaps 95% accuracy, that the pains are likely to be psychosomatic in origin. By contrast, the incidence of inflammatory bowel disease is quite low, for example: only 15% of all cases of ulcerative colitis occur before age 20, with an overall incidence of four to seven cases per 100,000. Crohn disease has an incidence of one to three cases per 100,000. "Common children and adolescents have common diseases" is an axiom useful in practice.

      Common organic causes of chronic abdominal pain include:

- *Constipation:* by far the most prevalent cause of chronic, organic abdominal pain, and easily diagnosable with a careful history and physical examination.
- *Lactase deficiency:* believed by many experts to be a very common cause of recurrent abdominal pain. A history of symptoms associated with milk ingestion **does not distinguish lactose malabsorbers** from others with chronic abdominal pain. Symptoms include bloating, increased cramping, and flatus but not

necessarily diarrhea. Lactase deficiency is more common among Asian, Mexican-American, Native American, Jewish, Mediterranean, and African-American populations, and lowest in Northern Europeans. A breath hydrogen test is an easy screening test for this disorder.

- *Irritable bowel syndrome (IBS):* a confusing disorder. Is IBS the equivalent of chronic abdominal pain in childhood or adolescence? Several studies indicate that there may, in fact, be significant overlap. But IBS requires not only recurrent pain but a dysfunctional pattern of elimination as well—diarrhea, constipation, or alternating diarrhea and constipation.
- *Gastroesophageal reflux:* usually responds rapidly to antireflux or antiacid medications.

Two disorders *not* on the list are chronic appendicitis and *H. Pylori* infection. Although appendicitis is often the *first* disorder that parents will think of when their teenagers have abdominal symptoms, people carry only a 7% *lifetime* risk for it, and it should not be considered in the differential diagnosis of chronic abdominal pain. Since *H. Pylori* is now known to cause peptic ulcer disease, researchers have tried to link it with chronic abdominal pain as well, with no real success.

A basic workup should probably include a complete blood count (CBC), erythrocyte sedimentation rate, urinalysis, stools for occult blood and, in select cases, ova and parasites, and a pregnancy test for young women. Sexually active female adolescents should also be tested for sexually transmitted diseases (STDs) and have at least a bimanual exam because of the possibility of subacute or chronic pelvic inflammatory disease.

2. **Chronic chest pain:** Chest pains in teenagers are not as common as abdominal pains, but they do account for 650,000 visits annually for teenagers seen in primary care settings, or three per 1,000. In a one-year study of all children and teens seen in a busy emergency room of a large children's hospital, a total of 407 had chest pain, with a mean age of 12 to 14 years. The symptom was present for longer than 6 months in about one-quarter of them. Many prospective and retrospective studies have found the following distribution of diagnoses:
   - 35% Musculoskeletal (including trauma and costochondritis)
   - 30% Idiopathic
   - 25% Psychosomatic (including hyperventilation)
   - 10% Miscellaneous (respiratory, cardiac, breast abnormalities, esophagitis)

   Hyperventilation can be a particularly difficult diagnosis to make because patients are completely unaware of their behavior. More than half report anxiety, paresthesias, or light-headedness, but few are aware of breathing too fast and too shallowly. Although having the patient hyperventilate to try to reproduce the symptoms is a common maneuver, it may take 20 to 30 minutes to reproduce the pains. Closely related to hyperventilation are panic attacks. These are characterized by a massive autonomic system discharge, associated with overwhelming feelings of anxiety. A predisposition to panic attacks may be inherited.

   Besides a careful history and physical exam, care should be taken to palpate all costochondral junctions using the firm pressure of two fingers, to elicit costochondritis. A basic workup might include a chest x-ray and electrocardiogram (ECG), depending on the type and severity of the symptoms.

   Given the benign nature of most of these diagnoses, it may be surprising to learn that teenagers take their chest pains very seriously: more than 50% fear heart disease, and 12% worry about cancer. How the clinician inquires about the pains may be extremely important (see Table 24-3).

Table 24-3. Importance of phrasing questions carefully when evaluating psychosomatic chest pain

	"What do you think caused your pain?"		"What were you afraid caused your pain?"	
Heart attack	4%	⎫	44%	⎫
Heart disease	6%	⎬ 12%	12%	⎬ 68%
Cancer	2%	⎭	12%	⎭
Gas	7%		0%	
Do not know	61%		23%	
Miscellaneous	20%		9%	

From Pantell RH, Goodman BW Jr. Adolescent chest pain: a prospective study. *Pediatr* 1983;71:881. Copyright © American Academy of Pediatrics. Reprinted with permission.

Table 24-4. Features of brain tumor headaches

- Recent onset of headaches (within past 4 months)
- Presence or onset of neurological abnormality, especially ocular findings (papilledema, decreased acuity, or loss of vision)
- Persistent vomiting
- Increased severity of headache
- Headache awakening patient from sleep

Adapted from Honig PJ, Charney EB. Children with brain tumor headaches. *Am J Dis Child* 1982;136:121.

3. **Chronic headaches:** Headaches are extremely common during childhood and adolescence, with incidences as high as 21% to 55% of all children and teens in studies. Migraine headaches affect 4% to 10%. Data from national surveys indicate that nearly 5% of teens suffer from frequent or severe headaches.

   The fear of missing an early brain tumor is nearly universal among practitioners. Yet brain tumors occur only rarely during adolescence, with an incidence of two to three cases per 100,000. Despite the availability of high-tech scans, the best screening test is still a careful neurological exam, which will identify all but 5% to 6% of patients with brain tumors (Tables 24-4 and 24-5). In one unique study of children with headaches secondary to brain tumors, 85% of them manifested neurologic or ocular abnormalities within 2 months of the onset of their headaches. Two-thirds of the patients were awakened from sleep with their headaches, and more than three-fourths had associated vomiting.

   Unlike with abdominal or chest pains, there is no basic workup here, and walking the tightrope between doing too few diagnostic tests and too many can be difficult. Asking the patient to keep a headache diary is useful (Figure 24-3). For example, headaches that remit on weekends or in different environments should lead to an investigation of situational stressors. Depressed teenagers may demonstrate other features, such as a decline in school performance, sleep difficulties, or an abnormal score on a depression inventory. On the other hand, simple disorders such as chronic sinusitis or refractive errors should also be considered. One series of patients with chronic headaches found a 10% incidence of abnormal sinus films, and the patients all responded to medical treatment for sinusitis. In general, neuroimaging [e.g., magnetic resonance imaging (MRI) and computed tomography (CT)] should be reserved for those patients with specific neurological signs or symptoms or those who have life-threatening or acutely reversible conditions.

III.   **Management:**
   A. **Treatment:** A carefully crafted initial workup, which includes some means of assessing the teenager and his or her family's psychological function, will serve as a prelude to successful treatment of psychosomatic disorders. A variety of treatment options are available.
   B. **Counseling and psychotherapy:** Primary care clinicians are often the ideal people to do counseling, which is quite different from psychotherapy (Table 24-6). Often,

Table 24-5. Differential diagnosis of headaches

History	Headache type		
	Migraine	Tension	Organic
Acute onset	+	−	±
Daily frequency	−	+	±
Nausea or vomiting	+	−	±
Fever	−	−	±
Neurologic signs	±	−	+
Family history of headache	±	±	±
Signs of depression	−	+	−
Stress at school/home	±	+	−
Appears ill during headache	+	−	+

Adapted from Olness KN, MacDonald JT. Recurrent headaches in children: diagnosis and treatment. *Pediatr Rev* 1987;8:307. Copyright © American Academy of Pediatrics. Reprinted with permission.

Date _____   Name _____

CIRCLE ANSWER

1. How long did headadache last?
   1   2   3   4   5   >6   hours
2. Vomiting?   How many times?
   Yes   No _____
3. Did child practice relaxation exercise?
   Yes   No
4. Child slept to relieve headache?
   Yes   No
5. Drug given during headache?
   Aspirin   Tylenol   Midrin   Fiorinal
   Cafergot   Other _____
6. How severe was the headache?
   0   1   2   3   4   5   6   7   8   9   10
7. If school day, did you stay home?
   Yes   No

Figure 24-3. Sample headache diary. (From Olness KN, MacDonald JT. Recurrent headaches in children. *Pediatr Rev* 1987;8:307. Copyright © American Academy of Pediatrics. Reprinted with permission.)

patients and their families will not accept a psychotherapist; but a clinician who has had a long-term relationship with the patient may be able to engage him or her quite easily. Counseling can focus on the source of stress and discuss alternative ways of coping with it (Table 24-7). To relinquish the symptom, the patient will require another strategy for dealing with the particular stress that is less costly psychologically. Patients with more severe personality disturbances or marked anxiety may require assessment or treatment by a skilled child and adolescent psychiatrist. Anti-anxiety medications should probably only be used in consultation with a psychiatrist unless the clinician is highly skilled in psychopharmacology.

1. **Relaxation training:** Highly motivated or suggestive teens can learn to identify certain bodily cues that signal tension and then relax the muscles involved. Relaxation training, guided imagery, or self-hypnosis all accomplish this. They are particularly useful for teens who have chronic tension headaches or migraines or who are undergoing chemotherapy.
2. **Biofeedback:** Teens who are particularly somatic or who are not insightful or verbal may find that biofeedback is ideal. It is also well tolerated by families who continue to deny the psychosomatic nature of their teen's symptoms but are desperate to see them brought under control. A machine that measures galvanic skin

Table 24-6. Counseling versus psychotherapy

Counseling	Psychotherapy
Primary care provider	Mental health professional
Short-term (<6 months)	Short- or long-term
Shorter visits	Longer visits
No transference	Transference and counter transference
Supportive	Insight-oriented
Can bill for additional face-to-face time	Billing more straightforward
More easily tolerated by adolescents	Sometimes difficult for adolescents, especially young males
No medications	Psychotropic medications may be needed

Table 24-7. Methods of coping with stress

* Anticipating the stress
* Understanding and accepting the stress
* Family and social support
* Rehearsing a response to the stress
* Conditioning/practice/relaxation response
* Biofeedback
* Controlled breathing
* Changing the stressful situation or environment

response or temperature is used, and the conditions of stress and of relaxation are systematically rehearsed. Teenagers with chronic headaches, chest pains, or abdominal pains may find this technique useful.

   C. **Behavioral and environmental interventions:** When stressors can be anticipated, or the stress can be rehearsed, the patient is less likely to experience distress. Clinicians can help teens with two different coping strategies, "emotion-focused" coping (dealing with one's feelings without changing the stressor) and "problem-focused" coping (changing the stress).

   1. **Changing a teen's environment:** It may be difficult, but sometimes a minor alteration can help—for example, speaking with a particularly difficult teacher, arranging for an alternative class or a tutor. In abusive situations, removing the teenager from the environment may be necessary.

   2. **Family therapy:** Severe symptoms, conversion reactions, and noncompliance with medical protocols may all necessitate family-oriented intervention. Family therapy will ordinarily require a skilled mental health professional (e.g., social worker, psychologist, or psychiatrist).

IV. **Clinical pearls and pitfalls:**

   * Teenagers with psychosomatic illness don't *present* with psychological symptoms: they present with organic symptoms, like headaches, chest pain, or abdominal pains.
   * Even the most gifted clinician will be unable to divine the psychological roots of the illness on the first visit.
   * The most successful approach to psychosomatic illness is to work up the organic and the psychological aspects *simultaneously.*
   * The extent of the organic work-up will vary from patient to patient, depending on the symptoms. Do whatever is necessary to rule out organic illness, but remember that "common diseases present commonly."
   * Referral to an organ-system subspecialist will usually result in major and expensive testing being done. They have what they consider to be an absolute duty to rule out organic illness in their particular specialty, and they will use all the means at their disposal to do so.
   * If chronic abdominal pains are "crampy" in nature, then a trial of Bentyl, 10 to 20 mg. PO q.i.d. may be useful as an antispasmodic.
   * Psychosomatic pains are as "real" as organic pains.
   * Although families may resist the diagnosis of a psychosomatic illness, they can usually be persuaded that stress-related headaches are far preferable to brain tumors or that stress-related abdominal pains are preferable to inflammatory bowel disease.

BIBLIOGRAPHY

For the clinician

Annequin D, Tournaire B, Massiou H. Migraine and headache in childhood and adolescence. *Pediatr Clin North Am* 2000;47:617–631.

Hyams JS. Irritable bowel syndrome, functional dyspepsia, and functional abdominal pain syndrome. *Adolesc Med* 2004;15:1–15.

Kinsman S. Caring for the adolescent with somatic concerns. *Adolescent Health Update* 2004;16:1–9.

Li B ed. Recurrent abdominal pain in children. *Pediatr Ann* 2004;33:78–148.

Liang S-W, Boyce WT. The psychobiology of childhood stress. *Curr Opin Pediatr* 1993;5:545–551.

Owens TR. Chest pain in the adolescent. *Adolesc Med State Art Rev* 2000;12:95–104.

Reeve A, Strasburger VC. Is it "real" or is it psychosomatic? Principles of psychosomatic medicine in children and adolescents. In: Greydanus D, ed. *Behavioral pediatrics*. Elk Grove Village, IL: American Academy of Pediatrics, 2005.

Silber TJ, Pao M. Somatization disorders in children and adolescents. *Pediatr Rev* 2003;24:255–264.

Slater JA. Deciphering emotional aches and physical pains in children. *Pediatr Ann* 2003;32: 402–407.

WEB SITES

www.headaches.org   Web site for the National Headache Foundation

www.iffgd.org   Web site for the International Foundation for Functional Gastrointestinal Diseases

www.merck.com/mrkshared/mmanual/section19/chapter26   Merck manual on recurrent abdominal pain

www.postgradmed.com/issues/2000/11_00/holloway.htm   Postgraduate Medicine online article about somatization disorder

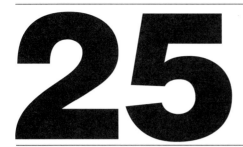

Adolescent Violence and Suicide

I hope I die before I get old.

—Lyrics from "My Generation" by The Who

I. **Violence**
  A. **Description of the problem:** Contemporary adolescents are experiencing one of the most violent cultures in the history of the United States. However, they are not just experiencing it: sometimes they are perpetrating it as well.
  B. **Epidemiology:** Violence among adolescents has become one of the most pressing issues in contemporary health care. Increasingly, clinicians who treat teenagers need to be aware of the public health aspects of adolescence, and the data are sometimes chilling:
    • Ten percent of American children report being **bullied** at school.
    • Homicide and suicide are the second and third leading causes of death among teenagers.
    • Many teens have either been victimized by violence or witnessed violence (Table 25-1).
    • More than 400,000 youth ages 10 to 19 were injured as a result of violence in the year 2000.
    • In the 2003 Youth Risk Behavior Survey, which surveyed more than 15,000 students in grades 9 through 12 in 150 schools throughout the US:
      • One-third reported being in a physical fight during the previous 12 months.
      • More than 17% had carried a weapon to school during the previous month. Ten percent of males had carried a gun to school.
      • Six percent of students who missed school in the month prior to being interviewed say that they felt unsafe, either at school or on their way to or from school.
      • Nine percent of students report being hit, slapped, or hurt on purpose by a girlfriend or boyfriend during the previous 12 months.
      • Nine percent of females and half as many males report ever being forced to have sexual intercourse when they did not want to.
    • **Homicide** is the second leading cause of death among older adolescents (after injuries, particularly automobile accidents). In the 15 to 24 year old age group, it is actually the leading cause of death among African Americans.

Table 25-1. Adolescents' exposure to violence

Type of violence	Cleveland		Small Ohio city	
	M	F	M	F
Victimized by violence:				
Threatened at home	24%	25%	29%	32%
Threatened at school	35%	31%	48%	39%
Beaten at home	9%	10%	6%	9%
Sexually abused/assaulted	7%	16%	4%	17%
Shot at or shot	33%	10%	19%	4%
Witnessing violence:				
Threat at school	82%	79%	89%	88%
Beating at school	75%	75%	82%	82%
Shooting	62%	49%	36%	25%

Adapted from Singer MI, Anglin TM, Song LY, et al. Adolescents' exposure to violence and associated symptoms of psychological trauma. *JAMA* 1995;273:477.

Table 25-2. Risk factors for violence in adolescence

Individual
- History of early aggression
- Beliefs supportive of violence
- Exposure to violent media
- Being male
- Bullying
- History of setting fires or cruelty to animals
- Use of alcohol or other drugs

Family
- Low socioeconomic status
- Exposure to violence at home
- Poor emotional attachment to parents
- Parental alcohol or drug use
- Access to firearms

Peer/school
- Poor school performance
- Association with problem peers

Adapted from "Youth Violence Facts," National Center for Injury Prevention and Control. Available at http://www.cdc.gov/ncipc/factsheets/yvfacts.htm. Accessed on March 8, 2004.

- In 1999, 4,998 youths aged 15 to 24 were murdered, an average of 14 per day.
- In 2000, 80% of murder victims ages 13 to 19 were killed with a firearm.
- **Suicide** represents the third leading cause of death among adolescents. In 1999, more young people died from suicide than from cancer, heart disease, AIDS, and birth defects combined.
- From 1952 to 1995, the suicide rate among adolescents has tripled. In 1998, 4,135 suicides occurred among 15 to 24 year olds. Younger teens, ages 12 to 15, accounted for another 514 suicides.
- Criminal arrests of youths were actually lower in 1999 than in 1983; however, rates for **aggravated assault** were nearly 70% higher.

C. **Role of the clinician:** Increasingly, clinicians are being asked to identify and to evaluate teenagers who have a potential for violence. Many risk factors are now known (Table 25-2), and health care workers need to be proactive in identifying susceptible youth and getting mental health and social services for them. Obviously, many of these factors would require a platoon of psychologists and social workers to make a successful intervention. But with others, the primary care clinician *can* have an impact. For example, aggressive counseling about television and other media with parents of infants can pay rich dividends later on:

- *Studies show that one-fourth of all very young children, one-third of all school-children, and one-half of all teenagers in the US have a television set in their own bedroom.* Parents of young children should be counseled to keep television sets out of their children's bedrooms, to limit total media time to no more than 1 to 2 hours per day, and to be very careful about letting young children view media violence.
- Of all of the areas of media impact, exposure to violence has been the best studied, with more than 3,000 studies finding that children learn violent attitudes and behavior from seeing them demonstrated on the TV screen.
- In the most recent content analysis of American television, involving nearly 10,000 hours of programming, 57% of the shows contained some violence, negative consequences were rarely portrayed (16% of the time), and only 4% of shows had an antiviolence theme.
- Although media violence is estimated to cause perhaps only 10% to 20% of real-life violence, changing the nature of programming seems far easier than eliminating poverty, racism, or the family and individual factors that probably play a greater role in fostering violence. The link between media violence and aggressive behavior is nearly as strong as the link between smoking and lung cancer (Figure 25-1).

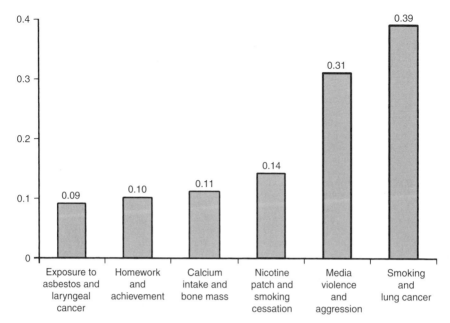

Figure 25-1. The connection between media violence and real-life violence is nearly as strong as the connection between smoking and lung cancer. (Bushman BJ, Huesmann LR. Effects of televised violence on aggression. In Singer DG, Singer JL, eds. *Handbook of children and the media.* Thousand Oaks, CA: Sage 2002:223–254. Copyright © 2002 by Sage Publications. From Strasburger VC, Wilson BJ. *Children, adolescents, and the media.* Thousand Oaks, CA: Sage 2002;382. Copyright © 2002 by Sage Publications. Reprinted by permission of Sage Publications.)

    D. Making the diagnosis:
       1. **Screening:** Clinicians can learn to do a **violence risk assessment,** ideally in the context of a comprehensive psychosocial screen. A simple checklist of questions may yield surprising results:
         • Does the teenager look toward the future?
         • Has the teenager been exposed to violence at home, in his neighborhood, or through the media?
         • How does the teenager typically cope with anger?
         • Does the teenager feel safe at home and at school?
         • Would the teenager ever consider fighting? (See Table 25-3).
         • Has the teenager ever been injured in a fight?

Table 25-3. Get out of my face

Violent interactions are characterized by four basic levels of escalating behavior:

Level 1: One teen calls another a name or says something insulting or disrespectful. If this doesn't get the desired response, the confrontation progresses to level 2.

Level 2: Insulting the target's mother or a family member. If the victim remains calm, the insulter moves to level 3.

Level 3: Invading body space ("getting in your face"). Finally, if the victim has not succeeded in de-escalating the exchange, the aggressor touches or pushes ("he was all over me").

Level 4: The aggressive response. Once an adolescent is touched, it is rare for them to walk away. Retreating means risking being labeled a punk or being repeatedly victimized.

From Ginsburg KR. Guiding adolescents away from violence. *Contemp Pediatr* 1997;14:101–111, with permission. Contemporary Pediatrics is a copyrighted publication of Advanstar Communications, Inc. All rights reserved.

II.   **Bullying**
  A. **Description of the problem:** Bullying has also come to the forefront in the past few years. It is defined as a form of aggression in which teens repeatedly and intentionally harm, harass, or intimidate a victim who is seen as unable to defend himself. The harassment can be physical or verbal.
  B. **Epidemiology:** Although studies cite 10% as the number of children who have been bullied in the US, other research suggests that the majority of teens face some sort of harassment during their school careers. Older children and teens may not report being bullied; instead, they may show signs of anxiety, depression, or school phobia or refusal.
  C. **Role of the clinician:** The role of the clinician in this area is 4-fold:
     1. Identifying the problem
     2. Counseling parents, patients, and school personnel
     3. Making mental health referrals when necessary
     4. Advocating for school violence-prevention programs
III.   **Management of adolescent violence and bullying:**
  A. **Educational/behavioral management:** Clinicians often reality-test teenagers in other situations (e.g., the teenager who thinks that she wants to get pregnant). Violence prevention can take a similar tack in the office setting. Ask high-risk teens, "What would you do if…?" Map out the long-range consequences of violent retaliation (Figure 25-2). One traditional office practice that is not likely to work is lecturing or offering facts about violence. Behavioral change requires not only that people recognize a problem and want to change it but that they possess the skills to change the problem as well.
  B. **Counseling on guns:** Probably the most important part of counseling teens and their families is to ask, "Is there a gun in the house?" This question should now be a part of every pediatric and adolescent health check-up. Guns—particularly handguns—play a key role in the cascade of violence:
     • America is the most heavily armed nation on earth, with more guns (230 million) than households (200 million). Approximately one-third of families with children or teenagers report owning guns.
     • Firearms—mostly handguns—are involved in two-third to three-fourths of all homicides. In 2001, there were nearly 30,000 firearm-related deaths in the US.

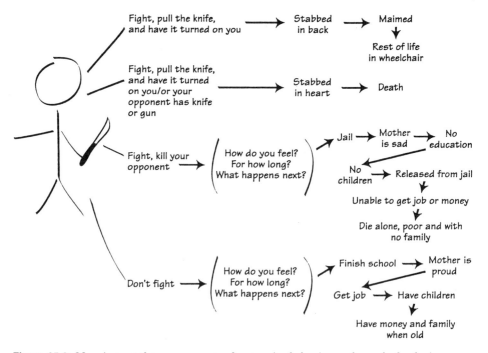

Figure 25-2. Mapping out the consequences of aggressive behavior—a form of role-playing—may be useful in persuading some teens in avoiding violence. (From Ginsburg KR. Guiding adolescents away from violence. *Contemp Pediatr* 1997;14:105. Contemporary Pediatrics is a copyrighted publication of Advanstar Communications, Inc. All rights reserved.)

- The US has the highest homicide rate among the 21 most industrialized countries. A child growing up in the US is 12 times more likely to die from a shooting than a child in 25 other Western countries.
- In 2000, 1,776 children and teens were murdered with guns, 1,007 committed suicide with guns, and 193 died in unintentional shootings. This makes a total of 3,042 young people who were killed by firearms in the US, an average of one every 3 hours.
- In 2001, suicides with firearms accounted for 54% of all suicides among 15 to 23 year olds. Guns are used in 88% of teen male suicides but only 12% of teen female suicides.
- For every child or teen killed by a gun, four are wounded.
- On primetime television, 25% of the violent episodes involve gunplay.

Admittedly, guns and gun control are "hot-button" topics. But from a purely public-health perspective, practitioners would do well to counsel families about firearms, particularly handguns. **The current epidemic of handgun injuries is ten times larger than the polio epidemic in the 1950s.** Specifically, patients and their parents need to know that:

- Although people say that they are purchasing handguns for protection, a gun in the home is 43 times more likely to kill a family member than an intruder.
- Adolescents and handguns do not make a good combination. Teen suicide is nearly 10 times more likely if a handgun is present at home. Guns are a particular risk in the suicide of teens who do not have any apparent psychiatric disorder.
- The Second Amendment of the US Constitution poses no obstacle to broad gun control legislation, according to several Supreme Court rulings.

IV. **Clinical pearls and pitfalls:**
- Consider the possibility that aggressive adolescents may be suffering from a "masked depression."
- Most violence represents a *learned behavior.* Minimizing exposure to violent media (especially first-person shooter video games and violent movies) at a young age is extremely important.

BIBLIOGRAPHY

For the clinician

American Academy of Pediatrics. The role of the pediatrician in youth violence prevention in clinical practice and at the community level. *Pediatr* 1999;103:173–181.

American Academy of Pediatrics. Firearm-related injuries affecting the pediatric population. *Pediatr* 2000;105:888–895.

Centers for Disease Control. Youth risk behavior surveillance—United States, 2001. *MMWR Morb Mortal Wkly Rep* 2002;51(SS-4):1–68.

Fleishman AR, Barondess JA. Adolescent suicide: vigilance and action to reduce the toll. *Contemp Pediatr* 2004;21:27–35.

Ginsburg KR. Guiding adolescents away from violence. *Contemp Pediatr* 1997;14:101–111.

Glew G, Rivara F, Feudtner C. Bullying: children hurting children. *Pediatr Rev* 2000;21:183–190.

Gutgesell ME, Payne N. Issues of adolescent psychological development in the 21st century. *Pediatr Rev* 2004;25:79–85.

Lyznicki JM, McCaffree MA, Robinowitz CB. Childhood bullying: implications for physicians. *Am Fam Physician* 2004;70:1723–1730.

Strasburger VC. Children, adolescents, and the media. *Curr Probl Pediatr Adolesc Health Care* 2004;34(2):54–113.

Teplin LA, McClelland GM, Abram KM, Mileusnic D. Early violent death among delinquent youths: a prospective longitudinal study. *Pediatr* 2005;115:1586–1593.

WEB SITES

www.cdc.gov/ncipc   Web site for the CDC's National Center for Injury Prevention and Control

www.bradycampaign.org   Web site for the Brady Campaign to Prevent Gun Violence

www.safeyouth.org   Web site for the National Youth Violence Prevention Resource Center

I. **Suicide**
A. **Epidemiology:**
1. **General:** Many people would be surprised to learn that adolescent suicide is relatively uncommon and that teenagers actually have lower rates of completed suicides than adults. In 2000, suicides among people under age 25 "only" accounted for 15% of the total. Yet teenage suicide is considered (rightfully) a serious and important health problem and is the third leading cause of death among adolescents.

Clearly, any loss of life during childhood or adolescence is tragic, given the potential for a full and productive lifespan of perhaps 70 to 80 years. Suicide does account for 12% of the overall mortality during adolescence. But completed suicides represent only the tip of the iceberg: for every completed suicide, there are an estimated 100 to 200 attempts. Female attempts outnumber male attempts by 4:1, but male adolescents complete suicide by a 6:1 margin. This is primarily due to their use of more lethal means (i.e., handguns and hanging).

One common misconception is that suicidal intent presupposes a mature view of death. In fact, in a classic study of nearly 600 13 to 16 year olds, researchers found that 20% thought that they would still be cognizant after death, 60% envisioned some sort of spiritual continuation, and only 20% thought death involved total cessation. Thus, it may be useful to ask teenagers who have made suicide attempts what they think would have happened had they succeeded. Such a question may tap into some substantial fantasies.

2. **Suicides:** From 1952 to 1995, the suicide rate for 15 to 19 year olds tripled. In 1999, more teens and young adults died from suicide than from all medical causes combined. Currently, the suicide rate for young people aged 15 to 24 is 11.1 per 100,000. For young people ages 5 to 14, the rates are considerably lower: 0.8 per 100,000. Estimates of the lifetime prevalence of adolescent suicide attempts range from 2% to 8% of all teenagers.

Suicide rates differ considerably by race, ethnicity, and sexual orientation. Certain Native American males have the highest rates (Arapahoe, Shoshone); African American females have the lowest rates. White males have higher rates than African American males. A large Minnesota study of students in grades 7 through 12 found that 28% of bisexual or homosexual males and 20% of bisexual or homosexual females had attempted suicide.

3. **Method:** Handguns have revolutionized teenage suicide. For both sexes, firearms are the most common method of completed suicide, particularly when alcohol is also involved, and the suicide rate by firearms remains higher than any other method (Figure 25-3). Considerable evidence now exists that the suicide rate is

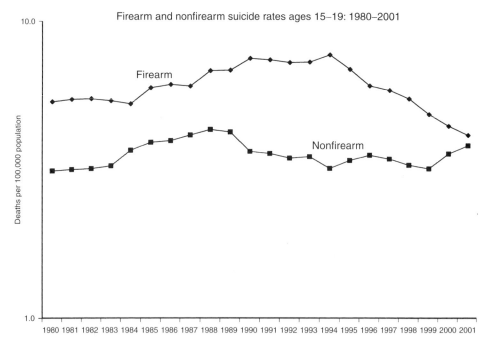

Figure 25-3. Firearm suicide among adolescents, 1981–2001. (From Fingerhut L, unpublished data, with permission.)

directly correlated with the sales and ownership of handguns and is inversely proportional to the restrictiveness of handgun control laws. One study in North Carolina found that half of all male adolescents own a gun. In another study of high-risk adolescents, as many as 20% report playing Russian roulette, usually in conjunction with use of alcohol or other drugs. Even when their teens have already made one suicide attempt, one-fourth of families who own guns refuse to get rid of them.

After firearms, hanging is the next most common method for male teenagers. Toxic ingestions and wrist slashing are the two most common methods for females attempting suicide.

4. **Suicidal ideation:** Adolescence can be a time of emotional shifts and turmoil; therefore, suicidal thoughts are not uncommon. According to the 2003 Youth Risk Behavior Survey:

- 29% of high school students felt sad or hopeless during the year prior to being surveyed
- 17% seriously considered suicide
- 17% made a suicide plan

Other studies have found rates of suicidal ideation as high as nearly half of teenagers surveyed, depending on their age and how the questions are asked. In addition, some teenagers go through a period of fascination with death. They may write about death in journals, wear black clothes, explore Satanism, and listen to heavy metal lyrics that are moody or violent. Distinguishing among those teens who are experimenting philosophically and those who are depressed and at risk can be difficult. According to the psychiatric literature, teens who escalate to suicide attempts appear to want help or attention, to escape a stressful situation, or to express anger or love. They have inadequate personal resources to cope with these feelings in alternative, nonharmful ways.

B. **Psychopathology:** Experts believe that as many as 90% of all adolescents who commit suicide and 80% of those who attempt suicide have had previous psychiatric symptoms. Using a technique called a *psychological autopsy,* researchers can piece together a full psychological profile of victims, even after their death. In most teenagers, significant symptoms have existed for months or even years, although the exact diagnosis was not apparent until too late in many cases. Most commonly, these psychological problems include depression, alcohol or substance abuse, aggressive behavior or conduct disorders, or anxiety disorders. Obviously, depression is of particular concern; 85% of depressed teens report having suicidal ideation, and one-third have attempted suicide during their adolescence. Similarly, approximately one-half of all male teens who commit suicide and two-thirds of female teens suffered from a depressive disorder. Of interest to clinicians: **half of all teenagers committing suicide have had contact with a mental health professional, and 35% to 45% have had a previous suicide attempt.** Of these, only 10% had received antidepressant medication.

Some researchers believe that there are four broad categories of adolescent suicide victims:

- 50%: Teens with a long history of school and behavior problems, fighting, and impulsiveness.
- 20%–25%: Depressed females.
- 20%–25%: Anxious, perfectionistic, rigid teenagers who are otherwise "model children," performing well at school.
- 1%–2%: Psychotic adolescents.

C. **Contributing factors:**
1. **Stress, loss, and conflict:** Traditionally, loss has been viewed as the cornerstone of suicide attempts. The loss could involve the loss of parents' divorcing, friends moving away, siblings dying, or "loss of face"—a previous honors student being caught shoplifting or getting an F on an exam, or facing a disciplinary crisis or humiliation. Environmental or family stress is important, as is interpersonal conflict or fighting. Hopelessness, impulsivity, and anxiety are also important antecedent psychological traits. However, adults need to be cognizant of the fact that adolescents may not share their parents' view of what actually constitutes stress (See Chapter 24, Tables 24-1 and 24-2). In one study of patients age 14 years and under admitted to a psychiatric unit after a suicide attempt, 80% had experienced a loss (death of a parent or sibling *or* loss of a possession!), and two-thirds had witnessed their parents fighting physically or had been physically abused themselves.

2. **Drugs:** Approximately half of all teen suicides involve the use of alcohol, which can increase impulsivity and impair judgment. Alcohol is particularly significant in the suicides of young male adults, ages 18 and older.

3. **Sexual abuse:** Physical abuse may increase the risk of suicide as much as 5-fold, and sexual abuse 3-fold.

4. **History of prior attempts:** *The single most significant predictor for suicide is a history of past suicide attempts.* This is one of many reasons why nonlethal attempts, self-inflicted wounds, and so-called "gestures" should never be underestimated.

5. **Contagion:** Epidemics of suicide have occurred throughout history—from the young women of Miletus in ancient Greece, to 665 A.D. when English people jumped from seaside cliffs to avoid catching the plague, to imitators of Goethe's *The Sorrows of Young Werther* in Germany in 1774, to present-day outbreaks in New Jersey and New Mexico. In Germany, a TV station broadcast a story about a teenager who committed suicide by lying on a railroad track. Several suicides by this method ensued. Although some critics were skeptical, when a TV program aired several years later highlighting this story, a recurrence of suicides occurred. Although teens seem to be uniquely susceptible to this type of imitative behavior, only 5% of suicides occur in clusters.

   Case-control studies have found that adolescent suicide victims are more likely to have been exposed to a suicide, either in real-life or in the media, than were their closest friends. Surviving friends and siblings of adolescent suicide victims also experience increased rates of depression and suicidal ideation. Such exposure probably serves as a catalyst for those teens already predisposed to making an attempt. Clinicians need to be aware of publicity surrounding suicides in their community or upcoming made-for-TV movies and be particularly vigilant for signs of depression or suicidal ideation in their adolescent patients.

6. **Homosexuality:** Several studies have found that gay, lesbian, and bisexual teens are at increased risk for suicide. In the previous year before being studied, up to 42% of these teens have suicidal ideation and more than one-fourth have made a suicide attempt. Gay and bisexual adolescents face considerable stigmatization surrounding their sexual orientation and have increased rates of substance abuse and depression as well, thus amplifying their risk of suicide.

7. **Biologic factors:** Research is beginning to establish a link between serotonin metabolism and the risk of depression and suicide. Adult studies have found that suicide victims have low levels of 5-hydroxyindoleacetic acid (5-HIAA), a serotonin metabolite, in their cerebrospinal fluid (CSF) and in prefrontal cortical tissue. In one study that looked at CSF samples in adult suicide attempters, researchers found a 10-fold increased risk of completed suicide within a year if levels of 5-HIAA were below 90 nmoles/L. Studies have also identified a peripheral marker of impaired serotonin metabolism in depressed or suicidal adults: increased platelet serotonin-2 receptor binding sites. Another test being studied is the Fenfluramine Challenge: Fenfluramine is a serotonergic drug that induces the release of prolactin. In a depressed patient, fenfluramine will yield only a small increase in prolactin 6 hours later rather than a large increase. It is entirely possible that, in the near future, a lumbar puncture or venous blood sample for serotonin metabolites will become part of the routine work-up.

II. **Assessing the suicidal teenager:** *All suicide attempts are serious and should be taken seriously.* The term "suicide gesture" is misleading, inappropriate, and should be avoided. Some have used it to try to designate a suicide attempt of high impulsivity and low lethality—in other words, one that, ostensibly, should not be taken seriously by the clinician involved. In fact, *any teenager who attempts suicide—even if he or she only swallows a handful of pills—deserves hospitalization in an adolescent medical unit, at least overnight.* Although this is not a popular recommendation by managed care standards, medico-legally it is one that will save a lot of time, trouble, and potential lawsuits. Even a 24- to 48-hour hospitalization accomplishes several important tasks:

   • It removes the teenager from his or her previously stressful environment.
   • It ensures that a reattempt will not be made immediately.
   • It serves as a signal to both the teenager and the parents that a serious threat exists to the teenager's health and well-being.
   • It allows the primary clinician and the mental health professional to make a joint assessment of the patient and determine if he or she requires further hospitalization in a psychiatric unit (this occurs only 10% of the time, according to the research).
   • It allows the mental health professional to make an initial contact with the teenager so that he or she will comply with outpatient treatment.

Hospitalization can be avoided only if a mental health appointment can be made for that same day, or the patient is already in therapy and the therapist is available that day. The choice is between gambling on giving a teenager an appointment with a mental health specialist that will be kept only 33% of the time versus keeping the teen in a protected environment for a full assessment. The former risks a completed suicide (and subsequent lawsuit); the latter ensures the patient's safety. Making a verbal or written contract with the patient not to commit suicide has traditionally been used and may give some insight into the patient's suicidal intent, but there is no evidence that contracts prevent future suicides.

What about suicidal ideation, or the teenager who may or may not be planning suicide? *All* teenagers should be asked about depression and suicidal ideation at routine health checkups. Research shows that teenagers *will* usually reveal suicidal thoughts if asked directly. In an otherwise healthy-appearing teenager, a single screening question might suffice:
• Have you ever felt so unhappy or depressed that you wished that you weren't alive?

If the answer is yes, or if the teenager shows evidence of being depressed or having a "masked" depression (with acting-out behaviors or psychosomatic symptoms "masking" the depression), then further relevant questions are:
• Have you ever thought about hurting yourself intentionally?
• Have you ever thought about trying to kill yourself?
• Have you ever made any suicide attempts in the past?
• Do you have a plan or means for trying to hurt yourself?
• Is there a gun at home, or do you have access to a gun?
• Do you know of anyone who has committed suicide recently? Is there a history of mental illness in your family?
• Do you use alcohol, marijuana, or other drugs?
• Has anything bad happened to you recently (e.g., a loss of any kind)?

There is no scientific evidence that asking about suicidal thoughts or behavior "puts ideas into the heads" of teenagers who are depressed or suicidal. In fact, suicidal adolescents are often relieved to know that someone will come to their aid. Obviously, if significant ideation or a plan is found, then confidentiality *must* be breached. Because suicide in adolescence is often impulsive, clinicians need to inquire about the availability of lethal methods at home (e.g., guns, medications, etc.). They also need to ask their depressed patients directly about suicidal thoughts and intent.

III. **Management:**
   A. **Prevention of adolescent suicide:** With one new exception, there is no evidence that specific suicide prevention curricula can predict or prevent adolescent suicide. In fact, giving lectures about suicide, encouraging suicidal students to identify themselves, or trying to teach students how to identify suicidal friends may actually undermine protective factors, according to some experts. Rather, prevention efforts need to focus on identifying youth at risk, limiting access to lethal agents, and restraining the media. On the other hand, data from the National Longitudinal Study of Adolescent Health demonstrate that perceived connectedness to parents and family, emotional well-being, and academic success serve as important protective factors against suicide (with a 70%–85% reduction if all three protective factors are present, across all groups). In addition, one study has documented that as antidepressant medications have been increasingly prescribed to adolescents, there have been corresponding declines in adolescent suicide rates.
   1. **School programs:** Only a few studies have examined the effectiveness of school-based suicide prevention programs, and the results are not encouraging. According to experts, attempts at school-based curricula must emphasize the following concepts:
      • Suicide is a permanent solution to a temporary problem that can be improved.
      • Death is permanent and final and does not allow the teenager any satisfaction from whatever ensues after his or her death.
      • Suicidal thoughts are common, but if they persist, help should be sought.
      • People who commit suicide are dysfunctional and, sadly, lack the ability to find help for problems that are usually solvable.

      Currently, researchers are pioneering a program that simply surveys students and asks them to identify themselves if they are suicidal (see www.afsp.org). Preliminary data from more than 1,500 students at five high schools show that 15.5% will do so. Of the students surveyed, approximately 4% were deemed in need of psychiatric referral. Few of those were receiving treatment, and half had not been picked out by school psychologists or social workers. The questionnaire takes 15 minutes to complete and is inexpensive. It may become the next important tool in reducing teen suicides.

2. **Hotlines:** Since the 1970s, suicide hotlines have been a traditionally popular strategy to try to prevent suicide. Unfortunately, when their effectiveness is studied scientifically, no impact on suicide rates is found. This may be because suicidal people do not actually use them, it is difficult to assess the situation by phone, or the interventions offered may not be useful.

3. **Restricting access to lethal methods:** Although this recommendation tends to get people fired up about handguns, decreasing any lethal means of suicide is effective. For example, Great Britain experienced a dramatic decrease in its suicide rates when highly toxic coal gas in ovens was replaced by nontoxic natural gas. New automobile emissions systems have decreased deaths by asphyxiation. But firearms do represent the most lethal and common method of committing suicide. Unlike toxic ingestions, firearms do not allow for a "second chance." Studies have documented reduced suicide rates in communities that have implemented strong antihandgun restrictions.

4. **Media:** Although research is limited, there is evidence that teenagers seem particularly vulnerable to media portrayals of suicide, both fictional and nonfictional. Imitation alone does not directly cause suicidal behavior, but media outlets need to be encouraged to avoid referring to suicides in headlines or in lead stories and avoid glamorizing celebrity suicides. For instance, the real headline "Boy, 10, Kills Himself Over Poor Grades" is problematic because it dramatizes the event. Even made-for-TV movies that want to deal with the subject sensitively and responsibly have been shown to have a boomerang effect. On the other hand, the media can be useful if they publicize:
   * Trends in suicide rates
   * Recent treatment advances
   * Stories of how individual treatment was life-saving
   * Myths about suicide
   * Warning signs of suicide

IV. **Clinical pearls and pitfalls:**
   * Teenagers who are being bullied may present with school phobia, depression, or psychosomatic pains.
   * Teenagers (and adults) are usually not aware that the media has any influence on them whatsoever.
   * Inquiring about suicidal thoughts does not predispose adolescents to committing suicide.
   * Breaching the confidentiality of a suicidal adolescent may be life-saving.

BIBLIOGRAPHY

For the clinician

American Academy of Child and Adolescent Psychiatry. Practice parameters for the assessment and treatment of children and adolescents with suicidal behavior. *J Am Acad Child Adolesc Psychiatry* 2001;40:24S–51S.

American Academy of Pediatrics. Suicide and suicide attempts in adolescents. *Pediatrics* 2000; 105:871–874.

Gould MS, Greenberg T, Vetting DM, Shaffer D. Youth suicide risk and preventive interventions: a review of the past 10 years. *J Am Acad Child Adolesc Psychiatry* 2003;42:386–405.

Hatcher-Kay C, King CA. Depression and suicide. *Pediatr Rev* 2003;24:363–371.

Fleischman AR, Barondess JA. Adolescent suicide: vigilance and action to reduce the toll. *Contemp Pediatr* 2004;21:27–36.

US Preventive Sciences Task Force. Screening for suicide risk: recommendations and rationale. *Ann Int Med* 2004;140:820–821.

For patients and parents

Mahler J. The antidepressant dilemma. *NY Times Mag* 2004;100:58–65, 118–119.

WEB SITES

www.cdc.gov/ncipc   Web site for the CDC's National Center for Injury Prevention and Control
www.apa.org   Web site for the American Psychological Association
www.afsp.org   Web site for the American Foundation for Suicide Prevention
www.surgeongeneral.gov/library/youthviolence/messages.htm   Surgeon General's Report on Youth Violence
www.mchlibrary.info   Maternal and Child Health Library
www.safeyouth.org   National Youth Violence Prevention Resource Center

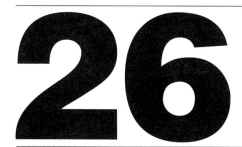

Adolescent Sexuality and Reproductive Health

ADOLESCENT SEXUALITY

I. **Description of the issue:** Adolescence is a time period of profound change in which sexuality is addressed directly in terms of its biologic, sociocultural, psychological, and spiritual components. Although adolescents may become sexually active, sexuality refers to a broader range of issues including comfort with physical changes and interpersonal relationships, as well as gender roles, identity, and sexual orientation.

A. **Definition:**
- **Gender identity** is the internal acknowledgement of being either male or female.
- **Gender role** refers to the overt outward expression of being male or female.
- **Sexual orientation** refers to physical and emotional attraction/arousal to another person. **Heterosexual** individuals are attracted to the opposite sex, **homosexual** to the same sex, and **bisexual** to both sexes.

In most cases, gender identity and role coincide with the individual's anatomic sex. However, **transgender** describes individuals who feel that their gender is different than their biologic sex and a **transvestite** is someone who finds gratification in dressing in clothes from the opposite gender. Transgender individuals and transvestites can be heterosexual, homosexual, or bisexual. Furthermore, **sexual orientation does not always coincide with an individual's actual sexual practices.** Individuals who self-identify as heterosexual may engage in sexual activity with those of the same sex while those that self-identify as homosexual may be sexually active with individuals of the opposite sex. It has been difficult to accurately quantify rates of sexual orientation because studies have frequently focused on sexual behavior rather than orientation.

B. **Etiology:** There is evidence that sexual orientation is established by early childhood and is determined by a combination of genetic, hormonal, and environmental factors. Concordance has been found among monozygotic twins, and there has been clustering within family pedigrees. There is also a possible relationship with prenatal androgens. There is no evidence that parenting issues, abuse, or other adverse life events are related to homosexuality.

II. **Recognizing the issue:**

A. **Sexual orientation during adolescence:** It is usually during adolescence and young adulthood that issues of sexual orientation are dealt with on a conscious level and self-identification of sexual orientation becomes clearer. A national survey of college students found that many self-identified gay, lesbian, and bisexual students reported knowing about their orientation in high school and some were aware as early as grade school. Studies in adults indicate that 3% to 10% of the adult population is gay or lesbian.

Several large studies of adolescents have shown that 1.1% to 4.5% describe themselves as being bisexual, gay, or lesbian while 1.3% to 10.7% are "unsure" about their sexual orientation. In general, the population self-identifying as predominantly homosexual increases with age. Description of sexual orientation does not necessarily coincide with sexual behavior. In one study, only about one-third of youth who engaged in homosexual behaviors self-identified as homosexual or bisexual, and heterosexual activity was seen with equal frequency among self-described homosexual and heterosexual youth. In another study, only 55% of subjects with same-gender sexual experience self-identified as gay, lesbian, bisexual, or unsure. However, those who did self-identify as gay, lesbian, bisexual, or unsure were more likely to report same-gender experiences (30.9%) compared to those who self-identified as heterosexual (0.9%).

B. **Risky outcomes:** Being aware if a youth is identifying as gay, lesbian, bisexual, transgender, and questioning (GLBTQ) is important because there is an increased risk for:
- Suicide
- Substance use and abuse

- Dropping out of school
- Being thrown out of their homes and living on the street
- Sexual activity including coercive sex
- Victimization and being threatened by weapons
- Disordered eating
- Body image dissatisfaction

III. **Management:** Nonjudgmental questions during the office visit including use of the term "partner" instead of "girlfriend" or "boyfriend" and asking if the adolescent is attracted to "men, women, or both" helps to facilitate the discussion on sexual orientation. Clinicians have an important role in providing supportive advice and referral to resources for both the adolescents and their families.

IV. **Clinical pearls and pitfalls:**
- Most adolescents self-identify their sexual orientation as heterosexual, but both heterosexual and GLBTQ youth may engage in sexual activity with same and opposite sex partners during adolescence.
- GLBTQ youth are a higher risk for significant morbidity and mortality.
- There is evidence that sexual orientation is in part determined by genetic factors.

SEXUAL ACTIVITY

I. **Description of the issue:** Approximately one-half of ninth to twelfth graders in the United States have been sexually active. Although the rate of sexual activity has fallen over the past decade, adolescents are still at significant risk for negative consequences of sexual activity including pregnancy and sexually transmitted diseases.

II. **Recognizing the issue:**
  A. **Global picture:**
   - **The median age** of first sexual intercourse in the United States is 16.5 years, with little difference between males and females.
   - **Almost one-half of adolescents in the ninth to twelfth grades have been sexually active** at least once, while one-third are currently sexually active.
   - **Most adolescents have similar age partners:** Among 15- to 19-year-old female adolescents, 63% have partners within 2 years of their age and 28% have a partner 3 to 5 years older. Among 19-year-old males, 76% have partners who are 17 or 18 while 13% are 16 and 11% are age 13 to 15.
   - **Sexual activity is not always completely voluntary:** One-third of adolescents report pressure to be sexually active. The younger the onset of sexual activity, the more likely there was coercion (see section IID on young adolescents). **Sexual activity is often mixed with other risk behaviors such as substance use.** In one study, approximately one-third reported doing more sexually than they planned because of the use of alcohol or drugs and approximately 20% reported lack of condom use because of concurrent use of these substances.
  B. **Sexual behaviors:** When discussing sexual activity, the clinician must consider a variety of behaviors other than vaginal intercourse.
   - **The 1995 National Survey of Adolescent Males** revealed that among 15 to 19 year-old male adolescents, 55% had engaged in vaginal intercourse, 53% had been masturbated by a female partner, 49% had received oral sex, 39% had given oral sex, and 11% had engaged in anal sex.
   - **The Kaiser Family Foundation Study** revealed further details about oral sex in adolescents. One-third of females and 40% of males in the 15- to 17-year-old age group reported having had oral sex and 46% considered oral sex to be "not as big a deal as sexual intercourse." Furthermore, one-third of females and one-fifth of males engaged in oral sex to avoid intercourse, and more than one-third of these youth considered oral sex to be "safer sex."
  C. **Overall trends:** Longitudinal trends in sexual activity among high school students in the United States are available for the past decade from the data collected in the Youth Risk Behavior Survey conducted by the Centers for Disease Control and Prevention. The latest data available are from the 2003 survey.
   - **Overall, rates of self-reported sexual activity have been falling.** Fewer adolescents initiated sexual activity prior to age 13 and they had fewer lifetime partners.
   - **Race/ethnic background:** Blacks (67.3%) were more likely to have ever been sexually active than Hispanic (51.4%) and white students (41.8%); Blacks (19%) were more likely to have first sexual intercourse before age 13 [Hispanic (8.3%);

Table 26-1. Longitudinal national data on sexual activity from YRBS

Year	Ever SA %	SA in past 3 mo %	SA before age 13%	Four or more partners%
1991	54.1	37.5	10.2	18.7
1995	53.1	37.9	8.9	17.8
1999	49.9	36.3	8.3	16.2
2003	46.7	34.3	7.4	14.4

YRBS, Youth Risk Behavior Surveillance; SA, sexual activity.
Adapted from Youth Risk Behavior Surveillance, *www.cdc.gov.*

white (4.2%)]; and Blacks (49%) were more likely to be currently sexually active [Hispanic (37.1), white (30.8%)].
- **Gender:** Male adolescents (48.0%) were more likely to ever have been sexually active than are female adolescents (45.3%).
- **Age:** When assessed by **grade** in school, sexual activity increased from ninth to twelfth grade, with 32.8% of ninth graders and 61.6% of twelfth graders reporting ever having been sexually active (see Table 26-1).
D. **Sexual behavior of young adolescents: The onset of sexual intercourse in young adolescents is particularly concerning since they are at higher risk for having more sexual partners, teen pregnancy, sexually transmitted infections, and coercion.**
   In the Kaiser Family Foundation study, among those who had sexual intercourse, 2% of 18 to 24 year olds reported that they first had sexual intercourse prior to age 12 while 25% had not experienced intercourse until age 18 or older. Among 15 to 17 year olds, 11% reported first intercourse at age 12 to 13, 44% at age 14 to 15, and 37% at age 16 to 17. The National Campaign to Prevent Teen Pregnancy report revealed that almost 20% of youth had sexual intercourse prior to age 15, with 2% to 4% of females and 6% to 8% of males being sexually experienced by age 12 and 14% to 20% of females and 20% to 22% of males experienced by age 14.
   Reasons for initiating sexual activity vary by age. In one study that examined predictors of sexual initiation, younger teens were more likely to report curiosity, a grown-up feeling, partner pressure, and friends having sex as reasons for having sexual intercourse while older teens reported being in love, physical attraction, having a partner who was drunk or high, and feeling romantic. Older age for sexual initiation was associated with a later age of menarche, and families who were expressive, provided a moral-religious emphasis and supervision, and had higher maternal education.
   The national studies provide additional **details about sexual activity in young teens.** Many (40%) of these younger teens had not had sex in the past 18 months and one-half were sexually active none to two times in the past year. One-quarter of sexually experienced teens between 12 and 14 reported multiple sexual partners. Although the nonsexual romantic relationships were short-lived, with 25% ending in 3 months and one-half ending in 6 months, those involving sex lasted longer, with one-quarter lasting at least 2 years.
   Partner age difference is a significant factor in the sexual behavior of younger teens. Twelve percent of romantic relationships in 12 to 14 year olds involved a partner who was 3 or more years older and 12% were with someone 2 or more years older. **This age difference was primarily seen in females—only 1% of males compared to 11% of females had a partner 3 or more years older.** This age difference is important because the likelihood of sexual activity increases as the age difference between the partners increases. While only 13% of relationships between same-age partners involved intercourse, 33% of relationships in which the partner is at least 3 years older involved intercourse.
   Sex among younger teens is not necessarily voluntary. The larger the age difference between partners, the less likely the sex was voluntary and the **younger the age at first intercourse the more likely that sex was unwanted or not voluntary.** Thirteen percent of females who first had sex at age 14 or younger reported that it was not voluntary.

Early sexual activity is also associated with more risk-taking behavior. While approximately one-half to three- quarters of youth reported contraceptive use the first time they had sex, 13% to 15% (1/7) 14 year olds who were sexually experienced had been pregnant. Younger teens who had been sexually active are more likely to smoke, use drugs and alcohol, and engage in delinquent behaviors.

E. **Sexual behavior and attitudes of virgins:** A survey conducted by Seventeen Magazine and the Kaiser Family Foundation among 15 to 17 year olds and published in 2003 revealed that **teens value virginity, with nine out of 10 saying that being a virgin is a good thing but difficult to do.** Most agreed that sex is most appropriate for those 18 and older, married, or in a committed relationship. Of teens who had not had sex, approximately 40% were waiting to be in committed relationship and approximately one-third were waiting for marriage. Over 90% were worried about pregnancy, sexually transmitted infections (STIs), human immunodeficiency virus (HIV) infection, or felt they were too young. Over 80% reported that they remained virgins because of their religious or moral beliefs. These teens endorsed the ideas that delaying sexual activity showed respect for yourself, allowed one to stay in control of the relationships, and resulted in respect from their parents.

Being a virgin and not having sexual intercourse, however, does not imply that adolescents are not engaging in sexual contact. Adolescents do engage in noncoital activities, and surveys have shown that they are unaware of the possibility of STI transmission.

- One study of 2,026 urban high school students revealed that among the 42% of male and 53% of female adolescents reporting that they were virgins, 29% had engaged in heterosexual masturbation of a partner, and 31% had been masturbated by a partner. They were also engaged in other forms of sex including 9% heterosexual fellatio, 10% cunnilingus, and 1% anal intercourse.
- In the Kaiser Family Foundation study, 10% of female adolescents and 15% of male adolescents age 15 to 17 who had not had sexual intercourse had engaged in oral sex and 21% of female adolescents and 39% of male adolescents reported they had been "intimate."
- In the 1995 National Survey of Adolescent Males, of those who had not had vaginal intercourse, one out of five male adolescents had been masturbated by a female partner and one in seven had received oral sex.

F. **Sexual abuse/assault:**
- **Adolescents have the highest rates of sexual assault and rape of any age group.**
- Female adolescents are more commonly victims than are male adolescents.
- In two-thirds to three-quarters of rapes and sexual assaults involving an adolescent, the perpetrator is a relative or acquaintance.
- **Rape** involves forced sexual intercourse (including penetration with a foreign object).
- **Sexual assault** involves sexual contact but not necessarily penetration.
- Older adolescents are commonly victims of **acquaintance or date rape** that occurs as part of a social encounter with the assailant. These situations can be confusing because there may have been consensual sex in the past or the situation may have begun with both parties seemingly in agreement.
- **Statutory rape** is defined as sexual penetration by an adult with a minor.

Clinicians should be aware of the laws in their state regarding sexual activity and minors. Sexual abuse involving a custodial adult and a minor is reportable to child protective services. However, sexual activity that does not involve a custodial adult may also be reportable. Various states have laws requiring mandatory reporting if one partner is below a certain age and/or if there is a minimum number of years of age difference between the partners. These laws may apply even when both individuals are under the age of 18.

Sexual assault patients should be evaluated for STIs and pregnancy. Prophylactic treatment for *C. trachomatis* and *N. gonorrhoeae* is recommended. Postcoital contraception should also be offered if the baseline pregnancy test is negative. Although HIV prophylaxis is not universally recommended, risk of exposure should be evaluated along with the risks and benefits of treatment. If the patient has not received the hepatitis B vaccine, the series should be started. Finally, since 80% of rape victims suffer from posttraumatic stress disorder, counseling is recommended.

III. **Management:** Sexuality education is a process that begins at birth and is a daily learning process in which parents teach children about relationships and caring. Honest open communication about sexuality issues throughout childhood and prior to adolescence can help create a solid framework for the future. **Children and adolescents consistently report that they want to discuss sexuality issues with their parents.** However, comfort levels among parents vary and youth get information from a variety of sources including friends, school, the media, and the Internet. **Studies have shown that parent–child communication on sexuality issues can decrease risk behaviors.**

School-based sexuality education has become a controversial topic. There are four types of programs:

- **Comprehensive:** Beginning in kindergarten, students are given factual information and taught skills to responsibly manage relationships. These programs include information on abstinence as well as contraception.
- **Abstinence based:** These programs emphasize abstinence but also include information on noncoital behavior, contraception, and STI prevention.
- **Abstinence only:** These programs discuss abstinence from all sexual behaviors and do not include information on contraception or STI prevention.
- **Abstinence only until marriage:** These programs present abstinence until marriage as the only correct moral context for sexual activity.

A. **Research findings: Comprehensive sex education** programs effectively help youth delay onset of sexual activity and do not hasten onset of sexual activity or increase frequency of intercourse or number of partners. **Furthermore, skill-based programs that teach contraceptive use and communication skills can reduce the frequency of intercourse, reduce the number of partners, and increase the use of condoms and other contraceptives.**

Abstinence programs vary in content and in the rigor of the evaluation process. **A 2001 report from the National Campaign to Prevent Teen Pregnancy found that most of the programs did not demonstrate a delay in the initiation of sexual activity or a reduction in the frequency of sexual activity.** One program did demonstrate a delay in the onset of sexual activity among younger teens (15 and younger) but not older teens. The conclusion in this report was that more research was needed to demonstrate whether abstinence-only programs will delay the onset of sex or have an effect on contraceptive use or teen pregnancy. More information was also needed to elucidate which factors of abstinence education are most effective. **Those abstinence programs that also encourage use of condoms and contraceptives if the adolescent is sexually active have demonstrated a delay in sexual intercourse, decreased frequency of sex, and an increase in condom/contraceptive use.**

IV. **Clinical pearls and pitfalls:**
- Rates of sexual activity among adolescents are declining but still high enough for continued concern about pregnancy and STIs.
- Teens who are not engaged in sexual intercourse may still be engaged in other noncoital sexual behaviors that place them at risk for STIs.
- Younger teens are more likely to be in coercive or unwanted sexual relationships with older partners.

ADOLESCENT PREGNANCY

I. **Description of the issue:** Pregnancy is a significant negative consequence of adolescent sexual activity. In the year 2000, there were approximately 841,450 pregnancies to individuals under the age of 20, resulting in 477,509 births and approximately 244,030 legal abortions, and 119,910 miscarriages. **Based on census year 2000 statistics, one in 12 15- to 19-year-old female adolescents in the United States became pregnant, with approximately one in five sexually active 15- to 19-year-old female adolescents becoming pregnant.** Among younger teens, nationally representative samples have shown that one in seven sexually experienced 14 year olds have been pregnant.

A. **Epidemiology:** Most teen pregnancies are unintended and unplanned and most occur outside of marriage. **Adolescent females are twice as likely as adolescent males to be involved in a pregnancy and three times more likely to become a teen parent.** The fathers of babies born to teen mothers are frequently older than the mothers. One in five infants of unmarried minors is fathered by individuals who are 5 or more years older than the teen mother. **The birth rate for 15- to 19-year-old male adolescents in the year 2000 was 20.2 in 1,000, which is about one-half of the rate for females in this age group.** Approximately one-quarter of teen mothers have a second child within 2 years.

The good news is that the rates of teen pregnancy, births, and abortions have fallen dramatically over the past decade in all age groups and among all racial/ethnic groups. These declines are in part due to decreased rates of sexual activity (25%) as well as more effective use of contraceptive methods (75%).

- In 2003, the birth rate for 10- to 14-year-old females was 0.6 in 1,000, representing a decline of 57% from 1991 and the rate for 15- to 19-year-old females was 41.7 in 1,000, representing a decline of 33% since 1991. Among 10 to 14 year olds, 97% of births are in the 13 to 14 year old age group.
- The rate of induced abortions for those under age 15 was 1.4 in 1,000 in 1991 and 0.8 in 1,000 in 2000 while the rate for 15 to 19 year olds was 37.4 in 1,000 in 1991 and 24.0 in 1,000 in 2000. These rates also fell for all racial/ethnic groups.

B. **Teen pregnancy outcomes:** Teen pregnancy in younger adolescents, particularly those under the age of 15, is associated with an increased risk of:
- Preterm birth
- Low birth weight babies
- Higher post-neonatal mortality rates
  - Low birth weight (four times higher than other ages)
  - Sudden infant death syndrome (SIDS) (2.7 times higher than for other ages)
  - Congenital malformations (1.5 times higher than other ages)

Teens and particularly those in the 10 to 14 year old age group are more likely to have delayed prenatal care, inadequate weight gain, and higher rates of pregnancy-associated hypertension, anemia, and eclampsia. Other factors associated with teen pregnancy include depression, which is twice as common as in adults, long-term socioeconomic disadvantage including lack of advancement in education, poverty, and less favorable outcomes in social and emotional development of the children. **Some of these negative outcomes appear to be related to inadequate prenatal care, nutrition, and poverty rather than age, and can be improved by individually tailored prenatal and postnatal services.**

C. **Comparison to other developed countries: Despite these dramatic declines in teen pregnancy in the United States, this country still has the highest rates of teen pregnancy in the developed world.** The rates of sexual activity are similar in these other countries but other Western countries have more open communication and dialogue about sexuality issues and are better at facilitating access to contraceptive services for sexually active teens. **Teens in the United States are less likely to use contraceptives and also use them less effectively.**

II. **Making the diagnosis:**
A. **Signs and symptoms:**
- **Most common sign:**
  - Overdue for menses
- **1 to 2 weeks post fertilization:**
  - Breast tenderness/nipple sensitivity
- **2 weeks post fertilization:**
  - Fatigue
  - Nausea
  - Urinary frequency

B. **Physical exam:**
- **2 to 3 weeks after implantation:**
  - Cervical and uterine softening
- **Uterine size:**
  - Out of the pelvis palpated at the pubic symphysis at 12 weeks
  - Midway between symphysis and umbilicus at 16 weeks
  - At the umbilicus at 20 weeks.

C. **Complications:**
- Lower abdominal pain and/or spotting could be a sign of ectopic pregnancy or threatened spontaneous abortion.
- Uterine size mismatched with expected dates could indicate ectopic pregnancy or incomplete or missed spontaneous abortion if too small; fibroids, twin gestation, uterine anomaly, or hydatidiform mole if too large.

D. **Laboratory diagnosis:** Pregnancy can be easily diagnosed in the office setting with use of immunometric urine pregnancy tests that are specific for the beta subunit of hCG. These tests are approved to detect hCG levels down to 10 to 25 mIU/mL and will identify a pregnancy 7 to 10 days after fertilization—in some cases before the next missed menstrual period. Ninety-eight percent of women will have a positive test within 7 days of implantation.

Serum hCG quantitative results can detect levels of hCG as low as 5 mUI/mL. They are rarely needed and usually reserved for cases of pregnancy complications such as ectopic pregnancy (in which levels will be lower than expected) or to follow declining levels in a suspected spontaneous abortion. They also are useful for molar pregnancies that have higher than expected levels of hCG.

III. **Management:** Once the adolescent is diagnosed as being pregnant, sizing and dates should be determined and **nonjudgmental options counseling** should be done to discuss potential options that include giving birth and raising the child, adoption, and abortion.
  • **Adoption has been the least popular option among adolescents.** Less than 1% chose this option in 1995. Discussion of adoption alternatives that are more open than in the past may be helpful in the decision-making process. In addition, adolescents are more likely to consider adoption if they themselves were adopted or know someone who was adopted.
  • Providers must understand their state laws regarding abortion in minors. **Approximately one-fifth of abortions in the United States are among adolescents.** Overall, 88% of all abortions are performed during the first trimester of pregnancy, with 54% in the first 8 weeks. Only 1% are performed at 21 weeks gestation or later. **Teens are at higher risk for delaying abortion because of problems with access.** Thirty-two states require parental involvement either in the form of consent or notification prior to obtaining an abortion. All of these states, except for Utah, have a judicial bypass procedure that permits a minor to obtain consent from the court if they cannot involve their parents. The ease of this process varies by jurisdiction. In some states a grandparent or other adult relative can take the place of a parent.
  • **Adolescents should be encouraged to begin prenatal care as soon as possible to help prevent negative pregnancy-related outcomes.** Primary care physicians can give pregnant teens a prescription for prenatal vitamins while waiting for the first prenatal care appointment as well as counsel them on healthy diet and avoiding alcohol and drugs. Some prenatal programs have special programs for teens and interventions with visiting nurses who provide support throughout the pregnancy and postpartum period. These programs have been beneficial for low-income unmarried women. One intensive short-term program with teens did show improvement in parenting skills, decreased risk of being on welfare, and better cognitive skills and fewer behavioral problems in their children. **However, no programs to date have eliminated the long-term effects of poverty.**
IV. **Clinical pearls and pitfalls:**
  • Rates of teen pregnancy, birth, and abortion have been steadily declining in all age and racial/ethnic groups.
  • Teens particularly those under age 16 are at higher risk for pregnancy-related complications.
  • Prompt referral for services helps diminish negative pregnancy outcomes.

CONTRACEPTION

I. **Description of the issue:** Consistent use of effective contraception by adolescents who choose to be sexually active is crucial to prevent pregnancy. Options such as the patch, vaginal ring, and medroxyprogesterone injection provide longer-acting options that do not require daily or coital dependent compliance. There are few, if any, contraindications to use of hormonal contraception in healthy adolescents. Of the available barrier methods, condoms are the most widely used method in this age group and reported use has dramatically increased over the past decade.
  A. **Epidemiology:** Data from the 2002 National Survey of Family Growth show that rates of contraceptive use increased between 1995 and 2002 for both the first and most recent episodes of intercourse among 15- to 19-year-old unmarried males and females. Approximately 74% of females and 82% of males used a method of contraception for their first episode of intercourse and 83% of currently sexually active females and 91% of males used a method at last sexual intercourse. Use of dual methods (a condom along with a hormonal method) increased between 1995 and 2002. Oral contraceptive pills and condoms are the most common methods used in this age group. Data on use patterns is found in Table 26-2.

Table 26-2. Percent of 15- to 19-year-old adolescents using a contraceptive method, 2002

Method	% Using at first intercourse		% Using at last intercourse[a]	
	Female	Male	Female	Male
Pill	16.5	14.9	34.2	31.0
Other hormonal[b]	—	—	9.1	6.3
Male condom	66.4	70.9	54.3	70.7
Dual Method[c]	13.1	10.4	19.5	23.9
Withdrawal	7.5	9.8	—	—
All other methods[d]	—	—	1.6	2.0
No Method	25.5	18.0	16.8	9.3

[a]Percent of never married 15- to 19-year-olds who had sexual intercourse in prior three months.
[b]Other hormonal: Depo-Provera, Lunelle, Norplant, emergency contraception, patch.
[c]Dual method: condom and hormonal method.
[d]All other methods: spermicide, periodic abstinence, vasectomy, female sterilization, and "other" methods.
Adapted from Abma JC, Martinez GM, Mosher WD, Dawson BS. Teenagers in the United States: sexual activity, contraceptive use, and childbearing, 2002. National Center for Health Statistics, *Vital Health Stat* 2004;23(24).

One other source of national longitudinal information on contraceptive use is found in the Youth Risk Behavior Survey. As shown in Table 26-3, condom use at last sex among currently sexually active students has steadily increased among male and female high school students and reported use of OCPs by female adolescents for the past 4 years has remained fairly constant. This study does not distinguish between use of condoms as a primary method of contraception and dual use of condoms for STI/HIV protection with another contraceptive method for pregnancy prevention.

A third source of recent national data is found in the Kaiser Family Foundation Survey published in 2003. Condom and OCP use was even higher in this study than in those previously discussed. More than 90% of 15 to 17 year olds reported using some method of contraception, at least most of the time, and 70% reported use all of the time. Furthermore, in this study, adolescents were found to use condoms more consistently and regularly than were young adults and were also more likely to report that they use "birth control or protection" all of the time. As in the other studies, the Kaiser data did not account for dual use of condoms and another method. Issues regarding contraceptive choice that were important to adolescents in this study included protection from STIs/HIV and pregnancy, partner's preference, weight gain, access without parental consent, not needing to discuss the method with a partner, and cost (see Table 26-4).

II. **Recognizing the issue:**
   A. **Contraceptive efficacy:** To be effective, contraceptives must be used correctly and consistently. Consistent use of contraception among adolescents has been associated with being older, white, having working parents with higher levels of education, being college bound, academic success in school, having a steady sexual relationship, contraceptive method satisfaction, and suburban residence. Methods such as an IUD that require no compliance have comparable values for theoretical and actual efficacy. A method like the condom that requires correct use for each coital act has a much larger discrepancy between theoretical contraceptive efficacy and failure rates with actual use (see Table 26-5).

Table 26-3. Percent of high school students reporting use of condoms at last intercourse and OCPs

	Male	Female	
Year	Condom use	Condom use	OCP use
1991	54.5	38.0	—
1995	60.5	48.6	—
1997	62.5	50.8	—
1999	65.5	50.7	20.4
2001	65.1	51.3	21.1
2003	68.8	57.4	20.6

OCP, oral contraceptive pills.
Adapted from Youth Risk Behavior Surveillance, *www.cdc.gov*.

Table 26-4. Contraceptive use among 15–17 year olds, Kaiser Survey

Method	Male%	Female%
Any method		
All of the time	65	76
Most of the time	25	16
Condoms		
Regularly	85	72
Last time had sex	86	71
Birth control pills		
Ever	—	46
Regularly	—	40
Withdrawal		
Ever	41	38
Regularly	1	4
Rhythm		
Regularly	14	13

Adapted from National Survey of Adolescents and Young Adults: Sexual Health Knowledge, Attitudes and Experiences. Kaiser Family Foundation, 2003.

When used correctly, hormonal contraceptives are a safe and effective contraceptive method in healthy adolescents. However, failure commonly occurs when the patient forgets to take a pill or replace a patch, or starts a new pill pack, patch cycle, or ring cycle late so that more than 7 days have passed since the last dose of hormones.

Reasons for condom failure include lack of consistent and correct use, breakage or slippage, poor withdrawal technique after intercourse, and use of an oil-based lubricant with a latex condom. Male condoms reportedly break or slip approximately 2% of the time. However, with proper use, these problems are uncommon. Female condoms have a higher failure rate in part because it is harder to use them correctly.

Anticipatory counseling about contraception should include a review of common side effects, the correct way to use the method, and thinking through the logistics about where the method will be kept and how the adolescents will remember to follow specific method instructions.

B. **Hormonal contraceptives:** Hormonal contraceptive choices currently available in the United States include combined hormonal contraceptives that contain both estrogen

Table 26-5. Failure rate during first year of contraceptive use

Method	Perfect use%	Actual use%
None	85	85
Withdrawal	4	27
Male condom	2	15
Female condom	5	21
Spermicide	18	29
OCPs	0.3	8
Evra patch	0.3	8
NuvaRing	0.3	8
Depo-Provera	0.3	3
Norplant	0.05	0.05
Diaphragm	6	16
Cap Nulliparous	9	16
Cap Parous	26	32
IUD Copper T	0.6	0.8
IUD Mirena	0.1	0.1

OCP, oral contraceptive pills.
Adapted from Hatcher RA, Trussell I, Stewart R, et al. *Contraceptive technology,* 18th ed. 2004; New York: Ardent Media, Inc.

and progesterone [oral contraceptive pills (OCP), the contraceptive patch (Ortho Evra), the vaginal ring (NuvaRing)] and progestin-only methods [progestin-only pills (POP, minipill) and injectable medroxyprogesterone acetate (Depo-Provera)]. Another progestin-only method, the subdermal implant Norplant, is currently not available, but a new formulation with one implantable subdermal progestin-containing rod is currently being evaluated. The expected product is named Implanon and has been shown to be very effective—providing higher rates of ovulatory suppression than Norplant.

1. **Method of action:** Hormonal contraceptives work by:
   • Inhibiting ovulation (primary mechanism)
   • Thickening cervical mucous to prevent sperm penetration
   • Incapacitation of sperm
   • Slowing tubal motility
   • Disrupting ovum transport
   • Inducing endometrial atrophy
2. **Formulation:** Combined OCPs contain both estrogen and progesterone. Low dose pills contain 20 to 35 micrograms of ethinyl estradiol and various progestins. The different progestins have different intrinsic potency and varying levels of androgenicity. The third generation progestins (norgestimate and desogestrel) have the least androgenicity. A newer progestin, drospirenone, derived from spironolactone, has both antiandrogenic and antimineralocorticoid activity.

   OCPs can either be **monophasic** formulations, in which the hormone levels are constant for 3 weeks, or **multiphasic** (usually triphasic), in which the hormone doses change two to three times during 21 days of hormone dosing. Most pill packs are packaged as 28-day packs with 3 weeks of hormones and 1 week of placebo for a withdrawal bleed. There is also an extended dosing pill in which the same dose of hormones is taken continuously for 84 days prior to taking the seven placebo pills to induce a withdrawal bleed. The extended dosing regimens have been useful for some specific clinical indications including dysmenorrhea, menorrhagia, and premenstrual symptoms.

   The contraceptive patch releases 20 micrograms per day and the vaginal ring releases 15 micrograms per day of ethinyl estradiol. The progestins in these methods are derivatives of the third generation progestins found in OCPs. The doses of hormones in the patch and ring are lower than oral OCPs because they are more bioavailable. These methods also avoid the first pass hepatic affects because the hormones are absorbed directly from the skin or vaginal mucosa.

   For the purposes of contraception in healthy adolescents, the patch, ring, or any low dose OCP containing 20 to 35 micrograms of ethinyl estradiol in either a monophasic or multiphasic formulation will be an effective method of contraception if used correctly and consistently.
3. **Medical concerns:** The absolute contraindications for using hormonal contraceptives that would be applicable to adolescents and would preclude use and are listed as a category 4 in the WHO Medical Eligibility Criteria (see Table 26-6).
   • **Cigarette smoking** is not a contraindication for adolescents, although certainly prescribing combined hormonal contraceptives is an opportunity to discuss

Table 26-6. Absolute contraindications for hormonal contraceptive use by medical condition

Combined hormonal contraceptives
Thromboembolic disorder (current or past)
Known thrombogenic mutation
Cerebrovascular or coronary artery disease
Valvular heart disease with thrombogenic complications
Uncontrolled hypertension >160 systolic, >100 diastolic
Headaches with aura or focal neurologic symptoms
Major surgery with prolonged immobilization
Breast cancer
Acute or chronic liver disease with abnormal liver function tests, or hepatic carcinoma, adenoma
Diabetes with nephropathy, retinopathy, neuropathy

Progestin-only contraceptives
Current breast cancer

Adapted from Hatcher RA, Trussell I, Stewart R, et al. *Contraceptive technology,* 18th ed. 2004; New York: Ardent Media, Inc.

smoking cessation. Combined hormonal contraceptives are contraindicated in women aged 35 or older who smoke 15 or more cigarettes per day, because of the increased risk of stroke and myocardial infarction.

- **Migraine with aura** is a contraindication for combined hormonal contraception for all age groups. There is an increased risk of ischemic stroke in these patients.
- **Thromboembolic disorders** and a known thrombogenic mutation are absolute contraindication because estrogen increases liver production of clot-promoting factors and decreases production of clot-lysing factors. Certain inherited disorders such as Factor V Leiden mutation and Protein S and C synthesis disorders also promote increased risk of clotting. It is important to take a family history of deep vein thrombosis (DVT) and pulmonary embolism (PE) in first-degree relatives to determine if the patient requires further investigation for an inherited clotting abnormality.

  Current labeling of products with the progestin desogestrel indicates that these products may have a higher rate of thrombosis than other progestins. The extent of this association is unclear because there were confounding variables and possible detection bias in the studies. In addition, norgestimate was also found to have similar associations in later studies. The most important take-home message is that most healthy women without an inherited thrombogenic disorder will have no clinically significant adverse clotting problems.
- **Sickle cell disease** is not a contraindication for OCPs. There is no difference in coagulation studies, blood viscosity, or incidence or severity of painful sickle cell crises in OCP users.
- **Diabetes** is not a contraindication for use of combined hormonal contraceptives. The low dose OCPs currently available do not adversely affect carbohydrate metabolism.
- **Breast cancer** is not increased among 35 to 64 year olds who were current or former users of OCPs. Breast cancer is rare in adolescents and finding a breast mass on exam would not be an indication to stop or avoid use of hormonal contraceptives even while the mass is being evaluated.
- **Active liver disease** is a contraindication to combined hormonal contraception since combined hormonal contraceptives are metabolized in the liver. Patients with active liver disease and those with abnormal liver function tests should avoid their use. However, chronic hepatitis with normal stable liver function is not a contraindication. The risk of hepatic carcinoma does not increase over baseline in hepatitis B carriers.
- **Drug interactions:** Certain medications including anti-tuberculosis medications (rifampin), antifungal (griseofulvin), anticonvulsants, anti-HIV protease inhibitors, and St. John's Wort can decrease the efficacy of OCPs by increasing hepatic clearance. OCPs can also affect the metabolism and clearance of other medications and can either increase or decrease their serum levels. **It is a popular misconception that broad spectrum antibiotics reduce the efficacy of OCPs.** No backup methods are needed even for long-term antibiotic use unless there is a concern about absorption of the OCP such as in the case of a patient with vomiting or diarrhea. There are no significant drug interactions for injectable medroxyprogesterone acetate except for aminoglutethimide, which is used to treat Cushing disease.
- **Depression:** Studies have not demonstrated increased depression in OCP users. Similarly, the overall rates of depression are not increased with injectable medroxyprogesterone acetate. However, individual women may have an increase in depression with this injectable method. Since this is a medication that cannot be discontinued immediately, some clinicians recommend trying oral progesterone prior to giving the injection in patients with whom depression is a concern.
- **Osteopenia/Osteoporosis:** Studies have indicated that long-term users of medroxyprogesterone acetate can have a decrease in bone density. This is a concern in teens, who are accruing bone density. In adults, this loss appears to be reversible but it is not clear whether this is the case for adolescents. World Health Organization (WHO) guidelines consider this a category in which benefits outweigh risks. However, the Food and Drug Administration (FDA) recently issued a black box warning about the bone density issue.
- **Lipids:** Adverse affects on the HDL/LDL ratios have also been found in some users of medroxyprogesterone acetate. However, this is not a category 4 contraindication.

Table 26-7. Health benefits of hormonal contraceptives

Relief from dysmenorrhea
Decreased menstrual flow
Reduced PMS symptoms
Decrease in ovarian cysts
Reduced rates of endometrial cancer
Reduced rates of ovarian cancer
Decreased gonococcal PID
Suppression of endometriosis
Decreased iron deficiency anemia

PMS, premenstrual syndrome; PID, pelvic inflammatory disease.

4. **Health benefits of hormonal contraceptives:** (See Table 26-7) In addition to this list, combined hormonal contraceptives reduce development of fibrocystic breast changes, improve acne, decrease androgen levels, improve menstrual migraines, and have a favorable impact in HDL/LDL cholesterol levels. Injectable medroxy-progesterone acetate has been shown to decrease the frequency of grand mal seizures and sickle cell crises. OCPs seem to improve bone density. However, there are mixed results concerning prevention of osteoporosis by estrogen-containing methods, particularly at the lowest doses.

5. **Physical exam:** A good medical history followed by a blood pressure and weight are the crucial elements necessary before hormonal contraception is prescribed. **A gynecologic exam is not needed.** Although the exam is important for detecting STIs, diagnosing vaginitis, and performing Pap smears, none of these test results will lead a clinician to choose not to prescribe hormonal contraception to an adolescent.

6. **Laboratory evaluation:** If there is a concern that the patient may be pregnant, a urine pregnancy test can be performed prior to prescribing hormonal contraception. Some clinicians have the patient present for the first Depo-Provera shot within 5 days of the onset of menses and perform a pregnancy test prior to initiating the method. Unlike the combined hormonal methods or the minipill, which are readily reversible, a pregnancy might be discovered later in Depo-Provera patients because they can have prolonged amenorrhea and only need to see the clinician only every 12 weeks for the injection. None of the hormonal methods are teratogenic and if pregnancy is discovered after starting a method, there is no concern about harm to the fetus.

Patients with a family history of thromboembolism should be evaluated for thrombogenic disorders prior to starting hormonal contraception containing estrogen.

C. **Barrier contraceptives:**

1. **Medical concerns:**
   - Most **male condoms** are made of latex, but there are polyurethane condoms for those patients with latex allergy. **Female condoms** are made of polyurethane. Although oil-based lubricants are contraindicated with latex condoms because of increased failure and breakage, they can be used with those made out of polyurethane.
   - Spermicidal condoms offer no advantage and some people may be sensitive to the ingredients in the **spermicide.** Furthermore, spermicides do not protect from STIs or HIV infection. In fact, nonoxynol-9, the ingredient in most spermicides, may increase the risk of HIV transmission if used two or more times a day because of associated vulvovaginal epithelial disruption. If spermicidal use is desired, then a separate full dose in the form of foam, a suppository, or film should be used.
   - **Diaphragms and cervical caps** are not commonly used in adolescents. They have a higher failure rate than other methods and are difficult to use for those who are poorly motivated and not comfortable touching the genital area. There is an increase in urinary tract infections in diaphragm users because the spermicide used with this device can alter the vaginal flora, and the device itself can push against the urethra.

2. **Health benefits:** Barrier contraceptives help protect from transmission of STIs and HIV infection.

3. **Physical exam:** Physical exam and gynecologic exam are not needed for any of these methods except the diaphragm and cervical cap, which require fitting by an experienced clinician.
4. **Laboratory evaluation:** No specific laboratory evaluation is needed to prescribe barrier contraceptives.

D. **Intrauterine device:**

1. **Medical concerns:** There are two intrauterine devices (IUDs) available in the United States, the Copper T and the progestin-containing Mirena. IUDs have traditionally been avoided in adolescents because of concerns about risk of STIs and subsequent pelvic inflammatory disease (PID). This risk is more of a concern in individuals having multiple sexual partners. However, studies have shown that the risk of upper tract infection is at the time of insertion, and the risk does not increase simply because an IUD is in place. WHO guidelines do not recommend insertion at the time of active infection. But an STI or PID that occurred more than 3 months prior to insertion would not be a contraindication.

   The other significant issue regarding the IUD that applies to adolescents is expulsion. This is more common in nulliparous women and specifically in those who have never been pregnant. Enlargement occurs in the uterus even if the pregnancy ends in miscarriage or induced abortion, and this change helps successful retention of the device. The issue of nulliparity should be considered but is not a contraindication to insertion. A distorted uterine cavity due to a fibroid or congenital malformation would be another potential contraindication to use of an IUD.

   Other absolute contraindications, which carry the WHO rating of 4 on the medical eligibility criteria and would potentially apply to adolescents, include puerperal sepsis, post-septic abortion, malignant gestational trophoblastic disease, cervical cancer (awaiting treatment), endometrial cancer, and in the case of the progesterone IUD, current breast cancer.

2. **Health benefits:** IUDs protect against ectopic pregnancy compared to use of no contraception and also protect from endometrial cancer. The progesterone IUD decreases menstrual blood flow and helps prevent anemia.

3. **Physical exam:** A pelvic examination is needed to see if there are any anatomical contraindications to insertion.

4. **Laboratory evaluation:** No specific laboratory evaluation is needed unless there is a clinical suspicion of an STI.

E. **Emergency contraception:** Emergency contraception (ECP) is the use of hormones or the insertion of an IUD to prevent pregnancy after unprotected sex. Hormonal ECP is the method most likely to be used by adolescents. ECP containing only progesterone reduces the risk of pregnancy by 89%, and those with both estrogen and progesterone reduce the risk by 75%. The primary mechanism of action is hindering of follicular maturation and ovulation, but there may also be some affects on sperm migration and function, fertilization, uterine lining maturation, and development and transport of the fertilized ovum. **Once a pregnancy is established, ECP is ineffective and will not disrupt an existing pregnancy.** The only currently available ECP method available by prescription is the progestin-only method Plan B.
   - According to the package insert, ECP should be given within 72 hours of unprotected intercourse, but studies have shown they are effective for up to 120 hours.
   - Although the progestin-only method (Plan B) is usually given as two doses 12 hours apart, both doses can be given simultaneously.
   - The progestin-only method is much better tolerated and produces less nausea and vomiting. If an estrogen containing ECP is given, either a prescription antiemetic or an over-the-counter product such as meclizine hydrochloride or dimenhydrinate can be used. There are no contraindications to giving ECP, and some clinicians give their patients a prophylactic prescription so that they can have it readily available to take as soon as possible after unprotected intercourse.

   ECP has not always been available in pharmacies. Combinations of pills from standard OCPs can also be used. The OCPs that can be used should contain ethinyl estradiol and levonorgestrel, and multiple pills should be given as two doses 12 hours apart to equal 100 to 120 micrograms of ethinyl estradiol and 0.50 to 0.75 mg of levonorgestrel per dose.

III. **Contraceptive management:**

A. **Common side effects and management issues:**
   - **Weight gain:** There is no significant weight gain with low dose OCPs. Some females may experience fluid retention as commonly seen premenstrually. In those cases, the newer OCP that contains drospirenone may be helpful. Patients on this

pill, however, may be at increased risk of hyperkalemia if they are on other medications that increase potassium levels. Unlike OCPs, there is significant weight gain associated with injectable medroxyprogesterone acetate. Patients on this method must be counseled about healthy nutrition and exercise.

- **Vaginal spotting and bleeding:** Breakthrough bleeding can be seen in the first few months of OCP use and then usually resolves. It is important to be sure that the patient is not missing pills, which would also contribute to bleeding, and does not have an STI. Most patients have regular predictable menses after the first few packs. Medroxyprogesterone acetate is associated with irregular unpredictable bleeding. However, over time many patients become amenorrheic—30% to 50% by the end of the first year of use and 70% by the end of the second year.

B. **Specific method management issues:**

- **Patch:** Patch users may experience hypersensitivity and the patch itself can detach. An extra patch should always be available for replacement since the hormones are embedded in the adhesive, and there will be reduced efficacy if the entire patch is not attached to the skin. Patch users also report more breast tenderness, vaginal spotting, and dysmenorrhea than OCP users for the first few cycles. To prevent skin irritation, the patch should not be placed in the exact same location each time. This method is also less effective for women who weigh more than 198 pounds.

- **Ring:** To use this method, the patient must be comfortable touching her body and inserting her fingers into her vagina. For this reason alone, the ring may not be a popular method with adolescents. Some patients complain about leukorrhea (4.6%), vaginitis (5.8%), and vaginal discomfort (.4%). The ring can be removed, if desired, for sexual intercourse, but if it is out for more than 3 hours, contraceptive effectiveness is compromised.

- **Minipill:** Compliance, including taking the pill at the same time every day, is particularly important for the progestin-only pill.

- **Female condom:** Users of this method must be comfortable touching the genital area and inserting their fingers in the vagina. The device can be noisy but extra lubricant can be used. An advantage of the female condom is that it can be inserted ahead of time, even hours before intercourse, and because it is made of polyurethane it has good heat transfer qualities. Female condoms have a higher failure rate than male condoms because it is more difficult to use them correctly. However, if a male condom is not being used, this is a viable alternative particularly to help prevent STI/HIV transmission.

C. **Prescription and follow up:** Clinicians should review the various contraceptive options available and help the adolescent decide which method he or she would be most likely to use properly and consistently. Clinicians should also emphasize the need for adolescents to protect themselves from STIs/HIV as well as pregnancy and that use of dual methods that include condoms is important.

There should be an anticipatory discussion about potential side effects of the chosen contraceptive method and an easy process in place in the office for patients to call and ask questions. Encouraging phone calls to troubleshoot problems can help prevent adolescents from prematurely stopping the method. Close follow up (within 2–3 months) after initiation of the method may also help improve compliance and provide an opportunity to address questions and concerns.

Finally, there should also be a discussion about confidentiality and parental involvement, as well as payment for the office visits and the contraceptive method itself. Parental involvement is desirable since adolescents are more likely to be compliant if their parents know they are using contraception. If confidentiality cannot be maintained in the office or there are payment issues, the adolescent can be directed to a Title X funded site that has federal funding to provide free confidential contraceptive services to adolescents under the age of 18.

IV. **Clinical pearls and pitfalls:**
- All low dose OCPs are safe and effective in healthy adolescents.
- A pelvic exam is not necessary prior to prescribing hormonal contraception.
- Clinicians should emphasize dual methods to protect from STIs/HIV infection as well as pregnancy.
- Patients should be informed about the availability of ECP.
- The IUD may be used in adolescents.
- Clinicians should be aware about the concerns about possible lack of adequate bone mineralization with use of injectable medroxyprogesterone acetate.

PELVIC PAIN

I. **Description of the condition:** Pelvic pain, which can be acute, cyclic, or chronic, is a common complaint in adolescent women. There is long differential diagnosis encompassing both gynecologic and nongynecologic problems including musculoskeletal and psychogenic causes of pelvic pain. Laparoscopic evaluation of 11 to 17 year olds with acute pelvic pain at Children's Hospital of Boston in the 1980s showed that ovarian cyst was the most common diagnosis, followed by acute PID and then adnexal torsion. For those patients with chronic pelvic pain between the ages of 11 to 21, endometriosis was the most common diagnosis, followed by postoperative adhesions.

II. **Making the diagnosis:**
   A. **Differential diagnosis:** (See Table 26-8)

Table 26-8. Differential diagnosis of pelvic pain

Gynecologic causes
Pregnancy complication- ectopic, threatened/spontaneous abortion
Ovarian mass
Ovarian/fallopian tube torsion
Hydrosalpinx
Infection—endometritis, PID, tuboovarian abscess
Vaginitis/vulvitis
Mittelschmerz
Dysmenorrhea
Endometriosis
Obstructing mullerian anomaly
Pelvic adhesions
Chronic vaginitis/vulvitis
Fibroids

Gastrointestinal
Appendicitis
Gastritis
Ulcer
Cholecystitis
Gastroenteritis
Intestinal infections
Obstruction
Irritable bowel disease
Inflammatory bowel disease
Hepatitis
Pancreatitis
Constipation

Genitourinary
Pyelonephritis
Cystitis
Renal calculi

Musculoskeletal
Trauma
Tumors
Joint inflammation

PID, pelvic inflammatory disease.
Adapted from Emans SJ, Laufer MR, Goldstein DP. *Pediatric and adolescent gynecology*, 5th ed. 2005; Philadelphia: Lippincott Williams & Wilkins.

B. **History: Pain history should include:**
- Location
- Intensity
- Radiation
- Length and progression of symptoms
- Relation to menses
- Urinary symptoms
- Bowel patterns
- Presence of systemic symptoms such as fever
- Contraceptive use
- Sexual activity

Key points in sorting out the differential diagnosis include:
- Onset of pain is usually acute and abrupt with torsion, rupture of a cyst, or ectopic pregnancy.
- Mullerian anomalies usually present as cyclic pain with timing as would be expected for a menstrual cycle.
- Infectious processes such as PID usually worsen over several days.
- Appendicitis usually starts as periumbilical pain that migrates to the right lower quadrant.
- Endometriosis symptoms may be confusing because it can present with both cyclic and acyclic pain. Generally, the pain is most severe during menses.

Endometriosis is defined as having endometrial glands and stroma outside of the uterus. It is found in 4% to 17% of postmenarchal females and is a common cause of chronic pelvic pain. The etiology is multifactorial including retrograde menstruation, metaplastic transformation of totipotent embryologic cells, metastases of endometrial cells, and possible genetic predisposition. This condition can be associated with bowel and bladder dysfunction, and there is no relationship between the stage of the disease or the site of the lesions and the severity of the pain.

C. **Physical examination:** Physical examination to evaluate pelvic pain should include examination of the abdomen for evidence of masses, hepatosplenomegaly, and peritonitis. A bimanual exam should also be conducted as either a vaginal–abdominal, recto–abdominal, or rectovaginal–abdominal exam to evaluate uterine size and assess for the presence of cervical motion/adnexal tenderness and any masses. If the patient is sexually active, he or she should be tested for STIs. If urine-based nucleic acid amplification testing for STIs is not available, then a speculum exam should be performed to obtain cervical specimens. In a patient with cyclic pain, particularly in the presence of amenorrhea, examination of the lower genital tract is crucial. The clinician can start by trying to insert a cotton swab into the vagina to establish patency of the vagina as a first step toward ruling out a vaginal or Mullerian anomaly.

D. **Laboratory evaluation:**
- Pregnancy test
- STD testing: *C. trachomatis, N. gonorrhoeae, T. vaginalis*
- CBC differential and erythrocyte sedimentation rate
- Urinalysis
- Urine culture

When evaluating these test results, it is important to remember the following points. The white blood cell count may be elevated as a result of either the ischemia found in torsion or an infectious process. The hematocrit may be falsely elevated during an acute bleeding episode since it takes time to drop with equilibration. In addition, sexually active teens may have an STI along with another nongynecologic diagnosis such as appendicitis or constipation. It is crucial to closely follow the evolution of symptoms, particularly when there is acute pain, to avoid missing the correct diagnosis.

E. **Radiologic evaluation:** Ultrasound is a useful tool in the evaluation of pelvic pain. This technique allows for evaluation of an adnexal mass and can be used in patients where an adequate bimanual exam is not possible. It is important to remember that 1 to 2 cm follicular cysts are normal in adolescents and not considered pathologic. Use of Doppler techniques during ultrasound can also assess flow to the ovary, which is important in cases of suspected ovarian torsion. Ultrasound is not diagnostic for PID or endometriosis. However, it may detect a tubo-ovarian abscess—a possible complication of PID.

III. **Management:**

A. **Goals of treatment:**
- Treat acute and chronic pain symptoms
- Diagnose and treat underlying cause of pain

B. Treatment: Torsion, PID, and pregnancy complications need prompt diagnosis and intervention. Many primary care providers treat PID themselves but torsion and pregnancy complications should be referred to a gynecologist.

A simple ovarian cyst can be treated with nonsteroidal anti-inflammatory drugs (NSAIDs) for pain and OCPs to prevent formation of new cysts while observing for resolution of the current cyst. An ultrasound is usually repeated after one to two cycles to demonstrate resolution. A ruptured cyst is treated with NSAIDs and requires no further evaluation if symptoms resolve. A complex cyst that does not resolve or a solid mass should be referred for further evaluation by a gynecologist.

Patients with chronic pain are initially treated with NSAIDs but if the pain persists for 3 to 6 months, laparoscopic evaluation may be indicated to confirm or elucidate the diagnosis. Patients with endometriosis frequently will respond to OCPs in combination with NSAIDs. Immediate laparoscopy is not necessary unless medical therapy is unsuccessful in controlling the symptoms.

IV. Clinical pearls and pitfalls:
- Pelvic pain does not necessarily indicate a gynecologic diagnosis.
- Endometriosis is a common cause of chronic pelvic pain in adolescents.
- Gynecologic evaluation is part of the evaluation of pelvic pain.

BREAST DISORDERS

Female

I. Description of the condition: Breast disorders in females encompass a wide range of conditions from mastalgia, to masses, to developmental anomalies.

II. Making the diagnosis:

A. Signs and symptoms/differential diagnosis:

1. Anomalies:
- **Asymmetry:** Asymmetry is commonly seen as breast development begins; however, usually it resolves in later stares of development. Causes of persistent asymmetry include trauma and iatrogenic causes. When asymmetry persists or occurs later in breast development, examination should be performed to rule out a mass, cyst, or abscess. Once breast development is complete, surgical intervention can be considered to improve cosmetic deformity.
- **Hypertrophy:** Very large breasts can cause back pain, postural kyphosis, breast discomfort, intertrigo, and shoulder pain. Reduction surgery, if needed, is usually delayed until breast development is completed.
- **Tuberous breasts:** Tuberous breasts occur with overdevelopment of the nipple-areola complex and underdevelopment of the base, creating a tuberous shape. This is a cosmetic problem of unknown etiology.
- **Amastia:** Amastia usually occurs unilaterally and is rare. There can also be absence of the nipple that may or may not be associated with absence of breast tissue. One specific syndrome presenting with amastia is Poland Syndrome, which includes unilateral amastia with aplasia of the pectoralis muscles and rib deformity.
- **Hypomastia:** Small breasts may be normal in a patient with otherwise normal pubertal development and normal menses. However, the lack of breast tissue or a small amount of tissue can be associated with malnutrition, inflammatory bowel disease, radiation, excess androgens, and hypogonadotropic hypogonadism.
- **Accessory nipples (Polythelia) or breast tissue (Polymastia):** Accessory nipples or breast tissue can be found along the fetal milk line. They can sometimes cause pain or enough cosmetic deformity to warrant removal.

2. Nipple discharge: Nipple discharge can have various presentations including:
- Purulent discharge from infection
- Multicolored discharge as found in ductal ectasia
- Serosanginous discharge in association with intraductal papilloma and, rarely, cancer
- Clear-yellow serous discharge from fibrocystic breast disease
- Milky discharge from true galactorrhea in pregnancy or in hypothryoidism, prolactinoma, use of psychotropic medications, renal failure, or substance use

3. Breast masses: Breast masses may represent cysts or solid tumors. Primary breast cancer is rare in adolescents, with only 0.2% of primary breast cancer occurring prior to the age of 20. Malignant breast masses in this age group are frequently metastatic tumors from other locations. Common abnormalities causing breast masses in adolescents include cysts, fibrocystic breast changes, and fibroadenomas.

- **Breast cyst:** Cysts are common in adolescents and usually resolve within a few months. Ultrasound of the breast will demonstrate the presence of a cyst, which can be aspirated if it does not resolve.
- **Fibroadenoma:** Fibroadenoma is the most commonly excised breast mass in adolescents. They are rubbery, firm mobile masses with a distinct border representing stromal proliferation around elongated and distorted ducts. Fibroadenoma can either remain the same size or increase through successive menstrual cycles. They last for several months but frequently resolve on their own. Although they are usually benign, patients with fibroadenoma may have an increased risk or carcinoma in the future when there is a family history of breast cancer in association with a complex fibroadenoma or adjacent proliferative disease. One particular type of fibroadenoma is more concerning. Rapidly growing masses called giant fibroadenomas can compress normal breast tissue and require intervention.
- **Fibrocystic breast changes:** Fibrocystic breast changes are cordlike thickenings and lumps that can become tender prior to menses. These breast changes vary throughout the menstrual cycles and may resolve when the monthly menstrual cycle is complete. A proposed etiology for fibrocystic breast changes is an imbalance in estrogen and progesterone. Most women do not have an increased risk of breast cancer in the future, but those with proliferative disease and atypical hyperplasia are at increased risk.

4. **Mastalgia:** Mastalgia (painful breasts) can occur in response to hormonal changes during the normal menstrual cycle, with use of hormonal contraception, during pregnancy, as part of fibrocystic breast changes, and as a result of poorly fitting bras. Breast pain can also be a sign of an infectious process causing mastitis or an abscess. Infection occurs with breast feeding, ductal abnormalities, or from trauma during sexual play. The organisms commonly involved are staphylococci and streptococci. Finally, pain can result from trauma. Breast contusion, commonly caused by trauma during sports, can result in a poorly defined mass including fat necrosis. This mass can sometimes be confused later with a malignancy because it can take months to resolve. Nipple irritation/trauma can also occur in runners due to acute or chronic abrasion from repetitive motion.

B. **Physical exam:** Physical exam evaluated in conjunction with the history is usually helpful in determining the diagnosis. Infection usually presents with tenderness and erythema. A cyst will frequently resolve after the next menstrual period whereas a fibroadenoma usually remains the same or enlarges. The breast thickening and tenderness seen with fibrocystic breasts will usually improve at the end of the monthly menstrual cycle.

C. **Radiologic evaluation:** Ultrasound is helpful in defining whether a breast is solid or cystic. Mammogram should not be performed on adolescents because the breast tissue is too dense and the test cannot be accurately interpreted.

III. **Management:** Infectious masses should be treated with antibiotics to cover staphylococcal or streptococcal organisms. Noninfectious masses can be followed through a menstrual period and, if there is resolution, no further evaluation is needed. Masses consistent with a fibroadenoma can be followed by physical exam and ultrasound to evaluate for growth. Persistent masses that appear cystic can be aspirated, and if they do not resolve or cannot be aspirated can be removed surgically. A professional fitting of brassieres should be done if the patient's bra size might not be correct.

Self breast exam is an important component of preventive health in adult women. However, there is controversy about the utility of teaching self breast exam to adolescents because breast cancer is extremely rare. Many people would advocate teaching older adolescents this technique as they become more comfortable with their bodies and are able to participate actively in preventive health care.

Male

I. **Description of the condition:** Breast disorders in males range from normal physiologic pubertal gynecomastia to pathologic causes of breast enlargement and breast masses.

II. **Making the diagnosis:** Pubertal gynecomastia is a benign increase in the glandular and stromal tissue in the breast that is caused by an imbalance between estrogen and androgen activity. The condition peaks during genital stage 2 or 3 in up to two-thirds of male adolescents and usually resolves on its own within 1 to 2 years. A small percentage of male adolescents have gynecomastia that persists.

Table 26-9. Differential diagnosis of gynecomastia in male adolescents

- Testicular tumors
- Adrenal tumors
- Other hCG-producing tumors: liver, lung, stomach, kidney
- Hyperthryoidism
- Liver disease/cirrhosis
- Renal failure/dialysis
- Obesity
- Malnutrition with refeeding
- Hyperprolactinemia
- Hypogonadotropic hypogonadism
- Primary hypogonadism: Klinefelter syndrome, Congenital defect of testosterone biosynthetic pathway
- Excessive extraglandular aromatase activity
- Androgen insensitivity/resistance
- True hermaphroditism
- Drugs, e.g., spironolactone, marijuana, phenothiazines, digoxin, cimetidine
- Breast masses: neoplasia, dermoid cyst, lipoma, hematoma, and neurofibroma

hCG, human chorionic gonadotropin

A. **Differential diagnosis:** Other causes of gynecomastia include entities that cause an increase in estrogen production, decrease in serum androgens, or cause of problem at the level of the estrogen or androgen receptor. The differential diagnosis can be seen in Table 26-9.

B. **Physical exam:** In pubertal gynecomastia, there may be subareolar nodules and breast tissue extending beyond the areola. Usually gynecomastia is bilateral but it can begin or remain unilateral and the glandular tissue is symmetrical with the nipple-areolar complex. Other masses, which do not represent pubertal gynecomastia, are more likely to be present in a location eccentric to the areola. Adipose tissue can be distinguished from true gynecomastia because unlike gynecomastia, adipose tissue does not feel like firm rubbery tissue when palpated between the fingers.

Physical exam should include evaluation for findings consistent with liver disease, thyroid disease, kidney disease, or prolactinemia. An abdominal mass suggests the need to evaluate for an adrenal tumor. A testicular exam should be performed to evaluate for testicular volume/atrophy and the presence of any masses.

C. **Laboratory evaluation:** If gynecomastia is consistent with pubertal gynecomastia, then laboratory evaluation is not needed. Patients who are Tanner stage 1 or 5 should not present with gynecomastia, and in those cases hCG, LH, serum testosterone, and estradiol levels are useful in sorting through the differential diagnosis.

III. **Management:** If the adolescent is in the middle of puberty, and drug-induced gynecomastia, liver, thyroid, and renal causes are ruled out, and the physical exam is otherwise normal, the patient can be followed in 6 months without further evaluation. Tender and recent onset gynecomastia in a patient past the stage of pubertal onset gynecomastia or prior to the onset of puberty should prompt further evaluation. Patients with pubertal gynecomastia should be reassured. Surgical intervention for significant gynecomastia that does not resolve and is causing psychological sequelae may be indicated.

IV. **Clinical pearls and pitfalls:**
- Breast cancer is rare in male and female adolescents.
- The most likely cause of a solitary nodule that does not change with menses in a female adolescent is a fibroadenoma.
- Pubertal gynecomastia is common in male adolescents.
- All male adolescents with gynecomastia that is not consistent with pubertal gynecomastia should have a testicular exam.

MENSTRUAL DISORDERS

I. **Description of the condition:**
A. **Definitions/epidemiology:** Menstrual disorders are common among female adolescents. Clinicians caring for adolescents will encounter a patient presenting with

amenorrhea, dysfunctional uterine bleeding, or dysmenorrhea. To properly evaluate menstrual disorders it is important to understand the parameters of normal menstruation, which include:
- Median age of menarche is 12.4 years; 12.1 years in African-American females.
- Most females will have menarche within 2 to 3 years of thelarche, but the range varies.
- Approximately one-quarter of females have menarche by Tanner 3, and almost 90% by Tanner 4.
- Normal cycles occur every 21 to 35 days and last for 3 to 7 days.
- Approximately 50% to 80% of cycles in the first 2 years are anovulatory. By 5 years 10% to 20% are anovulatory.
- The later menarche occurs, the longer it takes to develop regular ovulatory cycles.
- On average, it takes 14 months from menarche to establishing regular cycles and 2 years for regular ovulatory cycles.
- Dysmenorrhea is usually associated with ovulatory cycles.
- Normal blood loss is 30 to 40 mL, which is equivalent to 10 to 15 soaked pads or tampons per cycle.

B. Phases of the menstrual cycle:
  1. Follicular:
    - GnRH stimulates production of LH and FSH from the pituitary.
    - FSH stimulates granulose cells, and there is a rise in estradiol and proliferation of the endometrium.
    - LH simulates the theca cells, which produce androstendione and testosterone.
    - A dominant follicle is identified by day 5 to 7 and is located in a more estrogen-rich environment.
    - An LH surge occurs with positive feedback from rising estrogen levels leading to ovulation.
  2. Ovulation:
    - With ovulation the corpus luteum forms, producing progesterone in addition to estrogen.
    - Ovulation occurs 2 weeks prior to menstruation.
  3. Luteal:
    - Progesterone inhibits proliferation of the endometrium and leads to coiling of the endometrial glands and increased vascularity of the stroma.
    - The endometrium is mature 8 to 9 days postovulation.
    - Without a pregnancy and hCG, the corpus luteum cannot be sustained; with the fall in estrogen and progesterone levels, the endometrium becomes necrotic, leading to menstruation.

II. Making the diagnosis:
A. Amenorrhea
  1. Definitions:
    a. Primary amenorrhea is the lack of menarche by age 16. However, there should be concern if 2 to 3 years have passed since thelarche or if the patient is Tanner 5. In general, there should not be more than 4 years between the start of Tanner 2 and menarche.
    b. Secondary amenorrhea is defined as missing three cycles in a row. It is common to miss cycles close to the time of menarche, particularly during the first year after menarche. However, most females will have cycles within the range of 21 to 45 days even in the first few years after menarche.
  2. Differential diagnosis: The differential diagnosis of amenorrhea is extensive, and some entities may present with either primary or secondary amenorrhea depending on timing in relation to puberty. For example, if ovarian failure occurs prior to menarche, the patient will have primary amenorrhea whereas if it occurs afterward, she will have secondary amenorrhea. On the other hand, a patient with an imperforate hymen or agenesis of the uterus and vagina will only present with primary amenorrhea.
    a. Anatomic:
      - Imperforate hymen
      - Transverse vaginal septum
      - Agenesis of cervix, uterus, vagina
      - Uterine synechiae
    b. Hypothalamus:
      - Deficiency of GnRH
      - Chronic or systemic illness
      - Familial
      - Stress

- Athletics
- Eating disorders (anorexia, obesity)
- Drugs (opiates, amitryptiline)
- Tumor

c. **Pituitary gland:**
- Hypopituitarism (congenital, head trauma, postpartum shock, necrosis)
- Tumor (prolactinoma, other pituitary tumor)
- Absence of LH or FSH

d. **Ovarian:**
- Gonadal dysgenesis (50% Pure 45X, 40%–50% 46XX/45X)
- Ovarian failure (autoimmune oophoritis, premature failure, radiation or chemotherapy)
- Tumor
- Resistant ovaries
- 17-hydroxylase deficiency 46XX, without secondary sexual characteristics
- Mixed gonadal dysgenesis (45X/46XY, 45X/46XX/46XY)
- XY gonadal dysgenesis

e. **Androgen excess:**
- Polycystic ovary syndrome (chronic anovulatory hyperandrogenism)
- Adrenal tumor
- Congenital adrenal hyperplasia (complete or partial deficiency 11-hydroxylase, 21-hydroxylase, 3-hydroxysteroid dehydrogenase)
- Ovarian tumor

f. **Other endocrine:**
- Thyroid (hyper- or hypothyroidism)
- Cushing syndrome

g. **Pregnancy**
h. **Hormonal contraception**

B. **Selected clinical entities:**
1. **Turner syndrome:**
- Gonadal dysgenesis.
- 45XO or mosaicism.
- Stigmata include webbed neck, wide set nipples, short stature, low hair line, cardiac abnormality, abnormal carrying angle of arms, autoimmune disorders, hearing impairment, and delayed puberty.
- Mosaics may not have typical phenotypic features.
- Usually presents as primary amenorrhea.

2. **Androgen insensitivity:**
- XY chromosomes with inability to respond to androgens because of a defect in the response of the androgen receptors.
- In the complete form there is no secondary sexual hair, external genitalia appear female, there is no uterus or vagina because of presence of mullerian inhibiting factor, good breast development because of estrogen dominance, and undescended or partially descended testes that are at high risk for carcinoma.
- The partial form may have varying stigmata.
- Primary amenorrhea in a phenotypic female.

3. **Mayer Rokitansky Kuster Hauser (mullerian aplasia):**
- XX chromosomes.
- mullerian aplasia with normal ovaries and normal breast and pubic hair development.
- Associated with renal and skeletal anomalies.
- Primary amenorrhea.

4. **Prolactinoma:**
- **Classic presentation: amenorrhea, galactorrhea, visual field cut, headaches.**
- Microadenoma may only present with amenorrhea.
- Presents with elevated prolactin levels, but not everyone with an elevated prolactin has galactorrhea or amenorrhea.
- May be primary or secondary amenorrhea but usually secondary.

5. **Polycystic ovary syndrome (PCOS):**
- Functional ovarian hyperandrogenism.
- Seen in 4% to 6% of adolescents and young women.
- Common cause of infertility in adult women.
- **PCOS is a spectrum of disorders beginning in the perimenarchal period associated with abnormal gonadotropin secretion (exaggerated**

release and tonic elevation of LH leading to an increase in ovarian androgens), increase in adrenal androgen production, and insulin resistance.
- PCOS presents as oligomenorrhea or amenorrhea with signs of elevated androgens including virilization, hirsutism, acne, and clitoromegaly and can be associated with anovulatory dysfunctional uterine bleeding. Over the years, ovaries become enlarged with multiple 2 to 8 mm small peripheral cysts and a thickened glistening ovarian capsule, but this usually is evident only after adolescence.
- Most patients are overweight, have irregular menses from the time of menarche, impaired follicular maturation from relative FSH deficiency, increased LH, elevated ovarian androgens, and a decrease in sex hormone-binding globulin (SHBG) leading to an increase in free testosterone and estrogen and peripheral conversion of androgens to estrogens. Acyclic estrogen causes unopposed stimulation of the endometrium, increasing the risk of dysfunctional uterine bleeding. PCOS is associated with insulin resistance and hyperinsulinemia. Insulin and insulin-like growth factor-1 (IGF-1) increase ovarian androgen production in thin as well as obese women. IGF-1 simulates the ovarian enzyme responsible for androgen production in the ovary, and women with PCOS have apparent dysregulation of this enzyme. Insulin also inhibits SHBG, leading to increased free testosterone. Acanthosis nigricans is a nonspecific marker suggesting possible insulin resistance. Insulin-sensitizing agents decrease hyperinsulinism along with LH and ovarian androgens.
- PCOS is also associated with an abnormal lipid profile as part of the metabolic syndrome.

6. **Athletic Amenorrhea:**
- **Strenuous exercise can cause dysfunction of the hypothalamic-pituitary axis** and amenorrhea including inhibition of GnRH pulses, decrease in LH pulse frequency, and effects on levels of neurotransmitters.
- Athletic amenorrhea can be associated with delayed menarche and/or puberty. Menarche is delayed by 5 months for each year of intense training prior to menarche.
- Up to two-thirds of all athletes in some studies have oligomenorrhea or amenorrhea.
- Clinicians need to be aware of the **female athlete triad: amenorrhea, osteoporosis, disordered eating.** The osteoporosis may not be completely reversible, and there is an increased risk of stress fractures in these patients.
- Athletes in certain sports where a thin body habitus is important are at increased risk including: ballet, runners, and gymnasts.

7. **Pregnancy:**
- Can present as primary or secondary amenorrhea depending on age of onset of sexual activity.
- Clinicians must always consider pregnancy as a cause of secondary amenorrhea, and must not forget pregnancy as a possible cause, albeit rare, of primary amenorrhea.

C. **Physical examination:** The evaluation should begin with a thorough history and physical examination. The assessment should consider chronic illness, signs of endocrine dysfunction consistent with thyroid disease or adrenal disease, pubertal development including the stage and sequencing, as well as the timing of puberty and whether menses would be expected at this pubertal stage. During the general examination, the clinician should look for signs of elevated androgens including hirsutism and acne. External genitalia should be examined to determine that the clitoris is not enlarged and that the hymen is patent. The vaginal mucosa should be assessed for estrogen effect and appear to be pink and moist rather than red and thinned as seen with inadequate estrogen. Patency of the vagina can be assessed by inserting a moistened cotton-tipped applicator into the vaginal opening. Vaginal–abdominal or recto–abdominal exam can also be performed to assess for the presence of the uterus and cervix.

D. **Radiologic evaluation:** A pelvic ultrasound will help define upper tract anatomy; a magnetic resonance imaging (MRI) procedure is the next step to further define a suspected upper tract anomaly. An MRI of the head with sella views should be performed for suspected prolactinoma.

E. **Laboratory evaluation:**
1. **Initial evaluation:**
- Pregnancy test
- TSH

- Prolactin
- FSH: FSH is high in ovarian failure (hypergonadotropic hypogonadism), low in hypothalamic-pituitary axis suppression (hypogonadotropic hypogonadism)
2. **If ovarian failure is found and there is no history of radiation or chemotherapy:**
   - Chromosomes to rule out Turner syndrome.
   - If chromosomes are normal, check anti-ovarian antibodies for autoimmune oophoritis.
3. **If PCOS is suspected add:**
   - Total and free testosterone: An elevated free testosterone is sufficient to make the diagnosis because the total testosterone may be normal secondary to varying levels of SHBG.
   - 17-OH progesterone: This test can be mildly elevated in PCOS, but marked elevation suggests 21-hydroxylase deficiency possibly presenting as late onset congenital adrenal hyperplasia.
4. **If PCOS proven:**
   - Check fasting lipid screen.
   - Check fasting glucose and insulin.
5. **If virilization is present or an androgen secreting tumor is suspected, add:**
   - DHEAS: Level greater than 600 to 700 μg/dL concerning for tumor.
   - Androstenedione: Level greater than 500 ng/dL concerning for tumor.
   - Testosterone: Level greater than 150 to 200 ng/mL concerning for tumor.
III. **Management:** Treat any identified underlying illness: that is, thyroid disease, prolactinoma, eating disorder, congenital adrenal hyperplasia, etc. If these treatable causes are ruled out:
   A. **Give an oral medroxyprogesterone challenge (10 mg a day for 5 or 10 days)**
      - If patient has withdrawal bleeding, that indicates an intact lower tract with appropriate estrogen stimulation of the endometrial lining and sufficient FSH.
      - If there is no withdrawal bleeding, that indicates insufficient estrogen/FSH or an abnormality of the uterus or outflow tract.
   B. **If patient has ovarian failure:**
      - She will need hormone replacement therapy.
   C. **If patient has hypothalamic-pituitary suppression from athletic amenorrhea:**
      - Clinician can prescribe OCPs to help prevent further bone loss.
   D. **If patient has hypothalamic-pituitary suppression from an eating disorder:**
      - Various studies have demonstrated that OCPs probably will not make a difference in bone density in this clinical scenario. Many clinicians do not prescribe them for patients with anorexia nervosa since return of menses is a marker for adequate weight gain and this is lost when OCPs are prescribed.
   E. **If the patient has anovulation without ovarian failure:**
      - Clinician can give progesterone to induce withdrawal bleeding and prevent endometrial hyperplasia (minimum every 3 months).
      - Patients can be also be prescribed OCPs to maintain menses and prevent endometrial hyperplasia.
   F. **If patient has PCOS:**
      - Clinician can give OCPs to suppress the hypothalamic-pituitary-ovarian axis, raise SHBG and bind up testosterone, lower adrenal androgen secretion, and protect from unopposed estrogen stimulation of the endometrium. OCPs should also improve acne and help decrease progression of hirsutism.
      - Additional therapy for hirsutism can include spironolactone.
      - Clinician can give drugs that improve insulin sensitivity. With reduced insulin levels there will be lower testosterone levels and there can be improvement in ovulation and decreased progression of hirsutism. At the time of publication of this manual, use of insulin-sensitizing agents may not be first-line therapy in adolescents. If the patient is sexually active, then contraception will also be needed since use of these agents may result in ovulation.

DYSFUNCTIONAL UTERINE BLEEDING

I. **Description of the condition:** Irregular and/or profuse menstruation is a common complaint in adolescents, particularly around the time of menarche. The most common diagnosis is dysfunctional uterine bleeding (DUB), which frequently occurs during the first year after menarche and is caused by a maturational defect in which rising levels of estrogen do not cause a drop in FSH. As a result, there is persistent elevation of estrogen and thickening of the endometrium. This is compounded by anovulation in which there is a lack of progesterone that would normally stabilize the endometrium. As previously mentioned, anovulation is common after menarche, but normally the negative feedback of estrogen on FSH results in a withdrawal bleed preventing excessive endometrial overgrowth.

A. **Definitions:**

DUB: Excessive, prolonged unpatterned bleeding not caused by structural or systemic disease.

Menorrhagia: Cyclic prolonged or heavy bleeding.

Menometrorrhagia: Irregular prolonged bleeding.

Polymenorrhea: Cyclic bleeding occurring less than 21 days apart.

II. **Making the diagnosis:**

A. Anovulation and a maturational defect are diagnoses of exclusion. The differential diagnosis of abnormal vaginal bleeding includes pregnancy-related complications, an underlying bleeding disorder, genital trauma, and other entities that cause anovulation including endocrine problems and PCOS.

B. **Differential diagnosis of dysfunctional uterine bleeding:**

1. **Hypothalamus:**
   - Chronic or systemic illness
   - Familial
   - Stress
   - Athletics
   - Eating disorders (anorexia, obesity)
   - Drugs

2. **Pituitary gland:**
   - Tumor (prolactinoma)

3. **Outflow tract:**
   - Trauma
   - Foreign body
   - Vaginal tumor
   - Cervical carcinoma
   - Polyp
   - Uterine myoma
   - Uterine carcinoma—rare in adolescents
   - Intrauterine device

4. **Ovary:**
   - Tumor
   - Cyst

5. **Androgen excess:**
   - Polycystic ovary syndrome (chronic anovulatory hyperandrogenism)
   - Adrenal tumor
   - Congenital adrenal hyperplasia (complete or partial deficiency 11-hydroxylase, 21-hydroxylase, 3-hydroxysteroid dehydrogenase)
   - Ovarian tumor

6. **Other endocrine:**
   - Thyroid (Hyper- or hypothyroidism)
   - Adrenal disease
   - Diabetes

7. **Hematologic:**
   - Thrombocytopenia
   - Clotting disorders
   - Platelet disorders (von Willebrand disease)
   - Anticoagulant meds

8. **Pregnancy:**
   - Ectopic pregnancy
   - Miscarriage
   - Molar pregnancy

9. **Infections:**
   - STIs
   - PID

10. **Hormonal contraception**

C. **History:** The history should include questions addressing other clinical entities listed in the differential diagnosis. Key questions should include:
   - Age at menarche
   - Menstrual pattern: duration, quantity, amount of flow, dysmenorrhea, dates of menses
   - History of sexual activity
   - History of genital trauma

- Use of contraception including condoms
- History of or symptoms of sexually transmitted diseases
- Associated abdominal pain
- Signs of hypovolemia: lightheadedness with standing, dyspnea on exertion, headache, syncope
- Signs of androgen excess: hirsutism, acne
- Presence of galactorrhea
- Signs of a bleeding disorder including other episodes of prolonged bleeding (tooth extraction, epistaxis, petechiae, bruises)
- Medications including anticoagulants
- Review of systems including: stress, chronic disease, weight changes, eating disorder, athletics, and visual disturbances

Understanding the pattern of bleeding—for example, whether it is cyclic or acyclic—is also helpful. Heavy cyclic bleeding is usually seen with a bleeding disorder or problem in the uterus itself. Normal cyclic bleeding that is accompanied by intermenstrual bleeding may be the result of a vaginal foreign body, infection, uterine polyp, congenital malformation of uterus with obstruction, a problem with the cervix, or a vaginal malignancy. Genital tract malignancy (uterine, cervix, or vagina) is rare in adolescents. The lack of any cyclic pattern suggests DUB and anovulatory disorders.

Patients with bleeding disorders may not have had a previous condition that caused an episode of prolonged bleeding. Menarche may be the first time a disorder such as von Willebrand disease presents. In addition to acquired problems such as thrombocytopenia, liver disease, or use of anticoagulant medication, and inherited clotting disorders should be considered in all patients who present with heavy prolonged bleeding at menarche.

D. **Physical exam:** The physical exam should include:
  - **Postural vital signs:** to exclude hypovolemia
  - **General habitus:** height, weight, body fat distribution to assess for Cushing disease/syndrome, PCOS
  - **Skin exam:** to look for hirsutism, acne, bruises, petechiae
  - **Thyroid exam**
  - **Breast exam:** to look for galactorrhea
  - **Gynecologic exam:** The pelvic examination may be skipped if the menstrual pattern is described as a few months of irregular bleeding at menarche that has resolved in a patient who is now having regular cycles. The pelvic exam can also be omitted in a patient who has a classic history for anovulation in the early postmenarchal time frame, is not experiencing significant pain, and has a negative pregnancy test. However, a pelvic examination would be indicated in patients who are sexually active and hemodynamically unstable. Pelvic exam should also be considered in patients who have a history of continued menstrual pattern disruption which does not respond to medical therapy to assess for vaginal or cervical abnormalities. Diagnoses to be excluded in this situation include polyps, cervicitis, and complex anomalies. If a vaginal exam is not possible, the clinician can perform a recto–abdominal exam to assess for a vaginal foreign body, or uterine or ovarian mass.

E. **Laboratory evaluation:** Laboratory evaluation should include:
  - **Pregnancy test**
  - **CBC with differential and platelets:** The Hgb should be interpreted in conjunction with the vital signs and bleeding history. A patient with a normal Hgb but postural changes will likely have a significant fall in the level on repeat testing once she is volume repleted and hemodynamically stable.
  - **Prothrombin and partial thromboplastin time**
  - **von Willebrand panel:** This should be performed in patients with heavy bleeding at menarche as well as a consistent history of heavy prolonged bleeding. Testing should be done prior to starting hormone therapy since estrogen will elevate the von Willebrand factor.
  - **TSH**
  - **Prolactin**
  - **If there is hirsutism, acne—PCOS labs:** Total and free testosterone, DHEAS
  - **STI testing:** If sexually active test for *N. gonorrhoaea, C. trachomatis, T. vaginalis.*
  - **Other:** Some clinicians will draw a PFA 100 to assess for platelet function problems including von Willebrand disease.

F. **Radiologic evaluation:** Ultrasound can help define the upper pelvic anatomy and measure the thickness of the endometrial stripe. An MRI of the pelvis can further define a suspected uterine anomaly.

III. Management:

A. Goals of treatment: The goals of treatment are to stop the acute bleeding and stabilize the endometrium to prevent further bleeding. This is usually accomplished by a combination of estrogen that heals the individual sites of bleeding in the endometrium by inducing proliferation and simultaneous use of progesterone, which stabilizes the endometrial lining. The evaluation should determine if there is a treatable underlying cause of the bleeding. If the bleeding episode is not simply DUB, additional specific treatment of that cause is needed to prevent recurrence (e.g., PCOS, thyroid disease, thrombocytopenia).

B. Treatment regimens:

1. **Mild DUB:** Patients with a normal hemoglobin who have only mild prolongation of menses or shortening of the cycle can be observed by following a menstrual calendar. Iron supplements can help prevent anemia and antiprostaglandin medications may decrease blood loss.

2. **Moderate DUB:** Patients showing more severe prolongation of menses with heavier flow or more extreme shortening of cycle length are considered moderate DUB. These patients will frequently present with anemia, and medical therapy to stop the bleeding would be indicated. The treatment regimen can include monophasic (30–35 µg OCPs) with a potent progestin (norgestrel, levonorgestrel), oral medroxyprogesterone, or other progestins such as norethindrone acetate. The combination of an estrogen and progestin together is consistently most effective and preferred over progestin-only therapy. Depending on the amount of bleeding, one to two OCPs a day for 3 to 4 days may stop the bleeding, and then the patient can be continued on one pill a day. However, with heavy bleeding or significant anemia, if may be important to stop the bleeding quickly—within 48 to 72 hours. In those cases, starting with four pills a day and tapering down to one pill over several weeks may be necessary. One possible regimen includes:

   - One pill four times a day for 4 days
   - One pill three times a day for 3 days
   - One pill two times a day for 2 weeks
   - One pill a day for 1 to 2 weeks depending on the level of Hgb

   Iron should be given to facilitate correction of the low Hgb and an antiemetic may be necessary during days of multiple pill use to prevent nausea and vomiting. This tapering regimen is followed by a week off pills to produce a withdrawal bleed and then cycling on any OCP for 3 to 6 months to ensure complete healing of the endometrium. In cases of von Willebrand disease, patients may elect to continue on OCPs to control bleeding. Other modalities for control of menses in coagulation disorders include use of DDAVP and Stimate; however, some patients prefer the cycle control of OCPs. Continuous OCPs is also an option, especially now that there is a 91-day pill pack approved for use.

   For patients who cannot tolerate estrogen or when estrogen use is contraindicated, alternative therapies include 3 to 6 months of cyclic medroxyprogesterone (10 mg) or norethindrone acetate (5–10 mg) a day for 14 days a month.

3. **Severe DUB:** Severe DUB is significant heavy prolonged bleeding usually accompanied by significant anemia (Hgb <9 g/dL) and/or orthostatic changes in vital signs. Most clinicians would admit patients with an Hgb less than 7 g/dL. Anyone with orthostatic changes regardless of their current measured Hgb should be treated as an inpatient. Different regimens are used to treat severe DUB:

   - Intravenous premarin at a dose of 25 mg IV every 4 to 6 hours for three to four doses, which is followed within 24 to 48 hours with combined OCPs. Some clinicians are concerned that intravenous estrogen may increase the risk of thromboembolism. However, in cases of severe hemorrhage, some clinicians prefer starting with intravenous therapy to stop the bleeding quickly.
   - OCPs starting at a dose of one pill every 4 hours and then tapering to every 6 hours after control of bleeding. This is followed by an OCP taper to one pill a day over several weeks.
   - Norethrindrone acetate: 5 to 10 mg every 4 hours and then tapering to every 6 hours with control of bleeding. This is followed by a taper to one pill twice a day to complete a 3- week regimen. An alternative is to use 5 mg four times a day for 4 days; then three times a day for 3 days, followed by twice a day for 2 weeks. If the patient can take OCPs, this regimen could be followed by cyclic OCPs or extended OCPs without withdrawal bleeding for several months.

   All of these regimes are accompanied by iron therapy. The patient should not be allowed to have a withdrawal bleed until the Hgb is in an acceptable range. The withdrawal bleed is followed by cycling on OCPs or a progestin-only product.

Most patients are successfully treated with hormonal therapy. Transfusion may be needed in severely anemic patients who are symptomatic. Rarely a dilatation and curettage may be performed to remove the blood clots that are distending the uterus and not allowing uterine contraction to stop the bleeding.

DYSMENORRHEA

I. **Description/etiology of the condition:** Dysmenorrhea is pain associated with menses. Twenty percent to 90% of adolescents suffer from this disorder.
   A. **Definitions:**
      1. **Primary dysmenorrhea** is menstrual pain not associated with pelvic pathology. This form of dymenorrhea is associated with ovulatory cycles and commonly begins 1 to 2 years after menarche. Prostaglandins formed in the endometrium during ovulatory cycles cause smooth muscle contractions as well as associated symptoms such as vomiting, diarrhea, and dizziness. Other symptoms can include headache, backache, and thigh pain.
      2. **Secondary dysmenorrhea** is menstrual pain associated with pelvic pathology such as endometriosis, uterine/genital tract malformation and obstruction, and PID. This pain may occur with either ovulatory or anovulatory cycles.

II. **Making the diagnosis:**
   A. **History:** History should include age of menarche, family history of endometriosis, and severity of the pain including any inability to go to school or participate in daily activities. Previous treatment, including response to therapy, should be assessed since a patient who has been unresponsive to appropriate doses of NSAIDs may require another treatment modality.
   B. **Physical examination:** A patient with mild symptoms and adequate response to NSAIDs can simply have an examination of the external genitalia to ensure patency of the hymen. For those with more severe symptoms or those that have a change in symptoms with onset of sexual activity, a pelvic examination including a speculum exam is helpful to define the anatomy and rule out STIs. If the patient is virginal and a speculum exam is not possible, inserting a cotton swab into the vagina to determine vaginal patency and performing a bimanual exam (possibly recto–abdominal) will help assess upper tract anatomy and pain symptoms.
   C. **Laboratory tests:** None are needed unless STIs or pregnancy need to be ruled out in sexually active patients.
   D. **Radiologic studies** are not usually necessary unless there is a need to assess upper tract anatomy, particularly in a patient where a pelvic examination cannot be completed.

III. **Management:**
   - Initial therapy involves the use of NSAIDs, around the clock, with the onset of menses to block the affects of prostaglandins. Possible regimens include:
   - Ibuprofen 400 to 600 mg every 6 hours
   - Naproxen sodium 250 mg every 6 hours or 550 mg every 12 hours
   - Mefenemic acid 250 mg every 6 hours
   Mefenemic acid works by a dual mechanism including preventing production of prostaglandins as well as blocking prostaglandin receptors.
   - If NSAIDs are not sufficient, adding OCPs is helpful. OCPs prevent ovulation and over time cause a decrease in menstrual flow. OCPs may be given as continuous hormonal therapy to prevent a withdrawal bleed for extended periods of time. Some clinicians have also used Depo-Provera for patients who cannot tolerate OCPs or have a contraindication to estrogen.
   - Patients who do not respond to the combination of NSAIDs and hormonal therapy may need a laparoscopy to evaluate for other causes of severe dysmenorrhea such as endometriosis.

PREMENSTRUAL SYNDROME

I. **Description of the condition:**
   A. **Epidemiology and etiology: Premenstrual syndrome** (PMS) is an array of predictable physical, cognitive, and behavioral symptoms that occur cyclically during the luteal phase of the menstrual cycle and resolve with the onset of menstruation. It is estimated that 85% of women have some symptoms prior to menses but that 5% to 10% have symptoms that affect their daily activities. Studies in adolescents have shown almost 90% report a PMS symptom, and almost two-thirds consider a symptom to be severe.

Premenstrual Dysphoric Disorder (PMDD) is defined in the DSM manual as feelings of depressed mood, hopelessness, self-deprecation, anxiety, affective lability, or marked anger or irritability that interfere with daily activities and are not an exacerbation of another underlying disorder.

The etiology of PMS is not completely understood but theories include estrogen excess or progesterone deficiency, vulnerability to normal fluctuations in hormones, and alterations in neurotransmitters such as opiates, monoamines, and serotonin.

II. **Making the diagnosis:**
A. **Symptoms include:**
1. **Emotional:** Irritability, depression, fatigue, lethargy, anger, insomnia, hypersomnia, mood lability, poor concentration, tearfulness, social withdrawal.
2. **Physical:** Headaches, swelling of legs or breasts, increased appetite, food craving, weight gain, abdominal bloating, muscle and joint pain.

To make the diagnosis, symptoms must be present and change by 30% in intensity between the follicular and luteal phases of the cycle and fall into the following pattern:
- Symptoms must occur in the luteal phase and resolve within a few days of onset of menstruation.
- Symptoms must be documented for several cycles and not be caused by other physical or psychological problems.
- Symptoms must recur and disrupt daily activities.

III. **Management:**
A. **Therapeutic interventions for PMS include:**
- Education on PMS
- Stress management
- Exercise
- Suppression of ovulation: OCPs (including extended regimens), medroxyprogesterone acetate
- Treatment of symptoms: NSAIDs, spironolactone
B. **Therapeutic intervention for PMDD:**
- Selective serotonin uptake inhibitors
IV. **Clinical pearls and pitfalls:**
- Polycystic ovary syndrome is a common cause of amenorrhea resulting in hyperandrogenic anovulation and signs of androgen excess including hirsutism, acne, and clitoromegaly.
- The most common cause of DUB in adolescents is anovulation.
- Primary dysmenorrhea is associated with ovulatory cycles.

MALE GENITOURINARY DISORDERS

I. **Description of the condition:** Genital disorders in male adolescents usually present as testicular or scrotal masses or lack of a testis in the scrotum. Urinary tract infection is rare in a healthy male adolescent with normal anatomy, and symptoms of dysuria commonly represent urethritis from an STI in a sexually active male adolescent (see Chapter 27 on STIs). Several clinical entities causing scrotal and testicular abnormalities commonly occur during adolescence and some represent true clinical emergencies requiring immediate intervention.

Normal genitourinary (GU) development in males includes the following:
- Testes begin development in the abdomen and begin descending into the scrotum through the inguinal canal at approximately 7 months gestation.
- Testes are covered by the processus vaginalis that eventually becomes sealed to obliterate the connection between the peritoneal abdominal cavity and the scrotum. The remaining portion is the tunica vaginalis. Failure to seal can lead to a hernia or hydrocele.
- The spermatic cord, which consists of blood vessels and the vas deferens, is connected to the base of the epididymis, which is located posterolaterally to the testicle.
- The gubernaculums attaches the testicle to the scrotum.
- Within the testicle, sertoli cells produce Mullerian inhibiting substance, which causes regression of the mullerian ducts. The appendix testis is a mullerian remnant. The Leydig cells produce testosterone leading to differentiation of the Wolffian structures (epididymis, vas deferens, seminal vesicles) and masculinization of the external genitalia. The appendix epididymis is a remnant of the wolffian system.
- Testosterone is involved in maturation of the spermatocytes and sertoli cells. Spermatogeneis in most male adolescents begins around the ages of 13 to 15.
- Testicular enlargement is the first sign of puberty in males. An orchidometer is a useful tool for measuring testicular volume. Testicular volume by age 18 in Tanner 5 males is approximately 15 to 20 cc.

II. Making the diagnosis:
  A. **Abnormalities of testicular size:**
    1. **Macro-orchidism** is defined as testes that are larger than normal.
       • **Bilateral enlarged testes** can be associated with **Fragile X** syndrome—a cause of mental retardation in males.
       • **Unilateral testicular enlargement** may be a compensatory response related to increased secretion of FSH because of a problem on the contralateral side. Other causes are discussed below including a malignant testicular mass, torsion, and hydrocele.
    2. **Micro-orchidism** is defined as testes that are smaller than expected.
       • Small testes can be found in **Kleinfelter syndrome.** The chromosomes are XXY, and there are small firm testes with hyalinized seminiferous tubules. These patients have low to low/normal testosterone levels and may have azospermia with infertility. Kleinfelter syndrome patients also can have gynecomastia and learning or behavior problems.
       • Another condition that can cause small testes is hypogonadotropic hypogonadism.
       • Unilateral small testes can result from cryptorchidism in childhood, varicocele, and previous testicular torsion.
    3. **Cryptorchidism** is defined as an undescended testis that cannot be drawn down into the scrotum.
       • After the first year of life, approximately 1% of males have cryptorchidism and spontaneous descent is unlikely. Early treatment to bring down the testis by 1 year of age is the standard treatment. An adolescent with an uncorrected cryptorchid testis is at risk for malignancy, infertility, and testicular torsion and should be promptly referred to urology.
  B. **Testicular and scrotal masses**
    1. **Differential diagnosis:** The differential diagnosis of testicular and scrotal masses can be separated into:
       Masses associated with pain:
       • Testicular torsion
       • Torsion of testicular appendage
       • Epididymitis/epididymoorchitis
       • Incarcerated hernia
       Masses that generally are painless:
       • Varicocele
       • Hydrocele
       • Spermatocele
       • Inguinal hernia
       • Testicular cancer
    2. **History:** History should include:
       • The presence of pain and whether it was acute in onset
       • History of sexual activity
       • Presence of dysuria or penile discharge
       • History of change in the size of the testicles or swelling in the scrotum
       • History of cryptorchid testes
    3. **Physical examination:** The physical exam should include complete inspection of the external genitalia including the penis, pubic hair, and inguinal nodes to evaluate for lesions, penile discharge, or inguinal adenopathy. The patient should be examined while he is standing to evaluate for varicocele that may not be apparent in the supine position. Testicular exam should assess for swelling or tenderness and there should be a comparison of the size between the right and left testis. The testicle itself should be smooth with a rubbery consistency, and the epididymis should be palpated in a posterolateral position. The spermatic cord should not demonstrate swelling. If a mass is felt, transillumination can help determine if it is cystic or solid. The abdomen should also always be palpated to evaluate for possible masses that could be affecting the scrotal contents.
    4. **Specific entities:**
       a. **Testicular torsion:**
          (1) **Clinical presentation:** Testicular torsion occurs most often among 12 to 18 year olds. It affects 1 in 4,000 males under the age of 25. Torsion occurs when the gubernaculum does not fix the testis well enough to the tunica vaginalis, causing twisting of the spermatic cord which results in arterial and venous obstruction and ultimately gangrene and necrosis. The Bell Clapper deformity is a common cause of torsion. Torsion can also occur between the epididymis and the testis or involve the testicular appendages.

The pain of testicular torsion is usually acute in onset and may be located in the testicle, scrotum, lower abdomen, or inguinal area. The pain may be accompanied by nausea, vomiting, and fever, and the testes may ride high in the scrotum with a transverse lie. There is absence of the cremasteric reflex. Torsion may be intermittent, and episodes of acute pain and swelling may be separated by long asymptomatic periods.

(2) **Diagnosis:** The diagnosis is made clinically and is further evaluated by radiologic studies. A Doppler ultrasound will demonstrate intratesticular anatomy and evaluate whether arterial blood flow is decreased or absent compared to the contralateral side. A nuclear medicine scan will also demonstrate the flow to the testicle. Decreased or absent flow would be expected in torsion while normal or increased flow would be expected with infection. However, decreased flow can also be seen with other diagnoses such as hydrocele, abscess, and hernia and ultimately surgical exploration may be necessary to accurately diagnose the problem.

(3) **Management:** Surgical exploration with derotation of the testicle is the treatment of choice. Ideally, this should occur within 6 hours to ensure viability of the testicle. The testicle probably is nonviable if the torsion has continued for 24 hours. Removal of the necrotic testicle is important because immune factors may affect the contralateral testicle and result in decreased fertility. The contralateral side is always evaluated during surgery since the Bell Clapper deformity is usually bilateral, so that the other side needs surgical correction to prevent future episodes of torsion.

b. **Torsion of a testicular appendage:**
(1) **Clinical presentation:** Torsion of a testicular appendage is more common between the ages of 7 and 12. When a testicular appendage is torsed, there may be a "blue dot" seen through the scrotum representing the twisted appendage. The most common appendage to torse is the appendix testes, which is located at the superior pole of the testicle. The pain of appendage torsion may be less severe than torsion of the entire testicle, and sometimes a normal nontender testis can be palpated separate from the appendage. However, the exam may also be difficult because of significant scrotal swelling. Other symptoms such as nausea and vomiting are not as prominent with torsion of an appendage.

(2) **Diagnosis:** The diagnosis is usually made clinically, but ultrasound or nuclear medicine scan may be helpful.

(3) **Management:** Intervention is not necessary since this type of torsion will resolve spontaneously with autoinfarction. Rest, scrotal elevation, and analgesics can be prescribed and symptoms usually resolve within a week.

c. **Epididymitis/orchitis:**
(1) **Clinical presentation:** Epididymitis is inflammation of the epididymis. In sexually active males, STI pathogens such as *C. trachomatis, N. gonorrhoeae,* and *Ureaplama urealyticum* are common causes. Pathogens such as mycobacterium and cryptococcus can also cause infection by hematogenous spread and coliform bacteria can be introduced during anal intercourse. A noninfectious cause of inflammation is reflux of urine. When the testicle also becomes involved there is concurrent orchitis. If only orchitis is present, without involvement of the epididymis, then a viral pathogen such as mumps or coxsackie A or B is more likely.

Symptoms include pain and swelling of the epididymis and or testicle. There may also be urinary frequency, urethral discharge, fever, and dysuria. The pain is usually more gradual in onset than with torsion and the cremasteric reflex is present. Pain frequently improves with elevation of the scrotum.

(2) **Diagnosis:** The diagnosis is usually made clinically, but an ultrasound or nuclear medicine scan demonstrating increased flow may be helpful in distinguishing inflammation/infection from torsion. A urine culture and urinalysis for leukocytes will be helpful in demonstrating infection, and testing for *C. trachomatis* and *N. gonorrhoeae* should be performed to rule out STI in sexually active male adolescents. Prehn sign may be positive, i.e., the pain may be relieved with support and elevation of the affected testis.

(3) **Management:** This condition is managed by rest, analgesics, and scrotal elevation. Antibiotics to treat STIs or other bacteria are needed when there is an infectious etiology. If the infection is STI related, the antibiotics of first choice are ceftriaxone and doxycycline. If there is an enteric organism,

ofloxacin or levofloxacin can be used. Quinolones can also be used for STI-associated infection if the patient is allergic to the first-line medication choices.

d. **Varicocelle:**
   (1) **Clinical presentation:** Varicocele is common in 10 to 20 year olds; it is found in approximately 20% of male patients. Varicocele is dilated tortuous veins in the pampiniform plexus and is probably caused by increased pressure from incompetent venous valves in the internal spermatic vein. Varicocele occurs on the left side 90% of the time because of the anatomical relationship between the left internal spermatic vein and the renal vein. However, it may be also present bilaterally. Usually a varicocele decreases in size when the patient is supine. If there is no change with position, or if it is only present on the right side, intra-abdominal pathology may be causing the increased pressure. When palpated, a varicocele feels like a bag of worms. It can be asymptomatic or cause a pulling or heavy feeling.

   Complications of varicocele include decreased size of the testicle on the side of the varicocele and infertility with alterations in spermatogenesis. Some of these abnormalities in spermatogenesis appear to be reversed with repair of the testicle. However, 80% of men remain fertile even without repair.
   (2) **Diagnosis:** The diagnosis is a clinical diagnosis. There are three grades of varicocele:
   • Grade I: small, palpable only with valsalva
   • Grade II: moderate, nonvisible, palpable with standing
   • Grade III: large, visible on gross inspection.
   (3) **Management:** Most patients are followed by observation. Indications for surgical repair include:
   • Pain
   • Massive distension
   • Decrease in testicular size of greater than 2 mL, which can be measured by ultrasound
   • Abnormal semen analysis (note that semen analysis is hard to evaluate during puberty)
   Referral to a urologist for consultation is recommended if there is any question about the need for surgery. A recent study suggested that early repair before the onset of infertility may be advantageous. In view of this finding, referral for a more in-depth discussion may be helpful. Repair is done by ligation of the internal spermatic vein or embolization.

e. **Spermatocele:**
   (1) **Clinical presentation:** A spermatocele is a painless cystic mass of the rete testis, ductuli efferentes, or epididymis that is filled with sperm and fluid. It is located superior and posterior to the testis and can be transilluminated to reveal a cystic structure. A spermatocele will feel like a smooth cystic sac that is separate from the testis.
   (2) **Diagnosis:** The diagnosis is usually made clinically, but an ultrasound can confirm the diagnosis.
   (3) **Management:** A spermatocele does not require intervention because it does not cause any problems.

f. **Hydrocele:**
   (1) **Clinical presentation:** A hydrocele is a painless fluid accumulation in the space of the tunica vaginalis that occurs when the processus vaginalis does not close. A hydrocele may also occur as a complication of torsion, trauma, a tumor, epididymitis, or orchitis. The typical presentation is a soft cystic anterior scrotal mass that may decrease in size overnight after the patient is in the supine position when there is communication with the intra-abdominal cavity.
   (2) **Diagnosis:** The diagnosis is made by physical exam and transillumination. However, an ultrasound can further define the anatomy.
   (3) **Management:** Surgical intervention is indicated for communicating hydroceles because they usually do not resolve and pose a risk of incarcerated hernia.

g. **Testicular Tumor:**
   1) **Clinical presentation:** Testicular tumors are the most common solid tumors in males 15 to 35 years old. Risk factors for testicular cancer are cryptorchidism and a personal or family history of testicular cancer.

Approximately 10% of cases of testicular cancer are found in patients with a history of cryptorchidism, and malignancy occurs 20% of the time in the normally descended contralateral testis.

Presentation includes a firm painless nodule that does not transilluminate or enlargement of the testicle sometimes associated with a change in consistency. There may also be fullness or a heavy sensation in the scrotum. In some cases there may be acute pain because of hemorrhage or necrosis. If the tumor produces hormones, there may be gynecomastia, change in sex drive, or premature growth of body hair. If the tumor disseminates, there may be systemic symptoms including hemoptysis, bone pain, abdominal mass, or supraclavicular mass.

Seminomas are a common tumor found in cryptorchid testes. They usually present as an enlarged testicle; three-quarters present in an early stage, and individuals with them have a greater than 95% survival rate. Nonseminomas present as smaller, more irregularly-shaped masses and are more likely to present with dissemination. The prognosis is excellent if tumors are detected at an early stage and prior to dissemination, but with current therapies even higher stage disease has a good prognosis.

(2) **Diagnosis:** Ultrasound is the first step to distinguish between a solid mass and other lesions such as a hydrocele, spermatocele, or torsion of a testicular appendage. Further evaluation of suspicious lesions includes blood work for tumor markers and surgery.

(3) **Management:** Treatment includes surgery, radiation, and chemotherapy. The most important strategy to prevent disseminated lesions is teaching male adolescents testicular self exam so that patients will detect abnormalities early. Testicular exam should be part of the general physical exam in all male adolescents.

III.   **Clinical pearls and pitfalls:**
- Testicular torsion is a surgical emergency that requires intervention within 6 hours to ensure testicular viability.
- Although they are associated with fertility issues, most men with varicocele are fertile.
- Varicocele is most common on the left side.
- Spermatocele is a benign lesion that does not require intervention.
- Seminoma is a common testicular tumor type associated with cryptorchidism.

BIBLIOGRAPHY

Abma JC, Martinez GM, Mosher WD, Dawson BS. Teenagers in the United States: sexual activity, contraceptive use, and childbearing, 2002. National Center for Health Statistics, Vital Health Stat 2004;23(24).

American Academy of Pediatrics. Care of the adolescent sexual assault victim. *Pediatrics* 2001; 107:1476–1478.

Bortot AT, Risser WL, Cromwell PF. Coping with pelvic inflammatory disease in the adolescent. *Contemp Pediatr* 2004; 21:33–48.

Belman AB. The adolescent varicocele. *Pediatrics* 2004;114:1669–1679.

Braunstein GD. Gynecomastia. *N Engl J Med* 1993;328:490–495.

Cromer BA. Bone mineral density in adolescent and young adult women on injectable or oral contraception. *Curr Opin Obstet Gynecol* 2003;15:353–357.

Emans SJ, Laufer MR, Goldstein DP eds. *Pediatric and adolescent gynecology*, 5th ed. Philadelphia, PA: Lippincott Williams & Wilkins, 2005.

Frankowski BL. Sexual orientation and adolescents. *Pediatrics* 2004;113:1827–1832.

French L. Dysmenorrhea. *Am Fam Physician* 2005;71:285–291.

Gates GJ, Sonenstein FL. Heterosexual genital sexual activity among adolescent males: 1998 and 1997. *Fam Plann Perspect* 2000;32:295–299.

Gillenwater JY, Grayhack JT, Howard SS, et al. eds. *Adult and pediatric urology*, 4th ed. Philadelphia, PA: Lippincott Williams & Wilkins, 2002.

Halpern-Felsher BL, Cornell JL, Kropp RY, Tschann JM. Oral versus vaginal sex among adolescents: Perceptions, attitudes, and behavior. *Pediatr* 2005;115:845–851.

Hatcher RA, Trussell J, Stewart R, et al. eds. *Contraceptive technology*, 18th ed. New York: Ardent Media, Inc., 2004.

Kaiser Family Foundation. National survey of adolescents and young adults: Sexual health knowledge, attitudes, and experiences, 2003.

Kaiser Family Foundation. Virginity and the first time, 2003.

National Campaign to Prevent Teen Pregnancy. Do abstinence-only programs delay the initiation of sex among young people and reduce teen pregnancy? 2002.

National Campaign to Prevent Teen Pregnancy. 14 and younger: The sexual behavior of young adolescents, 2003.

Perez-Brayfield MR, Baseman A, Kirsch AJ. Adolescent urology. *Adolesc Med Clin* 2005;16:215–227.

Remafedi G, Resnick M, Blum R, et al. Demography of sexual orientation in adolescents. *Pediatrics* 1992;89:7143–7721.

Rosenthal S, Von Ranson KM, Cotton S, et al. Sexual initiation: Predictors and developmental trends. *Sex Transm Dis* 2001;28:527–532.

Schuster MA, Bell RM, Kanouse DE. The sexual practices of adolescent virgins: Genital activities of high school students who have never had vaginal intercourse. *Am J Public Health* 1996;86:1570–1577.

Strasburger VC. Adolescents, sex, and the media: Ooooo, baby, baby—A Q & A. *Adolesc Med Clin* 2005;16:269–288.

WEB SITES

www.cdc.gov   Centers for Disease Control and Prevention: Information on youth risk behavior survey and national vital statistics reports

www.agi-usa.org   Alan Guttmacher Institute: Information on reproductive health issues

www.seicus.org   SEICUS, Sexuality and Information Council of the United States: Information on reproductive health issues

www.kff.org   Kaiser Family Foundation: Information on health care, including reproductive health issues

www.safeschoolscoaltion.org   Safe Schools Coalition of Washington: Information on sexual minority students

www.youngwomenshealth.org   Children's Hospital Boston Web site: Good patient information on reproductive and adolescent health issues

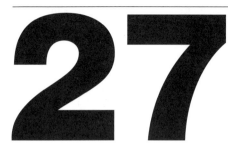

Sexually Transmitted Infections

I. Description of the condition:

A. Scope of the problem: More than 60% of adolescents become sexually active and about 25% acquire a sexually transmitted infection (STI) by the time they graduate from high school. Adolescents and young adults have the highest age-specific rates of infection for the majority of STIs in the United States, and this population serves as the reservoir for these infections in the community.

B. Risk factors:

1. **Young age:** Sexual activity at a young age places adolescents at high risk for STI. This reflects both **biologic and behavioral factors** that predispose young people to infection. The presence of columnar epithelial cells on the more external aspect of the immature cervix (cervical *ectropion*) increases risk because certain sexually transmitted pathogens, most notably *Chlamydia trachomatis*, preferentially infect these cells. Since adolescents have fewer ovulatory menstrual cycles than adult women, the cervical mucus may not confer the same degree of protection that is believed to be present in adults with regular ovulatory cycles. From a behavioral standpoint, limited skills at negotiating sexual activity and condom use with romantic partners and concurrent substance abuse may lead adolescents to make poor decisions and engage in risky sexual behaviors. Furthermore, younger adolescents often are incapable of foreseeing the future consequences of their decisions. Inconsistent or improper condom use, concurrence of sexual partners, and perceived or real barriers to confidential health care further increase the risk of contracting an STI.

2. **Female gender:** More female adolescents are diagnosed with STIs than are male adolescents. In part, this is due to the fact that asymptomatic female adolescents are much more likely than male adolescents to be tested for STIs during routine health encounters or when they present for other reproductive health care needs, such as contraception. Male-to-female transmission rates are higher than female-to-male transmission rates for certain infections as well; therefore, many STIs are truly more prevalent among female adolescents.

3. **Previous STI diagnosis:** The single greatest risk factor for a STI is history of prior STI or the current presence of another sexually transmitted pathogen. Therefore the presence of one STI should prompt the clinician to investigate for others. Coinfection is common.

II. Making the diagnosis:

A. Taking the history: History should be obtained from the adolescent in private after discussing confidentiality policies. In addition to eliciting particular symptoms of STI, a comprehensive sexual history includes the following elements:

- Age at first sexual intercourse
- Number of sexual partners (currently and total lifetime number)
- Types of sexual activity (vaginal, oral, anal intercourse)
- Gender(s) of sexual partners
- Condom use: consistency and appropriateness of use
- Use of contraception
- Current symptoms of STI
- History of prior STI
- History of abnormal Papanicolaou (Pap) smears
- History of sexual abuse or exploitation
- History of exchanging sex for drugs or money

B. Screening recommendations:

1. *All* sexually active adolescent females should be screened annually for *C. trachomatis* infection.

2. Most adolescent health professionals recommend annual screening for *Neisseria gonorrhoeae* and *Trichomonas vaginalis* as well.

3. For high risk adolescent females, such as those with new partners, multiple partners, or history of a prior STI, it is advisable to screen for *C. trachomatis* every 6 months, since reacquisition is common.
4. Although clear guidelines for STI screening in adolescent males have not been published, the authors recommend screening for *C. trachomatis* in those with a history of multiple partners and/or inconsistent condom use.
5. Annual Pap smears should be performed to screen for cervical dysplasia caused by human papillomavirus, starting within 3 years following the onset of sexual activity.
6. A rapid plasma reagin (RPR) or Venereal Disease Research Laboratory (VDRL) test may be indicated, based on the local prevalence of syphilis infection and personal risk factors.
7. Screening for Human Immunodeficiency Virus (HIV) in adolescents whose behaviors place them at increased risk of this infection should be considered.
8. Adolescents who are not immunized against hepatitis B may be screened for this STI (using anticore antibody); more importantly, they should be immunized.
9. Patients diagnosed with one STI should be screened for the presence of others.
10. The Centers for Disease Control and Prevention (CDC) recommends that the following screening protocol be performed at least annually for men who have sex with men (MSM):
    - HIV and syphilis serology
    - Urine/urethral testing for *N. gonorrhoeae*
    - Urine/urethral testing for *C. trachomatis* and pharyngeal culture for *N. gonorrhoeae* in men with oral–genital exposure
    - Rectal culture for *N. gonorrhoeae* and *C. trachomatis* in those who have had receptive anal intercourse.

C. **Types of testing available:**
   1. **Light microscopy** of vaginal or urethral secretions is useful for the identification of white blood cells, motile trichomonads, clue cells, and pseudohyphae in the evaluation of vaginitis or urethritis.
   2. **Urine leukocyte esterase** is an inexpensive screen for urethritis in male patients, with a negative predictive value of 97%. It is less useful as a screening test in female patients, in whom leukocytes may represent either vaginal or urinary tract inflammation.
   3. **Culture** is the gold standard for the diagnosis of most infectious processes. Sensitivity of culture is poor for the diagnosis of *C. trachomatis* (50%–85%) but somewhat better for *N. gonorrhoeae* (70%–93%). It remains the only approved method for identifying these organisms in rectal and pharyngeal specimens. Specimen processing may be laborious, and specimens should be transported to the laboratory as quickly as possible to maximize yield. Specificity is outstanding, making culture the only test admissible as forensic evidence in cases of sexual abuse or assault.
   4. **Antigen detection techniques** such as direct fluorescent antibody (DFA) and enzyme immunoassay (EIA) use antibodies to identify the presence of specific antigens on the pathogenic organism. They may be performed on endocervical or urethral specimens. Specimens are easy for the clinician to collect and transport to the laboratory. Sensitivity is 75% to 92%, with recently improved EIA having the best performance.
   5. **Nonamplified DNA probes** are widely used to diagnose *C. trachomatis* and *N. gonorrhoeae*. Endocervical and urethral specimens are easy to collect and transport, and cost is reasonable. Reported sensitivity is variable. A recent large, multicenter study that used independent reference standards found that the most widely used DNA probe product had a sensitivity of 61% to 72% for the diagnosis of *C. trachomatis*. Previous studies reported higher sensitivities.
   6. **Nucleic acid amplification tests (NAATs)** are able to detect tiny amounts of DNA or RNA and therefore offer superior sensitivity to the other methods described. A variety of NAATs are available to test for gonococcal and chlamydial infections, including polymerase chain reaction (PCR), ligase chain reaction (LCR), transcription mediated amplification (TMA) and strand displacement assay (SDA). Reported sensitivities for the various methods for cervical and urethral infections range from 85% to 99%, with specificity 97% to 99.9%. DNA from the pathogenic organism may persist in the vagina for several weeks following successful treatment; therefore, it is recommended that retesting (if indicated) not be performed for at least 3 weeks after therapy is completed. The greatest disadvantage of NAATs is the high cost. Still, their use may be cost-effective in higher-prevalence populations.

Sensitivities decrease slightly (particularly for female patients) but remain excellent when **first-void urine** specimens are tested rather than endocervical or urethral swabs. Several NAATs are approved by the US Food and Drug Administration (FDA) for use on urine. This allows for STI screening without performance of a speculum examination or urethral swab. It is likely that these tests will ultimately be approved for use on vaginal swab specimens as well.

III. **Management of sexually transmitted infections:**
   A. **Overview of treatment goals and strategies:**
      1. **Education:** Patients should be educated about the specifics of their infection and its natural history, their need for additional follow-up testing, if any, and their personal risk factors for future STI. Discussion of modifying these risk factors should be pursued.
      2. **Medications:** Single dose therapies are available for the treatment of several STIs. Advantages of single dose therapy include high efficacy, high patient adherence to therapy, and the ability of the provider to witness the patient completing therapy. Their use often obviates the need to perform "test of cure," since efficacy generally is excellent. Symptom relief with analgesics and other local treatments should not be overlooked when treating painful conditions such as pelvic inflammatory disease and genital herpes.
      3. **Counseling:** Patients should remain abstinent until both they and their partners complete therapy. Patients should be counseled about general sexual health issues and risk reduction for future STIs. Condom use should be encouraged with every sexual encounter, but it should be made clear that even perfect condom use does not completely eliminate the possibility of acquiring an STI. Sexually risky behaviors should be explored, including a discussion of choices of sexual partners. The concept of "secondary abstinence" should be introduced as a possible means of eliminating future STI risk.
      4. **Reporting:** STIs that are nationally reportable to the CDC are listed in Table 27-1. Local reporting requirements vary from state to state. Although some laboratories report directly to local health departments, it is the responsibility of the provider ordering the test to ensure that this result is communicated.
      5. **Partner services:** All recent sexual partners (arbitrarily defined as those within the past 2 months) should be informed that they have been identified as partners of a person with an STI. This may be done by the patient, the provider, or the local health department. The latter two can perform this while maintaining the patient's anonymity. Partners should be instructed to go to their health care provider or a local STI clinic to obtain *treatment* (not just testing) for the STI. Although patient delivered therapy, in which the provider prescribes treatment for both the patient and the partner, is an active area of research, this approach is not currently recommended.
   B. *Chlamydia trachomatis:*
      1. **Epidemiology:** *C. trachomatis* is the most common bacterial STI and the most common reportable infectious disease in the US. A recent STI surveillance project found an average chlamydia positivity of 11.3% for female adolescents attending school-based clinics. The rise in rates of diagnosis over the past decade reflects a greater awareness of the disease and the adoption of universal screening of sexually active young women, as well as the availability of more sensitive diagnostic techniques. Female adolescents 15 to 19 years of age have the highest age-specific incidence of infection, followed closely by women ages 20 to 24. No constellation of clinical and demographic factors has been identified that reliably

Table 27-1. STIs that are nationally reportable to CDC

Gonorrhea
Chlamydia
Syphilis
Chancroid
AIDS
HIV (Pediatric)
Hepatitis B

AIDS, acquired immunodeficiency syndrome; CDC, Centers for Disease Control and Prevention; HIV, Human Immunodeficiency Virus; STI, sexually transmitted infections.

predicts the majority of chlamydial infections among young women; it is therefore recommended that *all* sexually active females under 25 years of age old be screened annually for *C. trachomatis*.

2. **Clinical presentation:** Chlamydial infections are usually asymptomatic in both genders. Symptomatic female adolescents may present with cervical or vaginal discharge, urethritis, or pelvic inflammatory disease (PID). Women with tubal factor infertility are often found to have antibodies reflecting prior chlamydial infection, despite having no history of symptomatic infection. Up to 40% of untreated infections progress to clinically symptomatic PID. Male patients may have nongonococcal urethritis (up to 55% of which is caused by *C. trachomatis*) or epididymitis. Reiter syndrome, characterized by urethritis, conjunctivitis, and arthritis, usually is associated with chlamydial infection.

3. **Diagnosis:** Culture for *C. trachomatis* has a low sensitivity (70%–75%), and specimens sent for culture must contain epithelial cells (e.g., from the endocervix or urethra). Antigen detection techniques and nonamplified DNA probes have better sensitivity and are more easily processed. NAATs have the highest sensitivity, are easily processed, and may be performed using urine specimens as well as cervical and urethral swabs. Some NAATs may be approved for vaginal swab specimens as well.

4. **Treatment:**
   a. **Medication:** Treatments for *uncomplicated* cervicitis or urethritis include:
   - Azithromycin 1 g orally (single dose)
   - Doxycycline 100 mg twice daily for 7 days
     Patients with PID or epididymitis require additional therapy (see section IV).
   b. **Follow-up:** Test of cure is not necessary, but patients should be retested in 3 to 4 months, since reinfection within this timeframe is common. It is not necessary to treat all patients with chlamydial infections for *N. gonorrhoeae*.

C. **Neisseria gonorrhoeae:**
1. **Epidemiology:** Following a dramatic decline over the past 30 years, the incidence of *N. gonorrhoeae* infection is now declining at a slower rate. It is most commonly diagnosed in adolescent and young adult women. African Americans are disproportionately affected, although significant decreases in the incidence of gonorrhea in this population continue to be seen. The highest rates of infection are in large cities and in the southeastern US.

2. **Clinical presentations:** Gonococcal infection of the lower genital tract may cause purulent cervical, vaginal, urethral, or rectal discharge, dysuria, and local discomfort. Ascending infection can cause PID or epididymitis. Alternatively, *N. gonorrhoeae* may be completely asymptomatic, particularly in females. Persons who engage in oral sex may develop gonococcal pharyngitis, which typically is asymptomatic. *N. gonorrhoeae* is the second most common cause of septic arthritis in adolescents (after *Staph aureus*); it typically affects medium and small joints, and patients often present with polyarthritis. **Disseminated gonococcal infection (DGI)** may occur following gonococcal bacteremia. Symptoms include arthritis or arthralgias, tenosynovitis, and dermatitis. Multiple skin lesions often are present on the extremities; most commonly they are small macules and papules, but vesicles, pustules, and petechial lesions have all been described. Systemic symptoms may include fever and chills. Other organs (liver, heart, kidneys, central nervous system) are rarely affected. Although urogenital symptoms often are absent in patients with DGI, *N. gonorrhoeae* is more likely to be recovered from mucosal cultures (cervical, urethral, pharyngeal or rectal) than from skin or joint specimens. DGI is associated with complement deficiency (C5–8) in some individuals.

3. **Diagnosis:** Culture is the gold standard for diagnosis of gonococcal infections, with good sensitivity. Antigen detection tests and nonamplified DNA probes are widely used but offer few advantages over culture. NAATs offer improved sensitivity, but the biggest advantage of their use is for testing urine specimens.

4. **Treatment:** Single dose treatments may be used to treat *uncomplicated* cervicitis or urethritis:
   - Cefixime 400 mg orally
   - Ceftriaxone 125 mg intramuscular
   - Ciprofloxacin 500 mg orally
   - Ofloxacin 400 mg orally
     Although quinolones are not recommended for persons under 18 years of age, a great deal of clinical experience supports their safe use in adolescents, particularly

when given as a single dose; their use may therefore be considered if other treatment options are not available. Quinolone resistance is problematic in Asia and the Pacific islands (including Hawaii) and in California; cephalosporins are therefore recommended as first-line treatment in these regions. Elsewhere in the US, the prevalence of quinolone resistant *N. gonorrhoeae* is about 1%. Ceftriaxone or ciprofloxacin is recommended to treat gonococcal pharyngitis. Parenteral treatment and prolonged courses of antibiotics are required to treat arthritis and DGI. Treatment of PID and epididymitis are described below (Section IV). Since co-infection with *C. trachomatis* is common among patients with gonococcal infections, one should treat empirically for this infection as well.

D. Syphilis (*Treponema pallidum* infection):
1. **Epidemiology:** Although the US has seen dramatic decreases in reported cases of syphilis during the past several decades, the infection remains a significant problem in large urban areas and in the southeastern region of the country. African Americans and MSM have the highest rates of infection. These personal and geographic risk factors must be taken into account when choosing who to screen for this infection. Transmission occurs only when mucocutaneous lesions are present and is therefore unlikely to occur more than 1 year after the initial infection.
2. **Clinical presentation:**
   a. **Primary infection** is characterized by a single firm, painless ulcer (chancre) at the site of genital infection with *T. pallidum*. The chancre appears 10 to 90 days after exposure and resolves in 3 to 6 weeks.
   b. **Secondary infection** has numerous possible manifestations, including lymphadenopathy, mucocutaneous lesions, alopecia, condyloma lata, and rash. The rash of syphilis may vary in appearance; classically, it is present on the palms and soles. It is nonpruritic and resolves spontaneously. Constitutional symptoms of secondary syphilis include fever, malaise, and weight loss.
   c. **Latent infection** may persist for years without symptoms. "Early latent" infection is defined as the latent period within 1 year of initial infection. Latent infection beyond this point is "late latent" infection.
   d. **Tertiary infection** may include degenerative neurologic changes, blindness, and cardiac, auditory, or gummatous lesions.
   e. **Neurosyphilis** can occur during any stage of the disease. Patients with any evidence of central nervous system involvement should be evaluated with examination of the cerebrospinal fluid (CSF).
3. **Diagnosis:** Diagnosis during the primary infection is made by identifying *T. pallidum* in a sample of tissue or exudate from the chancre, using direct fluorescent antibody (DFA) testing or darkfield microscopy. All serologic tests have high false-negative rates during primary infection but excellent sensitivity during secondary infection. Nontreponemal tests (RPR and VDRL) have high false-positive rates (Table 27-2) but are appropriate for use as screening tests. They tend to correlate with disease activity and may be used to monitor treatment effect. Treponemal tests such as the fluorescent treponemal antibody absorbed (FTA-ABS) and T. pallidum particle agglutination (TP-PA) tests correlate poorly with disease activity and tend to stay positive despite adequate treatment. The two types of tests are therefore used together for diagnosis and management of syphilis. The VDRL-CSF may be used to diagnose neurosyphilis but has poor sensitivity.
4. **Treatment:**
   a. **Medication:** Syphilis is treated with parenteral penicillin G in all nonallergic patients, regardless of stage of infection. Primary, secondary, and early latent syphilis are treated with benzathine penicillin G 2.4 million units IM

Table 27-2. Possible causes of false-positive RPR or VDRL tests

Rheumatologic disease
HIV infection
Hashimoto thyroiditis
Lymphoma
Acute infection
Cirrhosis
Narcotic addition

RPR, rapid plasma reagin; VDRL, Venereal Disease Research Laboratory; HIV, Human Immunodeficiency Virus.

in a single dose. Late latent syphilis, latent syphilis of unknown duration, and tertiary infection (without neurosyphilis) are treated with weekly doses of benzathine penicillin G 2.4 million units IM for 3 consecutive weeks. Patients with neurosyphilis or eye disease require daily parenteral treatment in conjunction with oral probenecid for 10 to 14 days. Doxycycline has been used successfully in patients who are allergic to penicillin.

   b. **Follow-up:** Nontreponemal tests should be followed after treatment. Ideally they should be performed by the same laboratory each time. Titers should decrease four-fold within 6 months of treatment for primary or secondary syphilis and within 12 to 24 months of treatment for latent infection. The possibility of treatment failure should be considered if they do not decline appropriately. These patients may best be served by an infectious disease or STI specialist.

E. **Herpes Simplex Virus (HSV):**
   1. **Epidemiology:** HSV is the most common cause of genital ulcers in the United States. HSV-1 causes 30% to 40% of all genital outbreaks; HSV-2 causes the remainder and is associated with more frequent recurrences. Up to 20% of sexually active young adults are sero-positive for HSV-2, although the majority of these persons are asymptomatic and unaware of their status. Most infected persons acquire HSV from subclinical viral shedding by a sexual partner.
   2. **Clinical presentation:** Primary HSV infection classically is manifested by genital vesicles and ulcerations, inguinal lymphadenopathy, fever, malaise, and myalgias. Most patients do not experience all of these symptoms. Secondary genital outbreaks generally are less severe and include fewer systemic symptoms. The frequency of outbreaks diminishes over time: patients with HSV-2 experience an average of five to six outbreaks per year during the first 2 years; HSV-1 causes an average of one outbreak per year.
   3. **Diagnosis:** Mild cases of genital herpes are commonly misdiagnosed as a yeast infection, latex allergy, or folliculitis. A high index of suspicion is necessary for this prevalent condition. Viral culture is the gold standard for diagnosis. Early vesicular lesions that are unroofed by the clinician and scraped for culture have the highest yield. Older ulcers or crusted lesions may be tested by scraping the base of the lesion, but the likelihood of a positive culture is diminished. PCR is used by some centers in place of culture.

   Reliable HSV-2 type-specific serology testing, based on glycoprotein G2, has recently become available. Routine screening of asymptomatic persons is not currently recommended. Serologic testing may be appropriate in certain settings, such as in a patient who presents at the end of an outbreak when culture is likely to be negative, a patient who gives a history of recurrent genital irritation but who is currently asymptomatic, or a patient whose partner has HSV-2 who wishes to know his or her own status. Type-specific testing for HSV-1 is not useful because it may reflect prior oral, cutaneous, or genital infection.
   4. **Treatment:**
      a. **Medication:** Antiviral treatment regimens for primary outbreaks, recurrences, and daily suppressive therapy are listed in Table 27-3. Treatment of outbreaks within 24 to 48 hours of the onset of symptoms has been shown to decrease the severity and the duration of the outbreak. Patients should be given prescriptions with refills so they can initiate treatment of recurrent outbreaks as soon as possible.

      Daily suppressive therapy has been shown to decrease the rate of subclinical viral shedding and may be offered to any patient. It is particularly suitable

Table 27-3. Treatment regimens for genital herpes infections (all oral)

First clinical episode	Recurrent outbreaks	Daily suppressive therapy
Acyclovir 400 mg t.i.d. × 7–10 d	Acyclovir 800 mg b.i.d. × 5 d	Acyclovir 400 mg b.i.d.
Acyclovir 200 mg 5/d × 7–10 d	Acyclovir 400 mg t.i.d. × 5 d	Famciclovir 250 mg b.i.d.
Famciclovir 250 mg t.i.d. × 7–10 d	Famciclovir 125 mg b.i.d. × 5 d	Valacyclovir 500 mg q d
Valacyclovir 1 g b.i.d. × 7–10 d	Valacyclovir 500 mg b.i.d. × 3–5 d	Valacyclovir 1 g q d

for patients whose outbreaks are associated with significant morbidity (i.e., frequency, pain, school absence, psychological trauma) or patients with HSV-2 whose partners are known to be negative for HSV-2. The natural history of genital herpes is decreasing frequency of outbreaks over time; therefore, daily suppressive therapy should be discontinued after several months and the patient's need for ongoing therapy reassessed.

Pain management is a critical component of genital herpes treatment. NSAIDs used in appropriately high doses and sitz baths may provide significant relief. Severe pain may require oral narcotics. Topical lidocaine (2% viscous gel) can be quite effective, particularly in patients with dysuria caused by urine passing over ulcerative lesions.

b. **Counseling** should include the following elements:
- The adolescent is not alone: this infection is common, and lots of people have it but do not know it.
- Antiviral therapy should be started as soon as possible to reduce the severity of recurrences.
- Although the risk of transmitting the virus is highest during an outbreak, transmission may occur at any time.
- Future sexual partners must be informed of the diagnosis.
- Condoms do not effectively prevent transmission, but they should be used to reduce the risk.
- A woman who becomes pregnant must inform her obstetrician of the diagnosis in order to reduce the risk of transmitting HSV to the baby during delivery.
- Support groups (live and internet-based) are available for persons with herpes.

c. **Follow-up** includes:
- Monitoring the frequency and severity of outbreaks, and the effectiveness of treatment.
- Reassessing the need for daily suppressive therapy.
- Providing emotional support for this chronic illness.

F. **Chancroid (*Hemophilus ducreyi*):**
1. **Epidemiology:** This infection is relatively uncommon in the US but many experts suspect that it is underdiagnosed. It usually occurs in discrete outbreaks.
2. **Clinical presentation(s):** Patients with chancroid present with one or more painful genital ulcers and sometimes have tender inguinal adenopathy. A patient with painful genital ulcers and suppurative inguinal adenopathy most likely has chancroid.
3. **Diagnosis:** Culture of *H. ducreyi* requires a special medium that is not widely available. The diagnosis should be suspected if the above clinical findings are present and syphilis and HSV can be ruled out.
4. **Treatment** is with azithromycin 1 g given as a single dose. Other regimens are available as well. HIV testing should be performed. Some clinical improvement should be evident when the patient is examined 3 to 7 days following treatment.

G. *Trichomonas vaginalis:*
1. **Epidemiology:** Trichomoniasis ("trich") is one of the most common treatable STIs among adolescents. Its presence is associated with preterm delivery and increased risk of HIV transmission.
2. **Clinical presentation:** Infection with this single-celled, flagellated protozoan may cause a frothy, malodorous vaginal discharge and vulvovaginitis with an intense inflammatory reaction; alternatively, it may be asymptomatic. Punctate, hemorrhagic lesions on the cervix ("strawberry cervix") are present in only 2% of cases, but this finding is specific for trichomoniasis. Male adolescents rarely are symptomatic but may have urethritis.
3. **Diagnosis:** Diagnosis is most commonly made by visualizing motile trichomonads in vaginal fluid under regular light microscopy. Microscopy should be performed promptly after the specimen is obtained, since the trichomonads may become less motile as the temperature of their environment decreases to room temperature. Still, the sensitivity of this diagnostic method is only about 75% in symptomatic females. Culture is more sensitive but may take up to 5 to 7 days. The vaginal pH often is elevated, and a positive whiff test may be present.
4. **Treatment:** Due to the imperfect sensitivity of microscopy, empiric treatment should be considered if clinical suspicion is high and culture is not available, even if motile trichomonads are not visualized. Treatment is with metronidazole 2 g orally as a single dose. Alternatively, metronidazole 500 mg twice daily for 7 days has somewhat higher efficacy, but adherence to therapy is much less likely.

Tinidazole 2 g as a single dose was recently approved by the FDA for treatment of trichomoniasis, but it offers no clear advantage over metronidazole for first-line therapy. Topical treatment with metronidazole vaginal gel is inadequate for trichomoniasis, since organisms may be present in periurethral and perivaginal glands and thus are not exposed to the medication.

H. Bacterial vaginosis:
1. **Epidemiology:** Bacterial vaginosis (BV) results from the overgrowth of *Gardnerella vaginalis*, *Mycoplasma hominis*, and other anaerobic organisms in the vagina. Although the evidence for sexual transmissibility of BV is mixed, it is the most prevalent vaginal infection in sexually active adolescents and the most common pathologic cause of vaginal discharge in this age group. Douching and the use of other vaginal cosmetic or cleansing products may predispose to BV by disrupting the normal ecology of the vagina.
2. **Clinical presentation:** Persons with BV may be asymptomatic, or they may report dysuria, local genital itching and irritation, and a malodorous ("fishy") white or gray vaginal discharge. On exam, this discharge is homogeneous (rather than "clumpy") and adherent to the vaginal walls. Recurrence is common.
3. **Diagnosis:** Clinical diagnosis requires at least three of the following four criteria:
   • Homogenous, adherent white or gray vaginal discharge
   • Vaginal pH >4.5
   • 20% or more "clue cells" on saline wet mount
   • Amine ("fishy") odor released when 10% KOH added to vaginal fluid (positive whiff test).
   The vaginal pH should be measured from the distal lateral wall of the vagina rather than from the posterior fornix. Clue cells are squamous epithelial cells that are stippled with bacteria, giving the edges of the cells a "ragged" appearance. BV is a noninflammatory condition; therefore, the presence of excessive leukocytes on vaginal microscopy may indicate an alternative diagnosis. Microscopy also may be notable for a relative lack of lactobacilli, which predisposes to this condition. The diagnosis may also be made using a Gram stain. Several new products are now commercially available to assist with diagnosis; these detect the presence of amines and elevated vaginal pH.
4. **Treatment:** Treatment options include:
   • Metronidazole 500 mg orally twice a day for 7 days
   • Metronidazole gel 0.75%, one applicator (5 g) intravaginally once a day for 5 days
   • Clindamycin cream 2%, one applicator (5 g) intravaginally at bedtime for 7 days
   Metronidazole is more efficacious than clindamycin. Oral treatment is less expensive than topical therapy and often is preferred by adolescents. There is no demonstrated role for partner treatment.

I. Yeast vaginitis:
1. **Epidemiology:** Although not sexually transmitted, vaginal yeast infections commonly cause vaginal discharge and irritation. Up to 75% of females will have at least one episode of yeast vaginitis in their lifetime. Most vaginal yeast infections (80%–90%) are caused by *Candida albicans*. The remainder are caused by other candidal species and other yeasts such as *Saccharolyces cerevisiae*. Diabetes, HIV infection and other immunocompromised states, and recent antibiotic use are predisposing factors.
2. **Clinical presentation:** Women with symptomatic yeast infections complain of vulvar and vaginal itching and irritation. They report a clumpy vaginal discharge that is not malodorous. They may report dysuria from urine passing over excoriated skin and mucosa.
3. **Diagnosis:** Yeast vaginitis is a clinical diagnosis in most cases. The vulva may be erythematous and excoriated. A white clumpy discharge may be present in the vagina. The vaginal pH is normal (≤4.5). Pseudohyphae or budding yeast may be seen on saline microscopy or a KOH preparation, but these are only visualized in about half of all cases. When the diagnosis is in question, culture may be performed and/or empiric treatment may be prescribed. It is advisable to rule out other causes of vaginal discharge, such as BV or an STI, before treating empirically.
4. **Treatment:** Adolescents often prefer the simplicity of single dose treatment with oral fluconazole 150 mg. Fluconazole is particularly effective at treating infections caused by *C. albicans*. Topical azoles are effective as well. Several intravaginal agents are included in Table 27-4; some are available over the counter.

Table 27-4. Recommended intravaginal agents for the treatment of yeast infections

Over-the-counter preparations:
- Butoconazole 2% cream 5 g intravaginally for 3 days
- Clotrimazole 1% cream 5 g intravaginally for 7–14 days
- Miconazole 2% cream 5 g intravaginally for 7 days
- Miconazole 200 mg vaginal suppository, one suppository for 3 days
- Tioconazole 6.5% ointment 5 g intravaginally, single application

Prescription preparations:
- Butoconazole1—sustained release 2% cream 5 g intravaginally, single dose
- Clotrimazole 100 mg vaginal tablet for 7 days
- Clotrimazole 500 mg vaginal tablet, single dose
- Terconazole 0.4% cream 5 g intravaginally for 7 days
- Terconazole 0.8% cream 5 g intravaginally for 3 days
- Terconazole 80 mg vaginal suppository, one suppository for 3 days

---

These medications are oil based and may degrade a latex condom. Treatment of sexual partners is not recommended.

J. **Human Papillomavirus (HPV):**
   1. **Epidemiology:** HPV is believed to be the most common STI acquired by adolescents. It is estimated that as many as 50% of females under 25 years of age are infected; among sexually active adults, up to 75% have serologic evidence of a prior infection. The vast majority remain asymptomatic and undiagnosed.
      More than 30 serotypes of sexually transmissible HPV have been identified. They are further classified as "high-risk" types (e.g., types 16, 18, 31, 33, 35, and 45), which are associated with low-grade or high-grade squamous intraepithelial lesions and invasive anogenital cancers, and "low-risk" types (e.g., types 6, 11, and 42–44), which are associated with anogenital condyloma acuminatum (genital warts) but only occasionally with neoplastic lesions. In most infected persons, the infection will clear within 5 years (many within 1 year). High-risk serotypes are more likely to persist.
   2. **Clinical presentations:** Genital warts may occur on the perineal or perianal regions, in the vagina, on the cervix, or in the periurethral area. The warts themselves usually do not cause discomfort, but occasionally they may be painful, pruritic, or friable. Warts may be verrucous, flat, or papular. Untreated lesions may remain unchanged, spread, or resolve spontaneously, although this may take months or even years to occur. Asymptomatic HPV infection may manifest clinically as an abnormal Pap smear. Low-grade intraepithelial lesions frequently seem to follow new HPV infections, but the vast majority resolve spontaneously in adolescents.
   3. **Diagnosis:** Genital warts are typically diagnosed clinically, based on their characteristic appearance. If the diagnosis is in question based on unusual looking lesions or inadequate response to treatment, biopsy may be performed. Testing for high-risk HPV types using a nucleic acid hybridization with signal amplification process is now available. This may be used in the evaluation of certain abnormal Pap smears in adolescents, but routine screening in this population is not recommended at this time.
   4. **Treatment:**
      a. **Eradication of genital warts:** Treatment of genital warts is primarily for cosmetic reasons. No evidence clearly demonstrates that treating warts decreases the risk of transmission to sexual partners. A number of possible treatments are available, including patient-applied and clinician-applied therapies. Patient-applied therapies include imiquimod and podofilox. Imiquimod 5% cream is an immune stimulator that is applied to the genital lesions on alternate days, 3 nights a week (e.g., every Monday, Wednesday, and Friday), and washed off with soap and water in the morning (6–10 hours later), for up to 16 weeks. Podofilox 0.5% solution or gel is applied twice daily for 3 consecutive days, followed by 4 days of no treatment. This may be repeated up to four times. These therapies are efficacious in many people, but they require time and comfort visualizing and treating lesions in the genital and perianal area.

Clinician-applied therapies may be preferred by adolescents who want rapid resolution of their lesions and who are not comfortable applying their own treatment. These include trichloroacetic acid (TCA) 85% and podophyllin resin 10% to 25%. TCA causes local destruction of warts. It should be applied sparingly to lesions to protect surrounding skin from irritation. Repeat treatments may be needed every 1 to 2 weeks until lesions are destroyed; this may take several weeks for extensive lesions. Podophyllin resin 10% to 25% is applied in small amounts to warts, and may be repeated weekly. To avoid significant systemic absorption, a maximum of 0.5 mL of podophyllin or a maximum of 10 cm^2 should be treated at one time. Cryotherapy and surgical removal are other treatment options. Patients report significant discomfort from wart destruction.

Patients with cervical, deep vaginal, urethral, and rectal mucosal lesions should be treated by an experienced clinician. Overly aggressive treatment of these lesions may lead to fistula formation, scarring, or other complications. Perianal and vaginal introital lesions may be treated using the above patient- or clinician-applied therapies.

b. **Counseling of patients with HPV should include:**
- HPV is common and affects many people without them being aware of it.
- Most infections clear within 2 to 5 years; during this time, an infected person must assume that he or she can transmit the infection to sexual partners, and potential sexual partners must be informed of this possibility.
- High-risk HPV serotypes are more likely to persist than low-risk types.
- Elimination of warts does not "cure" the virus or decrease the risk of HPV transmission.
- Condoms should be worn with every sexual encounter, but they may not prevent transmission of the virus.

IV. **Approach to clinical conditions:** This section describes an approach to diagnosis in a patient who presents with a clinical syndrome or symptom. Please refer to the previous section for a more detailed description of each of the specific infections described.

A. **Genital ulcers:** Epidemiology is often the key to diagnosis in a patient who presents with genital ulcers. In most of the US, HSV is the most common cause of genital ulcers, but syphilis and chancroid are endemic in certain regions. Multiple agents may be present, complicating the diagnosis. Ideally, the evaluation of a patient with genital ulceration(s) would include culture for HSV, darkfield microscopy or DFA testing for *T. pallidum*, and culture for *H. ducreyi*. But since the latter two tests are not readily available to most providers, clinical diagnosis is sometimes necessary. Serologic tests for syphilis may be obtained, recognizing their limitations during primary infection. When the diagnosis is uncertain, when the patient's clinical course is inconsistent with the natural history of the presumptive diagnosis or they fail to respond to treatment as expected, biopsy may be performed to further clarify the diagnosis. Keep in mind that conditions such as Behcet disease and Epstein-Barr Virus infection may present with genital ulcers as well.

B. **Vaginal discharge** may be caused by mucopurulent cervicitis or vaginitis. Sexually active adolescents should be evaluated for both etiologies. The presence of itching and external vulvar irritation suggests vaginitis. Irregular vaginal spotting or postcoital bleeding is consistent with cervicitis. A speculum examination is useful to visualize the cervix for inflammation and mucopurulent discharge, to obtain a vaginal pH, and to collect a specimen for endocervical testing for *C. trachomatis* and *N. gonorrhoeae*. If endocervical testing is not necessary, a blind vaginal swab may be collected without the use of a speculum, and this may be examined using microscopy. Conditions commonly causing vaginitis may be differentiated from one another using physical examination, microscopy, and vaginal pH. Performance of microscopy is described in Table 27-5. Table 27-6 summarizes distinguishing features between the three most common causes of vaginitis. Keep in mind, however, that certain features are variable and may be absent in some patients. Consider obtaining vaginal cultures for yeast or *T. vaginalis* if the diagnosis is in question. Nonspecific vaginitis may also be caused by poor perineal hygiene or the use of irritating soaps or cosmetic products in the vaginal area.

C. **Pelvic Inflammatory Disease (PID)** is an inflammatory infection of the upper genital tract. Patients may have salpingitis, endometritis, oophoritis, pelvic peritonitis, or a tubo-ovarian abscess. Causative organisms include *C. trachomatis* and *N. gonorrhoeae*, but *Mycoplasma* sp. and anaerobic organisms often play a significant role in this polymicrobial infection as well.

Table 27-5. Performing microscopy on vaginal fluid

1. Collect specimen from vaginal secretions pooled in the posterior fornix, using a cotton-tipped swab.
2. Place in 1 mL of nonbacteriostatic 0.9% normal saline.
3. Place one drop of specimen onto a glass slide; cover with coverslip.
4. View first on low-power (10X) to scan entire slide, then high-power (40X) for better visualization of areas of interest.
5. Evaluate for presence of the following:
   - Clue cells ($\geq$20% of all epithelial cells is significant)
   - White blood cells (ratio of WBC:epithelial cells $\geq$1:1 represents significant inflammation)
   - Motile trichomonads
   - Pseudohyphae or budding yeast

Place another drop of specimen on the slide and add KOH 10%. Release of amine odor suggests presence of anaerobic bacteria (positive whiff test).

WBC, white blood cell.

Clinically, patients present with pelvic pain that is usually bilateral. They may report vaginal discharge, dyspareunia, irregular vaginal bleeding, and/or right upper quadrant pain as well. They may have pain with ambulation, which suggests peritoneal inflammation. Systemic symptoms include fever, nausea, and vomiting, but these may be absent. Onset often is within 1 week of menses.

Laparoscopy with intraoperative culture is the most definitive procedure for diagnosis of PID. In practice, the diagnosis is made clinically in most cases. Minimal **diagnostic criteria** endorsed by the CDC include abdominal or pelvic pain and the presence of cervical motion tenderness *or* adnexal tenderness (or both) on bimanual examination. It is acknowledged that the predictive value of these criteria is poor; nonetheless, when they are met the provider should strongly consider treating for PID, due to the significant morbidity associated with untreated disease. Further evidence supporting a diagnosis of PID includes leukocytosis, an elevated sedimentation rate or C-reactive protein, and positive genital cultures for *N. gonorrhoeae* or *C. trachomatis*. Most patients with PID have some evidence of lower genital tract infection, such as cervical inflammation, friability, or mucopurulent discharge on speculum exam, white blood cells on microscopy of vaginal fluid, or positive cervical cultures. It is not unusual for cervical cultures to be negative; this does not indicate that the diagnosis of PID is incorrect. Transabdominal ultrasonography may be used to identify tubo-ovarian abscess, but it is unlikely to be sensitive enough to detect milder tubal inflammation. Transvaginal ultrasound with an extrasensitive Doppler technique, which may identify tubal hyperemia, is currently under investigation as a diagnostic tool. Patients in whom gastrointestinal (GI) symptoms (nausea, vomiting, or diarrhea) dominate the clinical picture are likely to have a GI diagnosis; PID is much less likely. The differential diagnosis includes appendicitis, gastroenteritis, ovarian cyst, endometriosis, pyelonephritis, and ectopic pregnancy.

Table 27-6. Vaginitis: Distinguishing features

	Vaginal discharge	Vaginal pH	White blood cells	Amine release with KOH 10%	Additional findings
Yeast vaginitis	White, clumpy, odorless	$\leq$4.5	Rare to elevated	Absent	Pseudohyphae or budding yeast
Bacterial vaginosis	Gray or white, malodorous, homogeneous, adherent	>4.5	Rare	Present	>20% Clue cells
Trichomoniasis	White, gray, or green; frothy	Often >4.5	Often elevated	May be present	Motile trichomonads

Table 27-7. Suggested regimens for treatment of pelvic inflammatory disease

Inpatient therapies	Outpatient therapies
Cefoxitin 2 g IV every 6 hours	Ceftriaxone 250 mg IM, single dose
and	*and*
Doxycycline 100 mg orally b.i.d. x 14 days	Doxycycline 100 mg orally b.i.d. x 14 days
Clindamycin 900 mg IV every 8 hours	Ofloxacin 400 mg orally b.i.d. x 14 days
and	*and*
Gentamicin loading dose (2 mg/kg) followed by maintenance dose (1.5 mg/kg) every 8 hours	Metronidazole 500 mg orally b.i.d. x 14 days

The goal of **treatment** is to relieve symptoms and prevent long-term sequelae of infection. Several treatment regimens for PID are presented in Table 27-7. No evidence demonstrates the superiority of inpatient versus outpatient treatment. Inpatient treatment should be considered for severely ill patients, patients with vomiting who cannot tolerate oral therapies, patients who have failed a trial of outpatient therapies, and those who are otherwise unable or unlikely to adhere to outpatient regimens. Although many adolescent health experts recommend hospitalizing adolescent patients, insufficient data exist to support this practice. Nonetheless, hospitalization should be strongly considered when possible. Inpatients should receive parenteral antibiotics until significant clinical improvement is achieved; most can be changed to oral medications and discharged within the next 24 to 48 hours. Patients should be followed up within 72 hours of initiation of outpatient therapy. Patients who do not respond as expected to treatment should be evaluated with ultrasonography if this was not done as part of the initial evaluation. Adequate pain management usually can be achieved with aggressive use of NSAIDs.

Acute complications of PID include tubo-ovarian abscess (TOA), which occurs in 15% to 20% of cases. In most cases, this is a complex, inflamed, multiloculated mass involving the fallopian tube, rather than a discrete, walled-off abscess. TOA typically responds well to parenteral broad-spectrum antibiotics including anaerobic coverage, and the lesion may be followed to resolution with ultrasonography. In rare cases, surgical intervention is needed. A ruptured TOA is a surgical emergency with a 7% mortality rate. Due to the complex nature of the lesion, simple drainage of the abscess often is not possible, and salpingectomy is required.

Fitz-Hugh-Curtis syndrome is characterized by inflammation of the hepatic capsule and the adjacent peritoneum ("perihepatitis"); patients complain of right upper quadrant pain. It occurs in up to 20% of cases of PID. In rare cases Fitz-Hugh-Curtis syndrome may occur in the absence of clinical findings of PID (i.e., no pelvic pain). *C. trachomatis* or *N. gonorrhoeae* may still be isolated from the cervix or from cultures obtained laparoscopically. Standard PID treatment regimens may be used.

Long-term complications of PID include infertility, chronic pelvic pain, and an increased risk of ectopic pregnancy. The recurrence rate for PID is up to 30% in adolescents, and the risk of each of the above complications increases with subsequent infections. The risk of infertility is about 10% after a single episode of PID and increases to 50% after three or more episodes. "Silent PID" refers to PID in a woman who is asymptomatic or minimally symptomatic and is never treated. It is believed to be responsible for a large proportion of infertility caused by tubal obstruction.

D. **Urethritis** in male adolescents may cause dysuria, urethral pruritus, and urethral discharge that may be clear or purulent. Purulent urethral discharge most often is caused by *N. gonorrhoeae*; nongonococcal urethritis (NGU) is most commonly (50% or more) caused by *C. trachomatis*. Other possible pathogens include *Ureaplasma urealyticum*, *Mycoplasma genitalium*, and *Mycoplasma hominis*. Tests for these pathogens are not readily available, and they typically are susceptible to the antibiotics used to treat chlamydial infections. *T. vaginalis* and HSV may cause urethral symptoms as well. Asymptomatic NGU is common. A urethral swab may be obtained for Gram stain and culture/NAAT for *N. gonorrhoeae* and *C. trachomatis*; the presence of Gram-negative intracellular diplococci indicates gonococcal infection. Urine may be tested for leukocytes and NAAT, particularly if Gram stain and microscopy are not readily available.

Empiric treatment for chlamydial and gonococcal infection may be considered if symptoms are severe, rapid diagnostic techniques such as Gram stain are not available, or follow-up cannot be ensured. See sections III.B.4.a. and III.C.4. for treatment options. Patients with NGU who do not respond to treatment (after nonadherence to therapy and re-exposure have been ruled out) may be tested or treated empirically for *T. vaginalis*, or evaluated for HSV infection.

E. **Epididymitis** in adolescents is most commonly caused by *C. trachomatis* or *N. gonorrhoeae*. Persons who engage in anal intercourse may have sexually transmitted enteric pathogens. Patients complain of subacute onset of unilateral testicular pain and tenderness and may have associated edema. Dysuria, urethral discharge, and fever are sometimes present. On exam, it may be possible to localize the pain and swelling to the epididymis, which is at the superior, posterior aspect of the testis. Evaluation for urethritis should be performed, as described above; the presence of urethritis lends great support to the diagnosis of epididymitis. Perhaps the most important step in evaluation is to rule out testicular torsion, which is a surgical emergency in the differential diagnosis of epididymitis (see Chapter 26 on adolescent sexuality and reproductive health).

The clinician should treat empirically once the clinical diagnosis is made and not await culture/NAAT results. Recommended treatment is ceftriaxone 250 mg intramuscular plus doxycycline 100 mg orally twice a day for 10 days. An alternative regimen is levofloxacin 500 mg orally once daily for 10 days. Adjunctive therapy includes NSAIDs, bed rest, and scrotal elevation.

F. **Proctitis, proctocolitis, and enteritis** most commonly occur among persons who participate in receptive anal intercourse or whose practices include oral–fecal contact. Evaluation may include stool examination for leukocytes, stool culture, and anoscopy or sigmoidoscopy. These syndromes may be best managed by a clinician experienced with their evaluation and treatment. Proctitis is inflammation limited to the distal 10 to 12 cm of the rectum; patients may present with anorectal pain, discharge, or tenesmus. Gonococcal and chlamydial infections, HSV, and syphilis are the most common STIs causing proctitis. Proctocolitis presents with diarrhea or abdominal cramping in addition to the symptoms of proctitis; it is associated with colonic inflammation extending greater than 12 cm above the anus. It may be caused by *Campylobacter* sp., *Shigella* sp., *Entamoeba histolytica*, and rarely certain types of *C. trachomatis*. Enteritis usually manifests as cramping and diarrhea without signs of proctitis. *Giardia lamblia* is the most common cause among otherwise healthy people. Persons with HIV infection may have other pathogens involved as well. Pending laboratory results, treatment of acute proctitis may be prescribed with ceftriaxone 125 mg intramuscular once, and doxycycline 100 mg orally twice a day for 7 days. If HSV is suspected, antiviral treatment may be prescribed.

V. **Human Immunodeficiency Virus (HIV):** This section includes information for primary care providers on HIV testing and the initial management of an adolescent with newly diagnosed HIV infection. A complete discussion of the manifestations, complications, and management of HIV and acquired immunodeficiency syndrome (AIDS) is beyond the scope of this text.

A. **Definitions:** HIV-positivity represents a chronic RNA viral infection in the host. AIDS is defined in persons over 12 years of age when the $CD4^+$ lymphocyte count is less than 200 cells or when an opportunistic or other unusual infection is present. In untreated patients, the median time between infection and the development of AIDS is 10 years.

B. **Epidemiology:** Adolescents have one of the fastest growing rates of HIV infection in the United States. Due to the long and variable period of time between infection and diagnosis, as well as the lack of a national monitoring system for HIV infection among adolescents, the prevalence of infection is unknown. Some experts estimate that as many as 250,000 adolescents are infected. Most acquire HIV through sexual transmission. Almost half of adolescent HIV is diagnosed in male adolescents who have sex with other males. Compared to infected adults, female adolescents and ethnic minorities (African American and Hispanic) are disproportionately represented among HIV-infected youth. AIDS is now the seventh most common cause of death among people 15 to 24 years old in the United States. The vast majority of infections in the US are caused by HIV-1.

C. **Types of tests and their uses:** Initial screening tests identify antibodies to HIV-1 and HIV-2 (HIV-1/2) using EIA. EIA is positive in 95% of persons infected with HIV within 3 months after the initial infection. EIA is very sensitive, but false-positives may occur. Positive EIA must therefore be followed up with confirmatory testing such as Western Blot or an immunofluorescence assay (IFA). HIV viral load is determined using PCR to quantitate the number of HIV virions present in the plasma. This may be used for diagnostic purposes in some circumstances, but it is primarily used to monitor the efficacy of therapy; patients receiving optimal therapy will have a nondetectable viral load.

New rapid "point-of-care" HIV tests are now becoming available; they provide accurate results in as little as 20 minutes. These tests are performed on blood and oral fluid. Positive results still require additional confirmatory testing.

D. When to consider HIV testing: Early diagnosis and treatment of HIV infection may slow the decline of immune system function and decrease HIV-related mortality and morbidity. The CDC recommends offering HIV testing to all persons who seek testing for STIs and those who are diagnosed with STIs. Persons with high-risk sexual practices should be encouraged to undergo testing, as should adolescents with any history of intravenous drug use or sexual contact with persons who use intravenous drugs. MSM and females whose male partners have had other male partners should be tested as well. Local prevalence of HIV will also help dictate appropriate screening practices.

Adolescents with unusual (or unusually severe) infections should receive testing. This may include *Candida* esophagitis, oral thrush, or severe vaginitis, varicella zoster, or severe HSV recurrences, as well as opportunistic infections. Primary care providers should also recognize the features of acute retroviral syndrome, which may occur in the first few weeks following HIV acquisition. This mononucleosis-like syndrome is characterized by fever, lymphadenopathy, malaise, and a skin rash. It is seen in 30% to 70% of newly infected adolescents. During this time, antibody tests such as EIA are not yet positive, so testing for HIV RNA by PCR should be performed; a positive test should be confirmed by another HIV test since this nucleic acid testing is not approved for diagnostic purposes. These patients should be referred immediately for care, because early aggressive antiretroviral therapy may be beneficial. Patients may be candidates for clinical trial investigating this possibility.

Pretest and posttest counseling should be performed and informed consent obtained. Counseling should be "client-centered," focusing on the adolescent's risk factors and specific risky behaviors. Montefiore Medical Center's Adolescent AIDS program has developed an HIV testing protocol called ACTS: Assess, Counsel and Consent, Test, and Support. The protocol is practical for use by providers in a variety of settings including primary care and does not assume that comprehensive services are provided at the site of testing. More information on ACTS is available at www.adolescentaids.org. The protocol is summarized in Table 27-8.

Table 27-8. ACTS: A rapid system for HIV counseling and testing

Assess need for HIV testing, care, or prevention counseling
- Explain benefits of testing for patient's health and prevention.
- Discuss modes of HIV transmission (e.g., sex, needles, perinatal).
- Review risk assessment form or explain to patient that HIV testing is advisable if the patient has: (1) ever had sex, (2) has had intercourse without a condom, (3) has ever used recreational drugs intravenously, or (4) shared intravenous syringes and works.
- Recommend testing, discuss HIV prevention, and provide referrals as appropriate.

Counsel and obtain consent
- Clarify the meaning of positive and negative results and explore patient's potential reactions.
- Assess readiness for immediate testing, including patient's social support network.
- Review health department requirements, such as the difference between confidential and anonymous testing and names reporting, partner notification, and domestic violence screening.

Test
- Describe/provide HIV test (e.g., blood, oral, urine, rapid).
- Make appointment to deliver results in person, by phone, or have patient wait for rapid results.

Support during testing and afterward HIV-negative patients
- Clarify need to retest in 3 months (e.g., window period, based on risk assessment).
- Provide prevention strategies and referrals; HIV testing alone is not prevention.

HIV-positive patients
- Provide support and link to care and prevention.
- Review HIV reporting, partner notification, and domestic/partner violence issues.

ACTS, Assess, Counsel and Consent, Test, and Support; HIV, Human Immunodeficiency Virus.
Complete ACTS training materials are available at www.adolescentaids.org.
From Futterman DC. HIV and AIDS in adolescents. *Adolesc Med Clin* 2004;15(2):369–91, with permission.

E. **Managing a newly diagnosed HIV-positive adolescent:** Adolescents who have positive HIV test results must receive some initial counseling on-site at the time of diagnosis. Their acute distress should be acknowledged and emotional support provided. Since it is often unknown how long a patient has been infected with HIV, newly diagnosed patients should be reevaluated for the presence of signs or symptoms that suggest more advanced disease, such as fevers, weight loss, chronic respiratory symptoms, or oral candidiasis. They should be informed of what to expect as they receive care for the infection, including comprehensive physical examinations, STI testing and gynecologic care (for female patients), periodic blood testing, extensive psychosocial evaluation and risk-reduction counseling, and antiviral therapy. Patients should be promptly provided (or referred for) comprehensive medical, psychosocial, and mental health services. Centers that provide all of these services at one site are desirable but are not always available. It may then be the role of the primary care provider to coordinate these services and often to remain the primary provider of medical care.

F. **Overview of HIV management:** Investigators at many HIV treatment centers maintain a living document on the Web at www.aidsinfo.nih.gov/guidelines. This document is constantly updated as new findings or recommendations for HIV/AIDS treatment emerge.

Combination therapy remains a mainstay of HIV treatment, including the use of reverse transcriptase inhibitors (e.g., AZT, didanosine [ddI], lamivudine [3TC]), nonnucleoside analogue reverse transcriptase inhibitors (e.g., nevarapine, efavirenz, delavirdine), and protease inhibitors (e.g., nelfinavir, ritonavir, indinavir). Therapy is initiated based on clinical status, HIV viral load, and CD4$^+$ lymphocyte count. It is usually recommended to all HIV-positive adolescents, unless they have no evidence of immune suppression and are clinically asymptomatic. The goal of therapy is to reduce the HIV viral load to nondetectable levels quickly, and to maintain this suppression. Poor or intermittent adherence to drug regimens, relatively common among adolescents, leads to drug resistance.

Other important components of treatment include prophylactic therapy for the prevention of opportunistic infections such as *Pneumocystis carinii* pneumonia, cytomegalovirus infection, and *Mycobacterium avium-intracellulare*. Most childhood immunizations are recommended in adolescents with HIV, although live viral vaccines should never be given to persons with very low CD4$^+$ cell counts.

VI. **Clinical pearls and pitfalls:**
- The greatest risk factors for having an STI are young age and history of a prior STI.
- Most STIs are usually asymptomatic.
- All sexually active adolescent and young adult women should be screened at least annually for *Chlamydia trachomatis*, regardless of whether they are considered "high risk."
- Strong consideration should be given to screening adolescent females routinely for *Neisseria gonorrhoeae* and *Trichomonas vaginalis*.
- Pap smears should be performed annually beginning 3 years after the onset of sexual activity (in immunocompetent females) to evaluate for cervical dysplasia caused by HPV.
- Nucleic acid amplification tests (NAATs) provide the greatest sensitivity for diagnosing *C. trachomatis* and *N. gonorrhoeae*, but at the greatest cost.
- Urine testing using NAATs for *C. trachomatis* and *N. gonorrhoeae* may be used for screening asymptomatic patients, but symptomatic female adolescents should still be evaluated with pelvic exams to identify other infections.
- Single dose treatments should be used when available, in order to maximize the patient's adherence to therapy.
- Patients with pelvic inflammatory disease and epididymitis require prolonged treatment; single dose therapy is ineffective.
- Adolescents in all 50 states may provide their own consent for issues related to STI diagnosis and treatment, and their confidentiality should be respected with regard to these issues.

BIBLIOGRAPHY

For the clinician

American Academy of Pediatrics, Pickering LK ed. *2003 Red book: Report of the committee on infectious diseases*, 26th ed. Elk Grove Village, IL: American Academy of Pediatrics, 2003.

Braverman PK, Rosenfeld WD. Sexually transmitted infections. *Adolesc Med Clin* 2004;15: 201–428.

Burchett SK, Pizzo PA. HIV infection in infants, children, and adolescents. *Pediatr Rev* 2003; 24(6):186–194.

Burstein GR, Murray PJ. Diagnosis and management of sexually transmitted disease pathogens among adolescents. *Pediatr Rev* 2003;24:75–82, 119–127.

Centers for Disease Control and Prevention. Revised guidelines for HIV counseling, testing, and referral and revised recommendations for HIV screening of pregnant women. *MMWR Morb Mortal Wkly Rep* 2001;50(No. RR-19):1–57.

Centers for Disease Control and Prevention. Sexually transmitted diseases treatment guidelines 2002. *MMWR Morb Mortal Wkly Rep* 2002;51(No. RR-6). Also available online at www.cdc. gov/mmwr.

Futterman DC. HIV and AIDS in adolescents. *Adolesc Med Clin* 2004;15(2):369–391.

Holmes KK, Sparling PF, Mårdh P, Lemon SM, Stamm WE, Piot P, Wasserheit JN, eds. *Sexually transmitted diseases*, 3rd ed. New York: McGraw-Hill, 1999.

Institute of Medicine, Eng TR, Butler WT, eds. *The hidden epidemic: Confronting sexually transmitted diseases*. Washington, DC: National Academy Press, 1997.

For patients and parents

Haffner DW. *Beyond the big talk: Every parent's guide to raising sexually healthy teens from middle school to high school and beyond*. New York: Newmarket Press, 2001.

WEB SITES

www.aidsinfo.nih.gov/guidelines   A living document describing current HIV/AIDS treatment recommendations

www.ashastd.org   Web site of the American Social Health Association (ASHA) with excellent information for parents and professionals

www.iwannaknow.org   ASHA's Web site for teens

www.teenwire.com   Planned Parenthood's teen Web site, providing comprehensive information on reproductive health

www.goaskalice.columbia.edu   Question and answer format for teens regarding sexual health and other topics. Maintained by Columbia University's Health Education Program

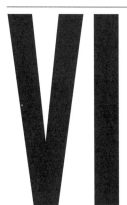

VI

Sports Medicine

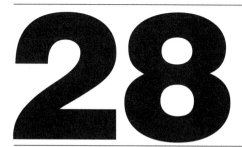

28 Sports Medicine

Adolescents comprise one of the most physically active of all age cohorts. Many adolescents participate in organized sports activities, and many more adolescents are involved in fitness activities on their own. It has been estimated that half of all 5 to 18 year olds participate in organized sports activities. That number translates into about 30 million school-aged participants.

Adolescents participate in sports for six primary reasons:

- To attain self-confidence and a feeling of personal satisfaction
- To combat boredom
- To socialize
- To satisfy peer and parental pressure
- To participate in socially acceptable risk-taking behavior
- To have fun

In this chapter we will discuss the evaluation of the adolescent prior to sports participation, sports nutrition and performance-enhancing substances (PES), issues for female athletes, and injury management by the primary care physician.

I. **The Preparticipation Examination (PPSE):** A physical examination to determine whether a child or adolescent is capable of participating safely in a particular sport is routine for scholastic sports and is highly recommended for voluntary sports.

A. **The goals of the PPSE** are:
- to assess the overall health of the young athlete
- to detect conditions that might compromise the adolescent's ability to participate
- to take anthropometric measurements
- to determine the athlete's level of fitness for the sport in question
- to provide an opportunity for counseling and education

The PPSE has a variable rate of detection of disqualifying conditions. Studies show a true positive rate of detection of from 0 to 12 out of 1,000 evaluations, but the detection of false positives in some studies is very high. Still, as a screening tool, the PPSE is effective. There are three **types of PPSE:**
- multiple examiner/station
- locker room
- primary care clinician

The station examination has been found to be the best at detecting possibly disqualifying conditions. The "locker room" examination is inadequate, and the examination by the primary care clinician can be deficient because the clinician may not be well versed in how to detect disqualifying conditions. However, with a primary care clinician trained in sports evaluation, the examination in the primary care office is the best type of examination because the clinician knows the adolescent well.

B. **History:** The history is the most important part of the PPSE. It is important to detect any past events that might be consistent with conditions that could result in sudden death with exercise, including syncope with exercise or early cardiac death in a first-degree relative. Also, old records of existing medical conditions can be reviewed. History of previous injuries is important because, for example, ankle sprains tend to not be rehabilitated adequately, and there may be a history of previous concussions. History of a chronic condition such as asthma is also important. Inadequate treatment of such a condition may prevent full participation by the adolescent. For females, history is important in ascertaining menstrual history and eating patterns since females who are highly trained are at risk for the **female athlete triad,** that is:
- disordered eating
- amenorrhea
- osteoporosis

A quick reference to which questions are important to answer at the PPSE can be found in the following list, which can be entered into any record of a PPSE:
- syncope with exercise
- chest pain with exercise
- history of recurrent concussion
- history of lower extremity injury
- problems with paired organs
- pre-existing illness/condition

The answers to these questions can provide most of the critical information needed in the PPSE.

C. **Anthropometric measurement:** Measurements of height, weight, blood pressure and, possibly, triceps skin-fold thickness are done next. Tanner stage can be assessed here as well, either by direct observation or by having the teens point to pictures of stages of development that are commensurate with their own level. Maturation assessment is very important in several sports. In collision sports, it is important to try to match contestants of similar developmental levels in order to help ensure fair competition. Also, in sports such as baseball, where throwing can stress growth plates, it is important to know if the athlete is fully matured. Athletes who are less than fully mature may be at increased risk for strains, sprains, and for overuse injuries. Table 28-1 shows the classification of sports by contact and by exertion. This is important because some teens who would not qualify for particularly heavy contact sports or ones with excessive exertion could be steered to ones in which they can participate.

D. **Physical examination:** For the PPSE, physical examination (PE) should be directed toward those body parts essential for participation. While a full examination can be done at this time, it is not necessary just for sports. The essentials of the PE for the PPSE are the cardiovascular examination, the assessment for musculoskeletal

Table 28-1. Classification of sports

Contact collision	Contact impact	Non-contact strenuous	Non-contact moderately strenuous	Non-contact non-strenuous
Boxing	Baseball	Aerobic dancing	Badminton	Archery
Field hockey	Basketball	Crew	Curling	Golf
Football	Bicycling	Fencing	Table Tennis	Riflery
Ice hockey	Diving	Field events		
Lacrosse	Field events	• Discus		
Martial arts	• High jump	• Javelin		
Rodeo	• Pole vault	• Shot put		
Soccer	Gymnastics	Running		
Wrestling	Horseback riding	Swimming		
	Skating	Tennis		
	• Ice	Track		
	• Roller	Weight lifting		
	Skiing			
	• Cross-country			
	• Downhill			
	• Water			
	Softball			
	Squash, handball			
	Volleyball			

From the Committee on Sports Medicine. Recommendations for participation in competitive sports. *Pediatrics* 1988;81:737, with permission.

integrity, strength, and flexibility, and the examination of paired organs. If a heart murmur is detected, then effort should be made to ascertain whether or not it is indicative of a problem that could increase the risk of sudden death. While sudden death in athletes is decidedly rare, any concern about a possible risk in an athlete should prompt referral to a cardiologist. The **most common cause of sudden cardiac death in youth sports is hypertrophic cardiomyopathy.** This condition is usually inherited, and it causes a distinctive murmur heard best when the patient is rising from a squatting position. **Sudden cardiac death** in this venue is described as death that is:

* nontraumatic
* unexpected
* due to cardiac arrest within 6 hours of a previously witnessed state of normal health

It occurs in approximately one in 200,000 high school athletes annually. The causes are shown in Figure 28-1.

Body habitus also should be observed, as patients with Marfan syndrome are at special risk for difficulties with sports. The **criteria for diagnosing Marfan syndrome** are:

* a family history plus phenotypic features in the skeletal and one other organ system, or
* negative family history and manifestations in the skeletal and two other organ systems
* the chief manifestations are tall stature with long limbs and fingers, ectopia lentis, dural ectasia, pectus excavatum, mitral valve prolapse, aortic dilatation, and aortic dissection

PE also should concentrate on the musculoskeletal system. **Risk factors for musculoskeletal injuries** include:

* body type
* ligamentous laxity or hyperflexibility
* muscle strength

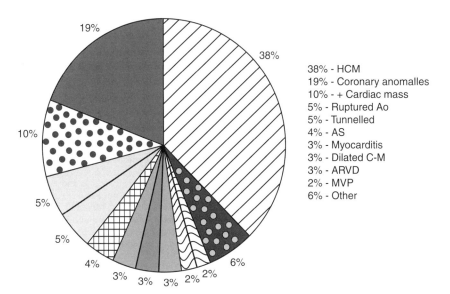

38% - HCM
19% - Coronary anomalies
10% - + Cardiac mass
5% - Ruptured Ao
5% - Tunnelled
4% - AS
3% - Myocarditis
3% - Dilated C-M
3% - ARVD
2% - MVP
6% - Other

Figure 28-1. Causes of sudden cardiac death in young competitive athletes (median age, 17 years), based on systematic tracking of 158 athletes in the United States, primarily from 1985 to 1995. Ao, aorta; LAD, left anterior descending coronary artery; AS, aortic ventricular dysplasia; MVP, mitral valve prolapse; CAD, coronary artery disease; HCM, hypertrophic cardiomyopathy; +, increased. (From Maron BJ, Thompson PD, Puffer JC, et al. Cardiovascular preparticipation screening of competitive athletes. *Circulation* 1996;94:850, with permission).

Table 28-2. Five basic musculoskeletal screening tests for sports

Ability to rotate the head painlessly in all directions
Ability to shrug both shoulders
Ability to place both hands together behind the head on the neck
Ability to bend forward, touching toes with knees straight
Ability to duck-walk with the buttocks on the heels

Adapted from Luckstead EF, Greydanus DE. *Medical care of the adolescent athlete.* Los Angeles, CA: Practice Management Information Corporation, 1993, p. 26.

- inadequate rehabilitation from previous injury
- skeletal anomalies and malalignment

A body that is too flexible or too stiff might predispose to injury. Strength in body parts essential to a sport can decrease risk of injury, for example, the neck in football and wrestling. Weak quadriceps can lead to increased incidence of patellofemoral disorders. One quick way of determining strength and flexibility is the **90 second orthopedic examination** (see Table 28-2).

For athletes with special conditions such as Down syndrome, attention should be paid to particular body parts. In Down syndrome, there is a 10% to 20% incidence of atlantoaxial subluxation, and this may predispose to catastrophic neck injury. Therefore, these athletes are urged to not compete in sports with significant hyperflexion or extension of the neck. Also, athletes with a 50% spondylolisthesis should not participate in vigorous sports because of the risk of further slippage.

E. **Counseling:** The final part of the PPSE should be a counseling opportunity with the examiner(s) so that any abnormalities found can be explained, any needed referrals can be made, and the essentials of good sports training and nutrition can be reviewed. If there are pre-existing conditions such as asthma or diabetes, proper care while involved in sports should be reviewed at this time.

F. **Clinical pearls and pitfalls:**
- The PPSE is a great opportunity to assess overall adolescent health when done by the primary care clinician. This opportunity is the only one the clinician may have to perform this necessary evaluation; therefore primary care clinicians should become competent in performing PPSEs.

II. **Sports nutrition:** Proper nutrition is important for all adolescents, but even more so for athletes. Nearly all adolescents ingest sufficient food to provide adequate calories and proteins, fats, and carbohydrates. The food that is eaten contains adequate vitamins. The substances that may be lacking are minerals, especially calcium and iron for young women. The other nutrient whose intake is very important for adolescent athletes is water.

A. **Food:** A typical athlete's diet should mirror a healthy diet for any adolescent. If the athlete is in intense training, then more calories will be needed. The following basic proportions should be maintained:
- protein (15%–20%),
- carbohydrate (55%–75%), and
- fat (10%–30%)

With a good selection of whole grains, fruits and vegetables, and animal protein, the athlete should be well nourished.

The primary sources of energy for competition are carbohydrates and fats. Carbohydrates are stored as glycogen in the liver and in muscle tissue, and are called on for intense exercise of relatively short duration. Fat is helpful for sustained lower-intensity exercise. Prior conditioning enhances the body's use of fat as an energy source. Some athletes will want to practice **glycogen—or carbohydrate—loading.** With this technique, athletes deplete their glycogen stores by exercising intensely a few days prior to their competition, and then they eat large amounts of carbohydrates in order to more than double their storage of glycogen. This can help in endurance events of longer than 1 hour duration but otherwise is of no use. Carbohydrate loading can have deleterious effects such as creating a feeling of sluggishness and diarrhea.

Dietary protein ingestion by athletes usually is adequate. Protein or amino acid supplements, therefore, are of no use and should be discouraged. The guiding light of athletic nutrition for adolescents should be common sense and overall good dietary habits. Elite athletes may get some benefit from amino acid supplements, but this is by no means proven. Table 28-3 shows some "do's and dont's" for sports nutrition.

Table 28-3. Do's and dont's of sports nutrition

Do's

Do eat a well balanced diet consisting of elements of the four basic food groups. Your diet should include dairy products, cereals and grains, meats and animal products, fruits and vegetables.

Do drink water at regular intervals during exercise.

Do monitor your weight before and after exercise to prevent dehydration.

Do drink 16 oz. of water for each pound of fluid lost through exercise.

Do drink water or beverages with small amounts of simple sugars or glucoses, polymers and no or small amounts of electrolytes.

Do follow a goal of achieving a certain percentage of body fat when trying to lose weight. You want to lose body fat, not lean body tissue or water.

Do reduce caloric intake to not less than 1,200 calories for women and 1,500 calories for men per day if you're trying to lose weight.

Do combine increased calories with muscle work, (such as weight training) to gain weight.

Do eat a pregame meal at least $2\frac{1}{2}$ hours before competition. The meal should be mostly carbohydrates. You should avoid slowly digested foods such as fats and desserts and those with a great deal of sugar.

Dont's

Don't return to exercise activity if you've lost more than 3% of your body weight (through fluid loss). Return only after the fluid is restored.

Don't take salt tablets. They are rarely needed and may actually be harmful and increase dehydration.

Don't engage in glycogen loading by consuming large amounts of foods high in carbohydrates (such as breads, cereals, and pasta) unless you are engaging in endurance exercise that takes more than an hour (marathons, cross-country ski racing).

Don't take amino acids or protein supplements. They are potentially harmful.

Don't take vitamin supplements. They are usually unnecessary and a waste of money, and excessive doses can be harmful. One daily multivitamin is not harmful and would be helpful if you are not eating a well balanced diet.

Don't take mineral supplements unless you have developed a specific deficiency, such as iron.

Don't lose more weight than 1–2 lb per week. Any more weight loss could be water or lean body tissue.

Don't gain more than 1–2 lb per week. Any more weight gain could be body fat.

Adapted from Primos WA Jr, Landry GL. Fighting the fads in sports nutrition. *Contemp Pediatr* 1989;6:14, with permission.

B. **Minerals and electrolytes:** Iron and calcium are the two minerals that are frequently underrepresented in the diet of the adolescent athlete, particularly in females. The **recommended dietary allowance (RDA) for iron in menstruating females is 15 mg per day.** Female track athletes ingest an average of only 10 mg per day without iron supplements. Iron deficiency anemia has been associated with decreased ability to do physical work. This may also be true for iron deficiency without anemia, but there are not many studies on this point. Recommending an over-the-counter iron supplement for female athletes therefore may be a good idea. Of course, those females who are actually anemic need iron replacement. Males usually have more than adequate iron stores, primarily due to their larger caloric intake.

Calcium is necessary for good bone strength. Adequate intake is considered 1,200 mg per day. Females may eat less than that, and therefore the female who is also an athlete needs to have even more attention paid to her calcium intake. Females should be urged to eat sufficient amounts of dairy products. If they are lactose intolerant, calcium supplements such as calcium carbonate antacid tablets should be recommended, as long as there is adequate hydration. Calcium adequacy is even more important in the highly trained female athlete due to the risk of female athlete triad.

C. **Water: Water performs three main functions pertinent to exercise:**
   • it helps to regulate body temperature
   • it is the transport medium for nutrients, oxygen, and waste in the plasma
   • it is a necessary component of biochemical reactions in energy production
   Water is lost from the body through urination, from the respiratory track during breathing, and, primarily, from perspiration. The greater the intensity of exercise

and the higher the environmental temperature, the more water is lost. As much as **1.0 L/m²/hour may be lost** through sweating in hot and humid weather with intense exercise. The amount lost may vary considerably among competitors with diverse body types. A thin soccer player may not lose nearly as much water when exercising as would a beefy interior football lineman. Body weight is the most sensitive indicator of water loss and, therefore, of water requirements. For each kilogram of weight lost through exercise, 1 liter of water needs to be ingested (or approximately 16 oz for each pound lost). Because athletes are not weighed during competitions, water must be supplied prophylactically throughout the activity. **The hotter and more humid the environmental conditions, the more fluids are needed.**

First it is important that athletes maintain good nutrition and hydration in the 24 hours prior to competition. A few hours before the event (or the practice) the athlete should drink 400 to 600 mL of water or sports drink. This amount of time allows excess fluid to be eliminated in urine. The athlete then should drink 180 to 240 mL of fluid approximately 10 to 20 minutes prior to activity and every 15 to 20 minutes during activity. After exercise, 600 mL of fluid should be consumed for every pound of weight lost during the activity.

The American College of Sports Medicine recommends 4 to 8 g per 100 mL of carbohydrates and 0.5 to 0.7 g of sodium per liter in rehydration fluids. This combination can be found in a variety of products. Because of the palatable flavors of these commercial drinks, adolescent athletes tend to use them more often than plain water. Although water has been the traditional replacement fluid of choice, modern sports drinks that use accessible carbohydrates and have the correct amounts of sodium and potassium are now preferred.

One of the consequences of inadequate hydration during sports performance is **heat illness.** Heat illness can be defined as an accumulation of body heat that results when the body's ability to cool itself is overwhelmed. Different **types** of heat illness include **heat cramps, heat stress, heat exhaustion, and heat stroke.** They are explained in Table 28-4. The likelihood of heat illness increases with conditions that are associated with excessive fluid loss, excessive sweating, diminished thirst, inadequate drinking, abnormal hypothalamic thermoregulatory function, and obesity.

Prevention of heat illnesses requires adequate hydration and mineral replacement and also awareness of environmental conditions. One way of assessing these conditions is by measuring **Wet Bulb Globe Temperature (WBGT).** This is an indication of climactic heat stress by use of a **psychrometer,** an apparatus composed of three thermometers. One has a wet wick around it to monitor humidity (wet bulb), another is inside a hollow black ball (globe) to monitor radiation, and the third is a simple thermometer (temperature) to measure air temperature. The heat stress index is calculated as WBGT = 0.7 WB + 0.2 G temp + 0.1 T temp. This points to the fact that the humidity is in many ways more important than is the actual temperature.

The body cools itself during exercise primarily via sweat evaporation. The risk of developing heat illness significantly increases in hot, humid environmental conditions because the evaporation of sweat and resulting heat loss are hindered. This is why it is so important, as stated above, for athletes to prehydrate, to regularly rehydrate with water or with appropriately formulated sports drinks, and to rehydrate after activity.

Dehydration is also often used **as a weight loss strategy,** particularly by wrestlers when they are trying to make weight for a meet. Wrestlers and their coaches and parents need to be firmly advised to **not** engage in such practices. As a rule,

Table 28-4. Heat illnesses

Heat Cramps: Represent the exercising muscle's response to fatigue; can be precipitated by the depletion of total body sodium due to excessive sweating or to intake of excessive amounts of salt-free fluids during prolonged endurance activities. Symptoms are cramps, fatigue, tachycardia, and weakness.

Heat Stress: This indicates a mild elevation of body temperature associated with tachycardia, increased blood pressure, fatigue, and mild dehydration. Thirst may or may not be present.

Heat Exhaustion: Main features are hypovolemia, body temperature between 38.5° and 40°C., with the following symptoms: orthostasis, profuse sweating, clammy skin, dizziness, syncope, headache, nausea, and lack of coordination.

Heat Stroke: A medical emergency! Body temperature is >40°C, hypovolemia, hypotension, loss of coordination and inability to walk, loss of consciousness, and ultimately shock.

wrestlers should compete at no less than 90% of their preseason weight, so the need for acute weight loss by dehydration should not occur. Even 2% dehydration can negatively affect performance.

D. **Dietary supplements/ergogenic aids:** Athletes of all ages and of all levels of competition seek an edge in order to win. This "edge" can be an extra hour of conditioning or extra time spent honing technique with an expert coach. The "edge" also can be sought through the ingestion (or injection) of supposed PES. **These substances can contain anything.** Their composition and the claims made for them are unregulated, and therefore **the athlete is at the mercy of the manufacturers and of those who have a financial or emotional stake in their use.** These substances can purport to be vitamins, protein supplements, amino acids, hormones, "energy" boosters, or any other substance that is currently in vogue.

The clinician needs to be informed about the substances that his or her patients might be using. He or she should be prepared to offer wise counsel about these substances without condemning them absolutely. Frequently it is parents or coaches who are urging the adolescent to take these items, and the clinician has to be sensitive to that. As stated above, no vitamins or minerals, when taken in excessive amounts, are helpful to athletes who are ingesting an adequate diet, nor are protein or other supplements needed.

There are dietary supplements that are purported to increase strength or reaction time, including androstenedione and ephedra. Both can be harmful and should never be used. Other illicit substances, such as anabolic steroids, growth hormone, erythropoietin, etc., should be discussed with the athlete and with the parents and should also never be used. Effects of PES are listed in Table 28-5, and some information about anabolic steroids is listed in Table 28-6.

Another substance used as an ergogenic aid is creatine. This is a nonessential amino acid found in large amounts in meat and fish. **Creatine** is created in the body as well as being a supplement. It serves as an available source of adenosine 5'-triphosphate (ATP) within skeletal muscle and has four **basic functions:**
- rephosphorylation of adenosine 5'-diphosphate (ADP) provides a substantial source of ATP during short-duration, high-intensity exercise
- it enhances the capacity for high-energy phosphate diffusion within the cells
- phosphorylated creatine hydrolysis consumes hydrogen ions contributing to the buffering of intracellular acidosis during exercise
- the products of phosphorylated creatine hydrolysis play a role in the activation of glycogenolysis and other catabolic pathways

The functional outcome of all this is that creatine does improve athletic performance with short-term use. It enhances muscular force and/or power output during short episodes of intense exercise, particularly in well-trained athletes, but creatine has not been proven to enhance aerobic activities. There is no information that creatine has harmful effects, but lack of information does not prove there are no negative effects. While creatine has not been shown to be harmful, its unmonitored use cannot be recommended as totally safe given some case reports of adverse effects.

1. **Ephedra** is a natural plant product that is a stimulant with potential negative cardiovascular effects. It has been banned in Olympic sports, and its use should be actively discouraged.

2. **Beta hydroxyl, beta methylbutirate, or HMB,** another ergogenic aid, does seem to have some beneficial effects, but there are risks associated with its use. It unequivocally increases strength and fat free mass. It even has positive effects on cardiovascular risks, for example, blood pressure and cholesterol. However, its safety is compromised in that at least **50% of the product available is contaminated** with an anabolic steroid, stanazole. And an athlete could unwittingly fail a drug screen and be banished from organized sports.

3. These and other **performance enhancing drugs,** especially anabolic steroids, central nervous system stimulants, insulin, and possibly erythropoietin **can be dangerous.** Athletes who take nutritional supplements should know that they may contain banned substances not listed on the label. While elite athletes may try to use these substances to get the edge they think they need to win at the international level, there is absolutely no reason for adolescents in voluntary or scholastic sports to even consider their use. Clinicians should actively educate their patients, the patients' parents, and school/sports administrators and coaches about the reasons to not use these substances. They should emphasize that if the adolescent wants a 5% improvement in performance, increasing training and conditioning is the way to get it.

Table 28-5. Performance enhancing substances

Name	Proposed effect	Adverse effects	Physical exam findings	Rules/legal issues
Anabolic-androgenic steroids	Increase muscle strength and mass at high doses	Endocrine/reproductive-testicular atrophy and irreversible gynecomastia in males and irreversible virilization in females	Testicular shrinkage Male pattern balding Striae	Illegal and punishable as a felony Schedule III controlled substances
	Do not increase endurance	Cardiovascular-adverse changes in lipid profile and elevation of blood pressure, cardiomyopathy	Gynecomastia Acne	Banned by major sports governing organizations
		Hepatic-enzyme elevation, jaundice, and possible malignancy		
		Musculoskeletal: epiphyseal fusion and decreased tensile strength of tendons		
		Psychiatric: multiple effects including potential addiction and dependence		
Prohormones, "natural steroids," androstenedione (Andro), dehydro-epiandrosterone (DHEA)	Do not increase testosterone at moderate doses	Same as anabolic-androgenic steroids	Testicular shrinkage Male pattern balding	Banned by major sports governing organizations
	Might increase testosterone at higher doses	Increased estrogen effect May increase hormone-sensitive malignancies	Striae Gynecomastia	FDA ban on manufacture, marketing, distribution of Andro (March 2004)
	May increase muscle strength and mass at high doses	Can lead to adverse ratio of total cholesterol to high-density lipoprotein		

	Claims	Adverse effects	Symptoms	Regulatory status
Ephedra	May burn fat (not proven by research) May delay fatigue (not proven by research)	Serious cardiovascular and central nervous system events including: Hypertension, heart attack, stroke, seizure (effects are potentiated by caffeine)	Feeling jittery Sweating Increased heart rate Increased blood pressure	Systematic use banned by major sports governing organizations FDA ban on sales of Ephedra (April 2004)
Creatine	Increases work capacity over brief, repetitive exertion May delay fatigue of workouts Does not improve endurance Does not increase strength or muscle mass Has responders/non-responders	Early weight gain from water retention Muscle cramping, stomach cramping, hydration issues Case reports of reversible renal problems Not tested in those younger than 18 years	Rapid early weight gain	Not banned from use NCAA prohibits distribution in training facilities Purchased over-the-counter as dietary supplement
Protein supplements	Case weight gain (especially in some "restricted diets") Increase strength/power Increase lean muscle mass Require both carbohydrate and protein intake for strength and muscle gains	Anecdotal reports of renal problems with protein overload	Variable weight gain	Not banned by major sports governing bodies Cost can be prohibitive

FDA, Food and Drug Association; NCAA, National Collegiate Athletic Association.
- "Random" drug testing is a deterrent in the International Olympic Committee, NCAA, and some professional sports, but it is probably too costly for widespread use in high school.
- Human growth hormone and erythropoietin are currently used in the setting of elite athletes; however, their use may be filtering down to adolescents. At this point, they have been controlled and protected well by the medical community.

From the American Academy of Pediatrics, Section on Sports Medicine and Fitness, November 2004, with permission.

Table 28-6.   Side effects of anabolic steroids

Although anabolic steroids have been shown to increase muscle mass and strength, they are
also associated with a long list of potential reversible and irreversible side effects including:
- Premature closure of growth plates (irreversible)
- Acne
- Testicular atrophy
- Clitoromegaly, hirsutism, and voice deepening in females (irreversible)
- Psychological changes, alterations in mood
- Hepatocellular disease
- Hepatocellular cancer
- Abnormal lipid problems
- Hypertension
- Gynecomastia (males)
- Alopecia

    E. Clinical pearls and pitfalls:
- A well-balanced diet is sufficient for the adolescent athlete.
- Prehydration and hydration during participation, as well as hydration after the activity, are necessary to avoid heat injury.
- Nutritional supplements and ergogenic aids should never be used by the adolescent athlete. The athlete, family, and coach should be cautioned about the risks of using these substances.

III.   **Issues for the female athlete:** One of the major changes in participation in scholastic sports in the last 30 years has been the major increase in the number of females who are involved in organized, school-sponsored athletics. This is a result of the passage of Title IX of the Federal Education Act of 1972, which mandated equal athletic facilities for males and females. Concomitant societal changes that have enhanced the opportunities for female participation in all areas of life have further facilitated female involvement in sports activities. The ratio of school-aged female to male athletes has increased from 1 to 27 in 1972 to 1 to 3 in 2001.

    Female adolescent athletes have special issues that are not pertinent to their male counterparts. As mentioned above, highly trained female athletes potentially are in danger of suffering from the **female athlete triad** of amenorrhea, disordered eating, and osteoporosis. This is a risk particularly in elite athletes who participate in long-distance running, in gymnastics, and in ballet. History of restrictive eating behavior and of oligomenorrhea should be elicited in the PPSE by clinicians and during the season by coaches and parents. Physical stigmata of hypogonadism should be noted. These include lanugo hair, parotid swelling, and tooth enamel changes from vomiting, very low Body Mass Index (BMI), etc. If a female athlete presents with a stress fracture or with significant menstrual irregularities, this problem should be considered seriously.

    Another issue particular to female athletes is iron and calcium nutrition. These are mentioned above, but one cannot emphasize enough the importance of adequate intake of each of these minerals for the adolescent female athlete.

    A. Clinical pearls and pitfalls:
- Amenorrhea in a female athlete first should be evaluated with a sexual history and a pregnancy test.

IV.   **Injuries and trauma:**

    A. Epidemiology: The incidence of sports injuries in adolescents is reported differently from study to study. Therefore it is best to try to report injury data as case rates per 1,000 athlete-exposures, where an **athlete-exposure** is defined as **one athlete's participation in one practice or game in which there is a possibility of sustaining an athletic injury.** A "**reportable injury**" should include all of the following:
- injury occurs in a scheduled practice/game
- injury requires medical attention
- injury results in restriction or exclusion of the athlete from the remaining practice or competition or the following 1 or more days

    One study estimated that there are approximately 2.6 million emergency department visits per year for sports injuries for persons 5 to 24 years old. The peak incidence for these visits is between the ages of 5 and 14 years. One estimate states that 34% of school-aged adolescents and 38% of high school-aged adolescents will sustain a physical activity-related injury that will be treated by a doctor or nurse. That figure does not include injuries that are not seen by a clinician. The yearly cost of treating these injuries is estimated to be $1.8 billion.

Few studies report injury rates reliably across all sports. Of those that do, one examined rates in college athletes and found that female cross-country had the highest rate (15.9 in 1,000 athlete exposures) followed by wrestling (12.8), female soccer (12.6), football (12.2), and female gymnastics (10.2). NCAA injury reports state that spring football had the highest rates (9.8), followed by wrestling (9.6), female gymnastics (9.3), and female soccer (8.6). The NCAA reported that spring football had the highest rate of injuries requiring more than 7 days to return to activity: 43%, a rate of 4.1 in 1,000 athlete exposures. When injuries are classified by those requiring surgical intervention, female gymnastics leads the field.

In high school athletes 25% of all injuries occurred about the knee and ankle, and those joints were most commonly affected in collegiate sports injuries. It is worth noting that more experienced athletes suffer fewer injuries than do less experienced ones.

B. **Injuries in younger versus older adolescents:** Younger adolescents are more likely to have immature epiphyses than are older adolescents. When the epiphyses are immature, they are more subject to trauma, given that they may be weaker than the surrounding muscles and ligaments. Therefore younger adolescents may experience a fracture where an older adolescent would have a sprain. The best way to assess the possibility of one versus the other is to assess Tanner stage and to image the affected area when in doubt. There are "rules," for example the Ottawa Ankle Rules, to guide the clinician.

The Ottawa Ankle Rules direct the clinician to x-ray the ankle if there is perimalleolar pain and one or more of the following:
- younger than 13 years old
- older than 59 years old
- if the patient cannot bear weight on the affected foot
- bone tenderness at posterior edge or tip of either malleolus

C. **Types of injuries:**
1. **Sprains and strains** are the most common of sports injuries. A **sprain** is a stretching and/or tearing of a ligament, while a **strain** is a stretching and/or tearing of a musculo-tendinous unit. A **Grade 1** sprain is a stretching of a ligament without much tearing; a **Grade 2** sprain is stretching and tearing of some fibers; a **Grade 3** sprain has gross instability, marked swelling, and usually severe pain of the ligament. Grade 1 sprains are most common and have little swelling and no instability. Grade 2 sprains may have some laxity and more swelling. There also may be ecchymoses present due to subcutaneous bleeding from the tear. A Grade 3 sprain is a full tear of a ligament.

The treatment of sprains and strains is based on limiting movement of the affected area for the immediate post-traumatic period, limiting weight-bearing, and decreasing the swelling. This is best accomplished by **RICE, that is, rest, ice, compression, and elevation.** Rest should be mandatory for Grades 1 and 2 for the first 2 to 3 days. The concept of "relative rest" should be used, as in Table 28-7.

Cryotherapy is effective in reducing the recovery time for sprains and strains. Chipped ice is the most effective source of cold, and this can be applied in disposable plastic bags. Cold packs should be applied intermittently for the first 48 hours after injury for 20 to 30 minutes per session, three to four times a day.

Compression by an elastic bandage assists in minimizing the amount of edema. The bandage should be worn for a minimum of several days. This is important because edema can be deleterious for three reasons:
- it may act as an insulator, keeping cold therapy from reaching deeper tissues
- it can mechanically decrease range of motion, thereby decreasing the effectiveness of rehabilitation exercises
- it can keep ruptured ligament fibers apart, thereby promoting fibrous scarring rather than ligament-to-ligament regrowth

Elevation can reduce edema, especially if the injured part can be raised at least to the level of the heart. Finally, alleviation of pain is a consistent goal of treatment. Nonsteroidal anti-inflammatory drugs (NSAIDs) or acetaminophen are the analgesics of choice.

Rehabilitation is the second phase of treatment. This phase is designed to restore range of motion and strength in the injured part, and it should begin 48 to 72 hours after injury except in the most severe injuries. Early mobilization is

Table 28-7. Relative rest and return to play

Skeletally immature (prepubertal and early pubertal) adolescent athletes should not play or exercise if there is pain or swelling during or after activity.

• Discuss pain thresholds and pain-free movement as they apply to rehabilitation.
• Explain that normal activities are allowed if they cause no pain at any time within the next 24 hours.
• Address pain-free alternatives to maintain strength and improve flexibility.

When an athlete fails to improve in a rehabilitative program, one of the three explanations is likely:

• The diagnosis is incorrect.
• The patient is not compliant with the rehabilitation or is not practicing relative rest.
• The rehabilitation program is not appropriate.

In rare instances, a mature, older adolescent at an advanced level of competition may be permitted to practice and return to play during rehabilitation. This is an exception to the rule, and assumes that the following conditions have been met:

• The diagnosis is correct.
• The athlete has complied with an appropriate rehabilitative program, and shown progress toward recovery.
• A sports medicine or orthopedic specialist has been consulted, if possible.

From Hergenroeder AC. Acute shoulder, knee, and ankle injuries: part 2, rehabilitation. *Adolescent Health Update* 1996;8:1, with permission.

desirable whenever possible since it helps to strengthen ligaments by encouraging proper deposition of collagen and alignment of elastin fibers. It also improves the chances of successful functional rehabilitation. Aerobic exercises can be started and balance and proprioception should be worked on at this stage. Once swelling and pain have decreased, sports-specific drills are prescribed to build on the functional rehabilitation started in the last phase.

D. Injuries of specific sites:

    1. Ankle injuries: Ankle sprains are said to comprise 25% of all athletic injuries, and nearly 85% of all ankle injuries are sprains. Younger adolescents may injure the distal fibular physis instead of having a lateral ankle sprain, but more physically mature adolescents do suffer these sprains. Most commonly (80% of sprains), the lateral ligamentous complex is the site of the injury. The most severe type of lateral sprain is a "high" sprain involving the lateral ligaments and the interosseous membrane. Grade 3 and interosseous membrane injuries are more prone to chronic instability and osteochondral fractures. Medial ankle sprains are rarer and seem to be more unstable.

    Most ankle injuries occur when the foot is slightly plantarflexed and inverted with internal rotation, damaging the anterior talofibular ligament. The injury is usually abrupt. Common scenarios for this injury include a poorly executed cutting move enhanced by inadvertent foot fixation, landing on an irregular playing surface, and uncontrolled landing from jumps. This type of injury is most common in basketball.

    When the possibly sprained ankle is examined, the normal ankle should be examined first to ascertain the patient's normal anatomy (see Figure 28-2), and then the bony structures should be palpated for evidence of fracture. The ligaments should be palpated for point tenderness, and the stability of the ankle should be determined. This is done by stabilizing the leg and pulling the ankle forward with the foot in neutral position. A positive anterior drawer sign is produced when the talus slides forward more than 4 mm. An anterior talofibular ligament tear can result in an anterior drawer sign of 4 to 16 mm. Differentiation between Grades 2 and 3 sprains is important because surgical intervention probably will be needed in Grade 3, and the latter sprains should be referred to an orthopedist. Reasonable rehabilitation programs for Grade 1 and 2 sprains are described in Tables 28-7 and 28-8.

    2. Knee injuries: Injuries to knees occur very often in sports. In the United States, these injuries usually occur in football. During each week of the football season, it is estimated that 6,000 high school and college players injure their knees, and

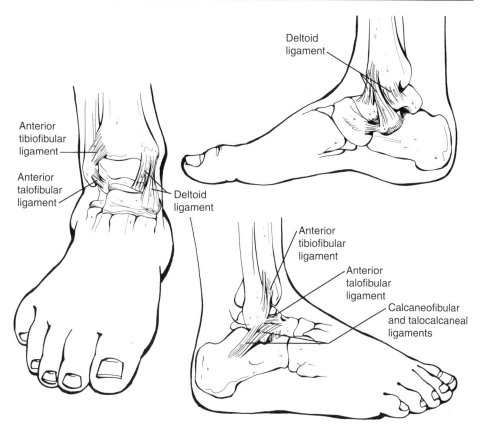

Figure 28-2. Ankle injury. Ankle ligaments. (From Harvey J. Ankle injuries in children and adolescents. *Pediatr Rev* 1981;2:217, with permission.)

Table 28-8. Ankle sprain rehabilitation: A walk/run program for transition from crutches to running

---

Patients recovering from ankle sprain can begin a rehabilitative walk/run program as soon as they can bear weight with minimal discomfort. Walk/run rehabilitation enables the athlete to build strength over a period of 2 to 3 weeks. Instruct the patient as follows:

- **Avoid bearing weight on the ankle until you can step down with minimal discomfort.**
- **Start a walking routine, beginning with 5 minutes per day, and increasing up to 20 minutes at a time, until you can walk for the full 20 minutes.**
- Begin to substitute 5 minutes of jogging for 4 minutes of walking at a time, until you are jogging for the full 20 minutes without pain.
- Begin straight-ahead sprints, then figure-eight sprints. Start with 20-yard figure-eights (e.g., figure-eights that are 20 yards long from top to bottom), and gradually restrict your running path to a 10-yard figure-eight.
- Once you are sprinting figure-eights without pain and swelling, it should be safe to return to play with ankle support.
- If pain or swelling occurs at any time, stop the regimen for a day or two, ice frequently, then resume your routine at the last comfortable level.

Athletes with Grade 3 sprains who follow this regimen (as tolerated) can expect to return to play in about 3 weeks.

From Hergenroeder AC. Acute shoulder, knee, and ankle injuries: part 2, rehabilitation. *Adolescent Health Update* 1996;8:1, with permission.

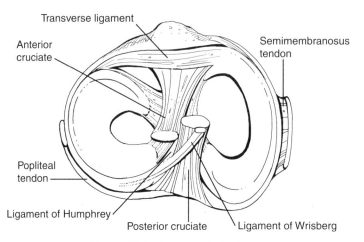

Transverse ligament

Anterior cruciate

Semimembranosus tendon

Popliteal tendon

Ligament of Humphrey

Posterior cruciate

Ligament of Wrisberg

Figure 28-3. Anatomy of the knee.

10% of these injuries require surgery. The most frequent injuries of significance are ligamentous injuries, meniscal (cartilage) injuries, and injuries involving the patellofemoral structures.

Ligamentous injuries occur when excessive rotatory, medial, or lateral force is applied to the knee. The most common ligaments affected are the medial collateral (MCLs) and anterior cruciate ligaments (ACLs) (see Figure 28-3).

The MCL is usually injured when there is a direct blow to the lateral aspect of the knee. The resulting medial stress can cause a first-, second-, or third-degree sprain. Because medial knee pain is felt at the time of injury, the knee may feel unstable when the player gets up and walks. Pain over the ligament or separation of the medial aspect of the joint when the abductor stress test is performed indicates a high probability that this structure is injured. A medial opening of more than 1 cm with the abductor stress test indicates possible damage to the anterior and posterior cruciate ligaments as well. If the knee is stable in extension but opens in 30 degrees of flexion, rotatory instability also should be considered (see Figure 28-4).

The **ACL** is the **site of the most serious injuries to the knee.** This injury usually occurs when the athlete is running and changes direction. A pop may be felt, and the player falls and is unable to continue playing. An anterior drawer test with the knee in 90 degrees of flexion and then with the knee in 15 degrees to 30 degrees of flexion—the Lachman test—should be performed as soon after the injury as possible because a bloody effusion will accumulate over the next 24 hours, making it difficult to assess the type or degree of injury. If the tibia moves anteriorly on the femur an anterior cruciate tear has occurred.

If the ACL is sprained but not ruptured, the athlete may be able to walk and even run but will hesitate to pivot, change directions, or jump. Tenderness on examination is usually due to concomitant injuries to the MCL and the meniscus. Radiographs are not routinely obtained. Magnetic resonance imaging (MRI) does not improve diagnosis for ACL injuries, but it is helpful for evaluating possible injuries to the menisci or articular cartilage. After initial treatment with RICE, referral to an orthopedic surgeon is advisable.

MCL sprains occur from a valgus stress to an extended knee. Frequently, a tearing sensation is reported followed by medial pain, swelling, stiffness, and instability with lateral movements. On physical examination there is tenderness over the MCL. If tenderness extends along the distal femoral physis, a physeal fracture may be present. The ACL should be assessed when there is injury to the MCL. Radiographs are only indicated if a fracture is suspected, and MRI is obtained when there is concern about meniscal injury.

Lateral collateral and posterior cruciate ligament injuries do occur, but they are much less common than the others mentioned above.

Injuries to **cartilage** in the knee may occur after a twisting impact, hyperflexion, or hyperextension. The medial meniscus is attached to the MCL and is frequently

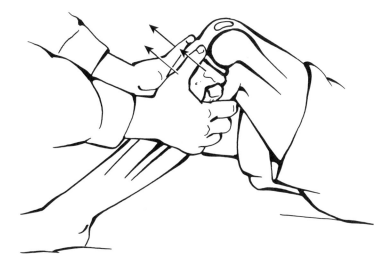

Figure 28-4. Anterior drawer test. The test may be falsely negative due to resistance from the meniscus or a tight hamstring.

damaged along with that ligament when a tackle hits the lateral side of the knee and produces external rotation of the tibia, stretching the MCL and rupturing the medial meniscus. The examiner finds tenderness over the medial or lateral joint line, pain at the medial or lateral joint line with hyperextension or hyperflexion of the knee, and pain with external tibial rotation when the knee is flexed to 90 degrees. Internal rotation produces pain with a lateral meniscus injury. Often, the examiner can feel a grating or crunch with fingers at the joint line when rotating the tibia in these maneuvers. If the primary care clinician feels that significant rupture has occurred, referral to an orthopedist should be made.

3. **Upper extremity injuries:** The most common upper arm injury that requires medical attention probably is the **dislocated shoulder.** This is usually anterior displacement of the humeral head with respect to the glenoid. This injury usually occurs as a result of a fall on the abducted or extended arm. Initial dislocations generate much pain and swelling and the appearance of a hollow on the lateral aspect of the shoulder as if the deltoid muscle has disappeared. The proximal arm and the clavicle should be palpated to detect a possible fracture, and a careful neurologic examination should be performed. Most commonly, decreased sensation in the axillary nerve distribution is found. Waiting to obtain radiographs should not delay treatment unnecessarily.

There are several methods for reducing the dislocation. Reduction should be attempted as soon as possible before significant muscle spasm has developed. It may take up to 5 minutes for steady traction to overcome the muscle spasm around the shoulder. There are several **reduction methods,** all of which can be effective. The Rockwood method can be seen in Figure 28-5.

If there is only one person to reduce the dislocation, a foot in the axilla can be used for countertraction. Once the dislocation is reduced, the arm is immobilized, usually with a sling and swath bandage, ice is applied on a regular schedule for 2 days, and analgesia is used. Once the arm can be carried out of the sling without pain, physical therapy is begun. Recurrent dislocations need surgical correction to stabilize the joint.

Acromioclavicular (AC) sprain or separation is a common injury that is due to falling on or a blow to the top of the shoulder. Severity of the pain varies with the degree of injury. The classification of this type of injury is based on radiographic appearance of the AC joint. The wider the separation of the clavicle from the acromion, the worse the sprain. With Grades IV, V, and VI, there is complete separation of the acromion from the clavicle. On examination, there is tenderness of the AC joint with a visible or palpable step off from the acromion to the clavicle

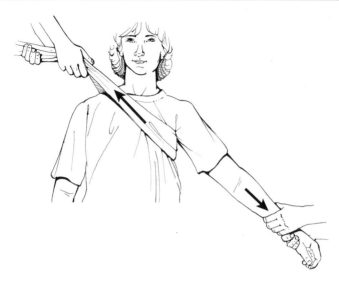

Figure 28-5. The Rockwood technique for closed reduction of left shoulder with traction against counteraction. (From Rockwood CA, Green DP, eds. *Fractures in adults.* vol. 1. 2nd ed. Philadelphia: JB Lippincott; 1984, with permission.)

in more serious cases. Grades I and II injuries can be treated with short periods of immobilization, physical therapy, and gradual return to activity. Grade III and higher should be referred to an orthopedist.

E. **Overuse disorders:**

   1. **Patellofemoral Disorders/Patellofemoral Pain Syndrome (PFPS):** The patella, the anterior shield of the knee joint and the fulcrum for quadriceps extension of the knee, can be injured in several ways. It can be fractured or, more commonly, it can be dislocated or subluxed. A twisting injury while the foot is planted and the knee is extended can cause the patella to sublux laterally or to dislocate. At the time of this type of injury, patients often report a ripping or tearing sensation in the knee. With either injury, an effusion occurs that makes the knee tense and tender. Gentle pressure on the medial patella laterally can produce pain and an apprehension sign. Patellar subluxation/dislocation can cause a shearing stress on the retropatellar cartilage, which can produce tenderness on the retropatellar surface, pain with patellar compression maneuvers, clicking, catching, or locking. Immediate treatment is RICE. Knee sleeves with lateral patellar buttresses can provide stability as activity is resumed.

   More commonly, knee pain is due to instability or anatomical abnormalities of the patellofemoral complex. This complex includes the patella, the quadriceps muscle, the patellar tendon, and its attachment on the tibial apophysis.

   PFPS is the term used when an athlete has a dull, aching knee without a clear etiology. The patient usually points to the patella as the source of pain, but the site of pain may be an immediately surrounding area as well. The onset is insidious, and the patient frequently says that the pain intensifies when sitting for a long time or when climbing down or up steps. Examination can reveal tenderness at the medial facet of the patella with or without patellar compression and pain with isometric quadriceps contraction with the knee in full extension. The clinician, when faced with a skeletally immature adolescent with knee pain of uncertain etiology, should always consider the possibility of slipped capital femoral epiphysis (SCFE) as the cause. This condition is more common in overweight, African American males. SCFE is a fracture of the femoral head that requires surgical intervention, as mentioned in Chapter 13, on musculoskeletal problems.

   Although there are several theories as to why PFPS happens, the prevailing view is that the cause is multifactorial with biomechanical problems, muscle dysfunction, and overuse. Poor tracking of the patella in the femur's patellar groove seems to be present, and this can be caused by problems with patella stabilizing mechanisms such as malalignment of the lower extremities, muscle weakness/ inflexibility, and foot problems, e.g., flat feet or high arches.

Treatment involves several methods such as analgesics, ice, relative rest, and quadriceps strengthening and stretching. We feel that **quadriceps strengthening is most important.** There are several exercises that can do this, such as partial knee bends with the patient sliding up and down with his or her back against a wall. Isometric quadriceps exercise work well. For these, the legs are fully extended and the patient is instructed to pull the kneecap toward the waist as hard as possible, hold it for 5 to 6 seconds, and then relax. Four contractions are done 15 to 20 times per day. Timing these episodes with other daily activities is a good way to have the teen remember to do them. The patient should be instructed to feel the correct muscle, that is, the vastus medialis, to be sure the contractions are working in the right place. Hamstring stretching and other stretches can be prescribed once strengthening is well underway.

2. **Osgood Schlatter disease:** Apophysitis of the anterior tibial tubercle, that is, **Osgood-Schlatter disease (OSD),** is another common cause of knee pain in the immature athlete. This problem presents with a report of anterior knee pain, with a swollen, tender anterior tibial tubercle, the site of insertion of the patellar tendon. Most probably, this is due to relative overuse of a strong muscle (quadriceps) on an immature bony union, that is, the physis, at that site. Treatment relies on rest, ice, and analgesics. Since the risk of rupture of the tendon from the tubercle is very slight, the athlete can be allowed to play if it is deemed important. Ice to the knee and analgesics before play and after play are helpful as are knee straps that can decrease the traction forces on the tubercle.

   PFPS and OSD are but two types of **overuse injuries** in adolescent athletes. Other types are spondylosis/spondylolisthesis, various stress fractures, iliotibial band syndrome, patellar tendonitis, rotator cuff tendonitis, little league elbow (extensor tendonitis), and medial tension/lateral compression syndrome. Conditions that must be referred to the orthopedic surgeon include:
   * anteromedial tibia fracture
   * femoral neck fracture
   * tarsal navicular fracture
   * proximal fifth metatarsal fracture (Jones' fracture)
   * spondylolisthesis

   The other conditions can be managed by the primary care clinician.

3. **Stress fractures:** Stress fractures occur due to overuse. The **most common** is the **proximal tibial stress fracture,** which accounts for more than 50% of these types of injuries. It usually occurs when there is an increase in the level of activity, particularly in high-impact sports such as gymnastics. They can happen in both legs simultaneously. This injury is **especially common in amenorrheic female athletes** who are suffering from the female athlete triad. Their osteoporosis puts them at much greater risk for this stress fracture. **Other stress fracture sites** can include the anterior mid-tibia, seen in jumping sports, and stress fracture of the proximal diaphysis of the fifth metatarsal and the femoral neck, seen in military recruits and runners. **A key emphasis** for athletes is that persistent pain for 3 weeks at a time is a sign that there may be a stress fracture.

4. **Shin splints:** Other stress injuries include the medial tibial stress syndrome, better known as **shin splints.** This is a periostitis that occurs along the posterior medial tibia due to repeated submaximal stress such as running or jumping, usually on a hard surface. Hyperpronation of the feet and genu varus are frequently found in athletes with shin splints. This problem usually occurs early in the season, is exacerbated by exercise, and if the athlete does not rest, the pain then persists when the athlete is at rest. Examination shows tenderness along the posteriomedial surface of the tibia at the junction of the middle and distal thirds of the bone. This is at the origin of the posterior tibial muscle. Radiographs can sometimes reveal small amounts of calcification in the area that hurts. **A bone scan frequently shows a long linear area of increased uptake along the medial tibial border dissimilar to the focal, dense uptake of a stress fracture.** Treatment involves rest, use of proper footwear, and gradual return to activity.

5. **Iliotibial band syndrome:** When the iliotibial band repeatedly rubs over the lateral femoral condyle as the knee flexes and extends, usually in runners, pain can occur. This is the **iliotibial band syndrome.** Factors that contribute to this problem include leg length discrepancy, excessive foot pronation, tibia varus, and

Table 28-9. Running injury analysis: Six "S's"

Shoes	Wear status or pattern
Surface	Uneven topography
Speed	Too much, too soon
Stretching	Flexibility
Strength	Muscle group imbalance
Structure	Anatomic malalignment

From Stanski CL. Overuse syndromes. In: Stanski CL, DeLee JL, Drez D Jr, eds. *Pediatric and adolescent sports medicine.* Philadelphia: W.B. Saunders; 1994:99, with permission.

scoliosis. Worn shoes, excessive running, running on banked surfaces (problem occurs in the down side leg), and extensive standing are additional factors. Pain is usually stinging and occurs over the lateral femoral epicondyle 3 cm proximal to the lateral joint line. Decelerating or running down a hill makes the pain worse. Treatment involves obtaining well-fitted shoes, iliotibial band stretching, rest, and slow return to activity. Other lower extremity overuse syndromes include **patellar tendonitis (jumper's knee)** and **osteitis pubis.** Table 28-9 shows how to analyze these conditions in runners, and Table 28-10 shows the routine treatment for overuse injuries.

6. **Compartment syndrome:** One more cause of lower extremity pain in an athlete is a **compartment syndrome.** There are four compartments in the lower leg: anterior, anterolateral, deep posterior, and superficial posterior. Characteristic symptoms include consistent onset of pain early in an activity, weakness of the involved muscles, tenseness on palpation, and paresthesias in the areas supplied by the nerves in that compartment. Symptoms occur only with exercise and are relieved shortly after the activity stops, especially if ice is applied. Rest and treatment for inflammation are usually sufficient, but occasionally the fascia of the compartment is tight, producing high intracompartmental pressure. This may require fasciotomy.

7. **Achilles tendonitis:** Achilles tendonitis also can occur. Pain emanates from the insertion of the Achilles tendon into the calcaneus. There is tenderness at that site along with crepitus and thickening of the tendon. Causes include a tight Achilles tendon, uphill running, and hyperpronation. Treatment consists of relative rest, ice, a temporary heel pad, stretching, and correction of the biomechanical problems. Included in the differential diagnosis for younger adolescents is **Sever Disease,** or traction apophysitis, at the insertion into the calcaneus. This is similar to OSD.

8. **Spondylolysis and spondylolisthesis:** These two conditions occur in the lumbar spine, usually at L5 or L5/S1. The cause is repeated hyperextension injuries to the pars intra-articularis. **A bony defect on one or both sides of a vertebra develops, and pain ensues. Spondylolysis** involves no forward displacement of one vertebrae over the inferior vertebrae. This forward displacement is **spondylolisthesis.** Those athletes who suffer from this most frequently are:
   • football linemen
   • basketball players
   • volleyball players
   • gymnasts
   • divers
   • tennis players

Table 28-10. Overuse treatment protocol

Identify risk factors
Modify offending factors
Institute pain control
Undertake progressive rehabilitation
Continue maintenance

Note: Phases are often concurrent (e.g., pain control and rehabilitation).
From Stanski CL. Overuse syndromes. In: Stanski CL, DeLee JL, Drez D Jr, eds. *Pediatric and adolescent sports medicine.* Philadelphia: W.B. Saunders; 1994:99, with permission.

The **typical history** is of insidious onset of back pain that begins around the time of the period of peak height velocity, that is, the growth spurt. The pain is exacerbated by strenuous exercise, twisting, and hyperextension when very active. The pain progresses and becomes more severe over time, occurring now with usual activities of daily living. Relief is obtained by rest. **Examination** shows lumbar spine and paraspinal tenderness. Relative hamstring tightness is present in 80% of the cases. Hyperextension of the lumbar spine while standing on the same side leg produces pain. There usually are no abnormal neurologic findings. Plain anterioposterior, lateral, and oblique **radiographs** show a fracture through the pars intraarticularis. When there is spondylolisthesis, the plain films also show the forward translocation of the superior vertebrae. A **bone scan** shows the pars intra-articularis lesion earlier. In spondylosis with or without spondylolisthesis, **treatment** is:

- restricting of activities
- immobilization for varying periods
- abdominal muscle strengthening
- pelvic tilts
- antilordotic and lower extremity flexibility exercises

When spondylolisthesis is greater than 50% of the lower vertebrae despite treatment or if pain persists, surgical intervention is advisable.

9. **Upper extremity overuse syndromes:** Upper extremity overuse syndromes include **extensor tendonitis of the elbow (tennis elbow), rotator cuff tendonitis/impingement syndrome,** and **medial tension/lateral compression syndrome of the arm. Tennis elbow,** or lateral epicondylitis, results from prolonged, repetitive use of the wrist extensors. This can occur with improper gripping of a tennis racquet. Lateral elbow pain occurs, and it is made worse by use of the wrist extensors. In addition to the usual overuse syndrome treatment, these athletes can benefit from adjustments in their racquet grip size, string tension, and backhand technique.

Rotator cuff tendonitis is common in young athletes involved in throwing, swimming, and racquet sports. These athletes present with aching pain of the shoulder made worse with overhead activity. They may have a history of shoulder dislocations. When combined with instability, there could be an **impingement syndrome. Swimmer's shoulder** is impingement of the structures in the subacromial space in swimmers. This presents with pain in the anterior and lateral aspects of the shoulder. The tendons of the supraspinatus and biceps muscles are most often involved. The problem is due to faulty stroke mechanics with either faulty technique or deterioration of technique as muscles fatigue. Relative rest, ice, and NSAIDs are used for the immediate symptoms followed by a rehabilitation period in which proper stroke mechanics are stressed.

Elbow problems are frequently encountered, particularly in pitchers. Most of these can be grouped under the term **little league elbow,** a group of disorders that result from repetitive valgus stress of the elbow as a consequence of throwing. These occur due to repetitive pitching and poor throwing mechanics by an immature arm. Valgus forces applied to the elbow create compression forces across the lateral structures (radial head and capitellum) and tension on the medial structures (medial epicondyle, MCLs). In immature arms, the tension forces can create chronic medial epicondylitis with overgrowth of the medial epicondyle from chronic traction. Occasionally an avulsion fracture of the medial epicondyle can occur. **Medial elbow pain is the most common presenting symptom.** Tenderness is elicited over the medial epicondyle. Rest, ice, and NSAIDs are the treatments of choice. The immature athlete should be instructed not to throw curve balls, not to throw with a sidearm motion, and not to pitch an excessive number of innings. These precautions will prevent the problem from recurring.

Common hand and wrist injuries include **finger sprains and dislocations.** Sprains should be evaluated for degree of injury. If they are not third degree, splinting for 7 to 10 days with ice and analgesia as necessary is usually sufficient. Dislocations of fingers should be assessed on the scene for functional impairment and for direction of the dislocation. The direction in which the finger is dislocated can suggest possible ligament tears. Once evaluation is complete, simple longitudinal traction with or without nerve block can reduce the dislocation. Splinting for a week or two and rehabilitation to return to previous flexibility is all that usually is required.

A **fracture of the navicular bone** in the wrist easily can be overlooked because the symptoms can mimic a sprain and radiographs may be negative for several days after the injury. Untreated navicular fractures can lead to nonunion and may require secondary surgery. This type of fracture is associated with tenderness in the anatomic snuffbox and pain at extremes of wrist motion. Standard treatment consists of using a long thumb spica cast for as long as 4 months until the fracture has healed.

F. **Concussion:** Concussion is the most common head injury in sports. The word "concussion" comes from the Latin *concussus* meaning "to shake violently." One **definition of concussion** is any alteration in cerebral function caused by a direct or indirect (rotation) force transmitted to the head resulting in one or more of the following acute signs or symptoms:
    *   a brief loss of consciousness
    *   light-headedness
    *   vertigo
    *   cognitive and memory dysfunction
    *   tinnitus
    *   blurred vision
    *   difficulty concentrating
    *   amnesia
    *   headache
    *   nausea
    *   vomiting
    *   photophobia
    *   balance disturbance

    Delayed signs and symptoms can include (and these may last a long time):
    *   sleep irregularities
    *   fatigue
    *   personality changes
    *   inability to perform usual daily activities
    *   depression
    *   lethargy

    Headache and confusion are the most typical initial symptoms.

    The First International Conference on Concussion in Sport in 2001 defined concussion as **"a complex pathophysiologic process affecting the brain, induced by traumatic biomechanical forces."** The statement went on to say:
    *   Concussion may be caused by a direct blow to the head, neck or face, or elsewhere on the body with an "impulsive" force transmitted to the head.
    *   Concussion typically results in rapid onset of short-lived impairment of neurologic function that resolves spontaneously.
    *   Concussion may result in neuropathologic changes, but the acute clinical symptoms largely reflect a functional disturbance rather than structural injury.
    *   Concussion results in a graded set of clinical syndromes that may or may not involve loss of consciousness (LOC). Resolution of the clinical and cognitive symptoms typically follows a sequential course.
    *   Concussion is typically associated with grossly normal structural imaging.

    Most concussions fit within the category of mild traumatic brain injuries (MLBI). An MLBI is defined as **head trauma with LOC, if any, lasting fewer than 30 minutes and post-traumatic amnesia lasting fewer than 24 hours.** A concussion can be considered simply as a bruise or contusion of the brain. Most frequently there is no significant cell loss or permanent damage, but occasionally there is. A small number of athletes who suffer a concussion take longer than the typical 5 to 10 days to recover. A few recover more slowly, and a small number suffer permanent brain damage.

    1. **Epidemiology/concussion facts:**
        *   20% of high school football players report having had at least one concussion.
        *   There are more than 300,000 concussions per year in the US.
        *   High school athletes are poor historians for reporting their own concussions.
        *   Fewer than 10% of concussions involve LOC.
        *   Once a concussion has occurred, a player is four to six times as likely to suffer a second concussion.
    2. **Outcomes:** It is very difficult to predict with any certainty what will happen with any one athlete who suffers a concussion of any sort. First, one may be unaware of any previous traumatic brain injury (TBI) that this athlete has suffered. To date, the **only prospectively validated signs and symptoms** are: amnesia,

LOC, headache, dizziness, blurred vision, attention deficit, and nausea. Attention deficit and amnesia are probably the most important of these. The delayed symptoms listed above have been jointly termed the **postconcussion syndrome.**

3. **Grading of concussion:** Most grading systems use LOC as the important marker for injury severity. LOC of less than a minute has been found not to reflect either severity or neuropsychological performance or to be associated with abnormal brain imaging. Orientation to person, place, and time has not been found to be very predictive of sequelae, but amnesia of recent events does seem to correlate to some degree. Duration of post-traumatic amnesia (PTA) does correlate with outcome of severe brain injury. With less severe injury, PTA is not so helpful. Retrograde amnesia, that is, loss of memory of events prior to brain injury, is also not a predictor of concussion severity or outcome. There is some evidence that there may be genetic predisposition to negative effects of repetitive TBI, that is, the punch-drunk syndrome.

   Second impact syndrome (SIS) occurs when an athlete sustains a second head trauma before the original concussion has healed. This leads to:
   - acute loss of autoregulation of cerebral blood flow with possible brain herniation
   - diffuse cerebral swelling

   SIS is predominately seen in children and adolescents. This is a rare but devastating condition that should be avoided at all costs.

   So what **guidelines** can clinicians use when confronted with the patient who has had a concussion? Unfortunately there are more than one set of guidelines. However, those issued by the most reputable organizations/experts agree on the following:
   - An athlete with a concussion should be removed from competition immediately and should be evaluated.
   - No athlete experiencing signs or symptoms at rest OR with exertion should be allowed back into play.
   - If signs or symptoms of concussion last longer than 15 minutes or there is PTA, the athlete should not compete for at least a week.
   - If there has been LOC, the athlete should be out of action for at least a week and must be asymptomatic at rest and with exertion to be allowed to resume activity.

   If you are the clinician at the event and a concussion occurs, the victim should have cervical spine stabilization, be removed from the contest, LOC should be ascertained, and evaluation on the sideline should be done. The athlete should be allowed to **return to play** in 15 minutes if there has been no LOC, symptoms have resolved, and the examination is normal. If there has been more than one light concussion, the athlete should be held out for a week. If symptoms last longer than 15 minutes, there should be no activity for a week. More than one of these types should keep the athlete out at least 2 weeks. If there is brief LOC (just a few seconds), the athlete should be held out for a week; if LOC lasts longer than a few seconds, the athlete should be held out 2 weeks; and if there have been more than one of the latter concussive episodes, the athlete should be held out at least a month.

   When should one recommend **neuropsychologic testing**? The answer is unclear, but this type of testing is recommended when post-concussion symptoms have lasted longer than a couple weeks, for the athlete who has had multiple concussions, as part of a head injury evaluation protocol, etc. One limitation of this type of testing is that there rarely is a baseline test available to which one can compare post-concussion findings.

   Urgent referral is needed when there is:
   - obvious skull fracture
   - deterioration of mental status following trauma
   - LOC greater than 5 minutes
   - confusion greater than 30 minutes
   - focal neurologic signs
   - seizure activity
   - the injured is a child
   - persistent nausea/vomiting or headache
   - inability to properly assess the injured
   - inadequate postinjury supervision
   - comorbid high risk medical conditions
   - high-risk method of injury (possibly penetrating, etc.)

One should use imaging if the injury has been severe, if symptoms progress, or for medicolegal reasons. MRI is developing rapidly, and there are new techniques that may be more helpful.

4. **Prevention:** Proper headgear, mouth guards, and proper technique all can lessen the chances of concussion. However, as long as there are sports in which any impact to or by the head is unavoidable, some concussions will be inevitable.

G. **Clinical pearls and pitfalls:**
   - Don't forget the Ottawa Ankle Rules for evaluating the young adolescent with an apparent ankle sprain.
   - RICE is the first treatment for almost any limb injury.
   - It is unusual for an adolescent athlete to suffer rotator cuff injury without having a shoulder dislocation.
   - Back pain in adolescents is not necessary analogous to that in adults. Consider the possibility of spondylolysis and spondylolisthesis.
   - When an adolescent has a concussion, err on the side of caution when considering return to action.
   - Adolescents with concussions may have post-concussive symptoms for several weeks afterwards; therefore, parents and schools should be counseled to expect possible cognitive problems.

BIBLIOGRAPHY

For the clinician

Adirim TA, Cheng TL. Overview of injuries in the young athlete. *Sports Med* 2003;33:75–81.

American Academy of Pediatrics, et al. *Preparticipation physical evluation*, 3rd ed. Columbus, OH: PSM, 2004.

American College of Sports Medicine, American Dietetic Association, Dietitians of Canada. Nutrition and athletic performance. *Med Sci Sports Exerc* 2000;32:2130–2145.

Bernstein J, ed. *Musculoskeletal medicine*. Rosemont, IL: American Academy of Orthopedic Surgeons, 2003.

Birrer RB, O'Connor FG. *Sports Medicine for the primary care physician*, 3rd ed. Boca Raton, FL: CRC Press, 2004.

Demorest RA, Bernhardt DT, Best TM, Landry GL. Pediatric residency education: Is sports medicine getting its fair share? *Pediatr* 2005;115:28–33.

Koester M, Mangus BC. Heads up for soccer injuries! What you need to know. *Contemp Pediatr* 2005;22:75–88.

Luckstead E. Pediatric sports medicine, parts I & II. *Pediatr Clin N Am* 2002;49:3–4.

McCrory P, Johnston K, Meeuwisse W, et al. Summary and agreement statement of the 2nd international conference on concussion in sport, Prague 2004. *Br J Sports Med* 2005;39:196–204.

Metzl JD. Preparticipation examination of the adolescent athlete. Parts 1 and 2. *Pediatr Rev* 2001;22:199–204, 227–239.

Putukian M, Madden CC, Mellion MB. *Sports medicine secrets*, 3rd ed. Philadelphia: Hanley & Belfus, 2002.

For patients and parents

Jennings DS. *Play hard, eat right: A parent's guide to sports nutrition for children*. Minneapolis, MN: American Dietetic Association, Chronimed, 1995.

Metzl JD, Shookhoff C. *The young athlete: A sports doctor's complete guide for parents*. New York: Time Warner, 2002.

WEB SITES

www.amateur.sports.com
www.teengrowth.com

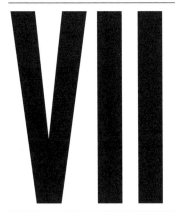

Common Legal Issues

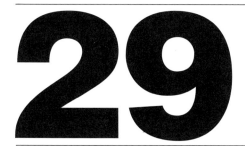

Legal Issues

I. **Description of legal issues:** Many physicians express hesitation or outright fear about the legal implications of treating adolescents. New Federal regulations have only made the situation more confusing. In a recent American Academy of Pediatrics' Periodic Survey of its membership, nearly two-thirds of the pediatricians surveyed said that the foremost obstacle to providing better adolescent health care was the lack of clearly defined state statutes on confidentiality, consent, and other legal issues.

Because state laws vary, this chapter will only feature general principles and guidelines. Specific situations regarding patients may require the services of a knowledgeable attorney.

II. **Maintaining appropriate standards of care:**

A. **Seeing teenage patients should not involve major legal risks unless physicians fail to observe a few basic rules:**

- Know your state law.
- Do not be hesitant about consulting with local attorneys and hospital attorneys when questions arise.
- **Document** information carefully and thoroughly in the patient's chart, with the exception of sensitive, confidential material. In malpractice cases, if something is not documented in the chart, it never happened!
- Never hesitate to obtain a second opinion if needed.
- When in doubt, **always do what is best for the patient.** Such a strategy is unlikely to result in legal difficulties because courts typically view this as the physician's appropriate role in treating patients.

B. **Confidentiality:**

1. **Relevance of confidentiality in treatment:** No single legal issue affects teenagers and clinicians more than the issue of confidentiality. It is paramount in the minds of adolescent patients, even if they are being seen for a trivial illness, and should be dealt with in a forthright fashion. In one survey of nearly 1,300 ninth to twelfth graders, 58% reported having health concerns that they wanted to keep private from their parents, and 25% said that they would forego health care in certain situations if it meant that their parents might find out. Nearly half would not go to their regular physician for pregnancy, acquired immunodeficiency syndrome (AIDS), or substance abuse concerns (Tables 29-1 and 29-2). Two-thirds had concerns about the privacy of a school-based clinic. Although physicians' assurances of confidentiality do increase teens' willingness to disclose sensitive information, **studies show that nearly half of primary care physicians fail to discuss the issue.**

Table 29-1. Perceptions of adolescents regarding health care

Survey item	Yes	No
"There are some health concerns that I would not want my parents to know."	58%	39%
"There are some health concerns that I would not want my friends and classmates to know."	69%	28%
"Would you ever not go for health care because your parents might find out?"	25%	73%
"Since becoming a teenager, when you have gone to get health care, has anyone talked to you about privacy?"	44%	54%

Adapted from Cheng TL, Savageau JA, Sattler AL, et al. Confidentiality in health care: a survey of knowledge, perceptions, and attitudes among high school students. *JAMA* 1993;269:1404.

Table 29-2. Attitudes of adolescents regarding confidentiality

Health issue	Yes, should keep private	No, should not keep private
Having sex	78%	19%
Homosexuality	57%	38%
Pregnancy	56%	40%
Sexually transmitted disease	46%	50%
AIDS/HIV infection	35%	60%
Alcohol/drug problem	35%	62%
Plan to run away	32%	66%
Sexual abuse	20%	77%
Physical abuse	18%	78%
Plan to commit suicide	15%	82%

AIDS, acquired immunodeficiency syndrome; HIV, human immunodeficiency virus. Adapted from Cheng TL, Savageau JA, Sattler AL, et al. Confidentiality in health care: a survey of knowledge, perceptions, and attitudes among high school students. *JAMA* 1993;269:1404.

2. **Numerous laws, public health regulations, and court decisions now recognize an adolescent's right to confidential health care:**
   - Nearly every state has consent laws that address the confidentiality of minors.
   - The US Supreme Court has ruled that a constitutional right of privacy exists and that it includes minors and their decisions regarding reproduction.
   - Lower courts have struck down laws that mandated parental consent for minors to obtain contraceptives.
   - In clinics that receive federal Title X (Family Planning) funds, minors are legally entitled to family planning services without parental consent.
   - The new Health Insurance Portability and Accountability Act (HIPAA) of 1996 states that minors have a right to confidential treatment if they can legally consent to health care or receive it without parental consent (or when a parent has agreed to confidentiality between the minor and the clinician). Whether parents can *access* this information depends upon "state or other applicable law."
3. **The physician's role in maintaining and breaching confidentiality:** Confidentiality is not absolute. Nor does it mean that clinicians should not encourage their patients to discuss sensitive medical problems with their parents. Clinicians need to be aware of the instances in which confidentiality must be breached:
   - If a teenager is in imminent danger of harming himself or herself *or* harming someone else. These two examples represent the only time where a clinician may have to phone the police (rather than a state agency).
   - If a teenager has been sexually or physically abused.
   - If a teenager has a reportable sexually transmitted disease (STD). Teens need to be informed that they are being reported to the public health department.
   - If there is a specific state statute that mandates disclosure.

   The easiest way to establish these principles in a clinical practice is to do it expectantly. When a child reaches age 10 to 12 years, a form letter can be sent to parents explaining that with the 12th birthday, confidential health care will be provided (see Figure 29-1). If established in advance, the concept of confidentiality does not alarm many parents. If the principle has to be raised first in the middle of an emergency (e.g., parents finding a teenager's packet of birth control pills), angry and threatening phone calls may ensue.

   Sometimes parents are delighted to have practitioners who will see their teenagers for confidential health care, but office personnel and administrators can undermine the clinicians' efforts (Table 29-3). A 2003 survey of 434 Washington, D.C., practices found that many offices do not offer confidential services to teenagers (especially pediatricians' offices) and that there was often considerable disagreement between what teens were told about confidentiality by physicians and by their office staff.

   In practice, the term "confidentiality" may actually never be used. Instead, clinicians can explain to teenagers: "Whatever you tell me will stay in this room, between us, unless you tell me that you are going to harm yourself or harm

Sample office policy

Consent and Confidentiality

Confidentiality is an ethical and legal concept that keeps a practitioner from revealing details about a patient without the consent of that individual. As physicians, we have obligations both to our adolescent patients and to their parents, and sometimes there can be a conflict regarding issues of confidentiality. Normally, the privilege of confidentiality belongs to the patient, but for minors (in Ohio, someone under the age of 18 years), the privilege of confidentiality belongs to the legal guardian. In Ohio, the law states that minors can consent to be tested and treated for venereal diseases, tested for the HIV (AIDS) virus, and for diagnosis and treatment of any condition believed to be related to alcohol or any other drug of abuse.

In many surveys of adolescents, a lack of confidentiality has been shown to be a significant barrier to seeking appropriate health care for situations that could have an important impact on their well-being. The American Academy of Pediatrics, American Medical Association, and the Society for Adolescent Medicine have all stated that adolescents should be entitled to confidentiality if they have the mental ability (capacity) to consent to treatment. Early in the adolescent years (age 10-14), parents should discuss health issues and access to medical care with their child, specifically, discussion regarding which conditions the adolescent could independently seek medical care in a confidential manner. Issues regarding sexuality, drugs including alcohol, smoking, depression, and weight control should be included since these are often mentioned as important issues to adolescents. These discussions should ideally include financial arrangements for the medical services. In other words, will the adolescent be expected to pay for the confidential care, or is there agreement for the parent to pay without asking the diagnosis? A "contract" can be established with the doctor defining the extent and limits of confidentiality that the adolescent may expect. The parents can help decide which services they would agree to have provided on a confidential basis.

There will be times when revelation of confidential information is necessary. These situations include physical or sexual abuse, or a situation in which there is a clear risk of harm to the adolescent or others. An attempt to gain the adolescent's agreement to reveal confidential information will usually be tried, but the need to protect the adolescent (and sometimes others) will be the deciding factor.

If you have any questions regarding the issues of consent and confidentiality, you are encouraged to bring this up during any office visit, or call by phone. Please discuss this important issue early in the adolescent years before a crisis situation arises, or management of important health problems is delayed due to reluctance to seek the appropriate care because of fear of lack of confidentiality.

Contract

As the guardian(s) for _____ , I (we) agree to allow him/her to consent to confidential care
 (patient)
from _____ , providing that Dr. _____
 (name of practitioner)
feels that _____ understands both the medical condition and the treatment being
 (name of patient)
offered. Exceptions to this agreement are _____
 (none or list exceptions)
I (we) also agree to financial responsibility without diagnosis disclosure.

Signed _____ (parent(s))   Signed _____ (adolescent)

I agree to provide confidential care to _____ . Exceptions to this confidential care would include
suspicion of abuse or if I have good reason to believe that there is imminent risk of personal harm to my patient or to others.

Signed _____ (practitioner)

Figure 29-1. Sample office policy for dealing with confidentiality. (From Falik HL. Beginning at ages 10–13, adolescent needs private time with physician. *AAP News*, April 2000:12, with permission.)

Table 29-3. Confidentiality in office practice

1. Routinely see teenagers alone, at least for part of each office visit, to periodically assess high-risk health behaviors.
2. Incorporate counseling on high-risk behaviors into routine visits.
3. Routinely discuss confidential health care with the adolescent and the possibility of parental involvement.
4. Establish office procedures that will:
   - Enable adolescents to make their own appointments
   - Provide for alternative billing and payment options
   - Ensure that office personnel will be sensitive to adolescents
   - Protect confidential information in the patient's chart, including the possibility of keeping dual records

Adapted from Hofmann AD. Consent and confidentiality: Critical issues in providing contraceptive care. In: Strasburger VC. *Basic adolescent gynecology: An office guide.* Baltimore, MD: Urban & Schwarzenberg, 1990.

Table 29-4. Recommendations for confidential health care for adolescents

- Confidential health care for adolescents is essential.
- Physicians should allow emancipated and mature minors to consent to their own treatment.
- Physicians should involve parents in the medical care of their adolescents when it is in the best interests of the adolescent. When it is not, parental consent or notification should not be a barrier to care.
- Physicians should discuss their policies about confidentiality with parents and the adolescent patient.
- State and county medical societies need to play a more active role in supporting confidential health care services for teenagers. They also need to work to eliminate laws that restrict such care.
- Medical schools and residency training programs need to educate students and residents about issues surrounding consent and confidential health care.
- Health care financers need to develop systems that preserve confidentiality for adolescents.

Adapted from Council on Scientific Affairs, American Medical Association. Confidential health services for adolescents. *JAMA* 1993;269:1420.

someone else." Clinicians can also use a variety of office practice techniques to ensure that confidential care will be provided and respected (Table 29-4).

C. **Emergency care:** All clinicians need to understand that emergency care can be provided to teenagers (or younger children, for that matter) without parental consent. Parents should be contacted as soon as reasonably possible. How an emergency is defined may vary from state to state, but in general, courts have given a wide latitude to health professionals, especially if efforts to contact parents have been documented. Emergencies may not necessarily be life-threatening; a teen with a broken leg or a bleeding laceration would almost certainly qualify under anyone's standards. Thirty-seven states have specific laws regarding emergencies; in the other 13, providing emergency care is still appropriate. In general, **when clinicians act in the *patient's* best interests, the law is not likely to object.**

D. **Issues of consent:** Every state has enacted statutes to address the issue of minors consenting for their own health care. Among the categories are:

1. **Emancipated minor:** At least 34 states have enacted legislation that allows emancipated minors to consent for their own health care. In the remaining states, the traditional criteria would usually apply—teens who are married, in the military, or living apart from their parents and self-supporting. Minors who are pregnant (35 states) or are parents (18 states) are often considered emancipated as well.

2. **Living apart from parents:** Even if they are not self-supporting, minors in 22 states can consent for their own treatment if they are living apart from their parents.

3. **Mature minors:** The mature minor doctrine has evolved in common law (which is case law). The doctrine generally means that a physician can provide medical care to a minor when that care is mainstream, not high risk, non-negligent, and the minor is capable of providing an informed consent. Often, this is a teenager who is near the age of consent (age 16, in many states). Only a few states have actually enacted specific legislation to accept this doctrine, but it has been acknowledged in Supreme Court rulings and many lower court cases. Currently, there is no help from case law with the issue of treating *immature* minors who may want or need confidential health care.

4. **General medical care:** At least 14 states allow for certain minors to consent for general medical care, depending on their age, high school graduation, or maturity.

5. **Incarcerated youth:** A few states specifically allow incarcerated youth to consent for their own health care.

6. **Sexually transmitted diseases:** *Every* state allows minors to consent for evaluation and treatment of STDs. This is an example of how concern for public health trumps parents' right to know about their teens.

7. **Treatment for drugs or alcohol:** Again, nearly every state has passed laws enabling minors to consent for treatment related to the use of alcohol or other drugs. Only two states do not have specific legislation.

8. **Outpatient mental health services:** At least 31 states have laws that allow minors to consent for some outpatient mental health services. Some limitations regarding number of visits, which health professionals are involved, and the type of care may apply. Special laws regarding confidentiality apply to programs that meet the federal definition of an alcohol or drug treatment program.
9. **Pregnant minor:** At least 35 states have legislation that allows minors who are pregnant to consent for their pregnancy-related care.
10. **Contraception:** At least 34 states have specific statutes which allow minors to consent for contraceptive care. A few of the statutes include qualifiers, including that the minor would suffer harm without the services being provided. If no state law exists, a minor may still be able to consent, based on the mature minor doctrine, the constitutional right to privacy, if the services are being provided at a federal Title X site, or if the minor receives Medicaid. In fact, **no physician has ever been successfully sued for providing contraception to a minor, nor is there a record of any such suits even being brought.** (This may be because a lawsuit is a matter of public record, and no parent wants to advertise that his or her teenage daughter has been seeking contraceptives.) Finally, there are several Supreme Court and lower court decisions that support provision of contraceptives to a minor:
    a. Minors have the same constitutional right to privacy as adults.
    b. Minors have a specific right of access to contraceptives, which falls within the right of privacy.
    c. Lower courts have struck down statutes that attempted to require parental consent for the provision of contraception. This is particularly fortunate, given a 2002 study of more than 1,100 teenage girls seeking contraceptive services at Planned Parenthoods in Wisconsin, which found that nearly 60% would stop using medical services if their parents had to be notified.

    The issue of what to do with immature minors is usually moot: When 12- and 13-year-old girls are sexually active, it is most often in the context of severe family dysfunction and adolescent acting-out behavior, and often the mother is suspicious. But, theoretically, if a 13 year old came by herself to see a clinician for contraception, that in itself would constitute evidence for applying the mature minor doctrine. Furthermore, few could question that providing contraception for her would be in her best interests (rather than becoming pregnant), unless she had a severe underlying medical disorder.
11. **Abortion:** This is the single most contentious issue in the interface between adolescent medicine and the law. Currently, about two-thirds of states have enacted legislation mandating either parental notification or parental consent before an adolescent can undergo an abortion. According to the Supreme Court, parental consent laws *must* include a judicial bypass route whereby a superior court judge can rule that a minor is mature and able to make her own abortion decision. Parental notification laws may include bypass procedures as well. Statutes sometimes include exceptions for emergencies, incest, or abuse, or provisions for other adults to consent or receive notification. In the other third of states, teens may obtain abortions on their own consent, either by statute or according to the mature minor doctrine or the constitutional right to privacy.

III. **Clinical pearls and pitfalls:**
- Always do what is best for the patient. Although there is no guarantee that you will not be sued (anyone can sue anybody for anything), you will at least be on solid footing.
- In an emergency, treat the patient first, then worry about the legalities.
- Providing contraception to a mature minor is legal.
- Providing contraception to an immature minor is an issue that does not usually arise, since very young teens who are sexually active are often brought in by their suspicious parents.
- No physician has ever been successfully sued for prescribing birth control to a minor.
- Find a good local lawyer whom you can consult with frequently, as needed.

BIBLIOGRAPHY

Akinbami LJ, Gandhi H, Cheng TL. Availability of adolescent health services and confidentiality in primary care practices. *Pediatrics* 2003;111:394–401.

Boonstra H, Nash E. Minors and the right to consent to health care. *Guttmacher Rep Public Policy* 2000;3:4–8. Available online at http://www.guttmacher.org/pubs/ib_minors_00.html.

Brindis CD, English A. Measuring public costs associated with loss of confidentiality for adolescents seeking confidential reproductive health care. *Arch Pediatr Adolesc Med* 2004;158:1182–1183.

English A, Ford CA. The HIPAA Privacy Rule and adolescents: Legal questions and clinical challenges. *Perspectives on Sexual and Reproductive Health* 2004;36:80–86.

English A, Kenney KE. *State minor consent laws: A summary*, 2nd ed. Chapel Hill, NC: Center for Adolescent Health & the Law, 2003.

English A, Simmons PS. Legal issues in reproductive health care for adolescents. *Adolesc Med State Art Rev* 1999;10:181–194.

Ford CA, English A. Limiting confidentiality of adolescent health services: what are the risks? *JAMA* 2002;288:752–753.

Reddy DM, Fleming R, Swain C. Effect of mandatory parental notification on adolescent girls' use of sexual health services. *JAMA* 2002;288:710–714.

Society for Adolescent Medicine. Position paper on confidential health care for adolescents. *J Adolesc Health* 2004;35:160–167.

WEB SITES

www.guttmacher.org   The Alan Guttmacher Institute. Information on state policies related to adolescents' access to reproductive health services

www.cahl.org   The Center for Adolescent Health & the Law. Many resource materials on a variety of legal issues relating to adolescents

www.healthprivacy.org   Health Privacy Project, Institute for Health Care Research and Policy, Georgetown University. Information on federal and state laws related to health privacy, including the HIPAA Privacy Rule

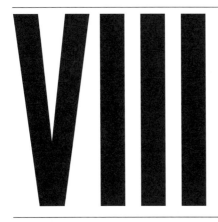

Appendix: Commonly Prescribed Medications

The following medications, formulations, and recommended doses are provided as a convenient reference for the user. Comprehensive prescribing recommendations including indications, contraindications, precautions, adverse effects, dose adjustment, drug monitoring, and drug interactions are not included. The user should refer to product labeling for complete prescribing information or if any questions arise with regard to the information presented here.

All doses provided are for adults and/or fully mature adolescents. Consult product labeling for pediatric dosing.

Adjust doses as needed for patients with renal or hepatic impairment.

Many of the medications listed *have not been approved by the US Food and Drug Administration for use in persons under 18 years of age.* The prescribing clinician should use his or her own clinical judgment when deciding whether the potential benefits of using these medications outweigh the associated risks.

All formulations are for oral administration unless otherwise specified.

Product	How supplied	Dosing	Comments
Acetaminophen	325 mg, 500 mg tabs	650–1000 mg q 4 h	Sedating. High abuse potential. Avoid with acute or severe asthma.
Acetaminophen + codeine (Tylenol with codeine No. 3)	300 mg + 30 mg tabs	1–2 tabs q 4 h as needed	
Acyclovir (Zovirax)	200 mg caps; 400 mg, 800 mg tabs	See Chapter 27 for dosing in genital herpes infections	For Acne: See Chapter 3. Reduce dosing frequency if irritation develops. Avoid sunlight and/or use sunscreen.
Adapalene (Differin)	0.1% cream (15 g, 45 g), gel (15 g, 45 g), solution (30 mL), pledgets (no. 60)	Apply small amount to clean, dry skin once daily at bedtime	See Chapter 7.
Albuterol (several)	0.63 mg/3 mL, 1.25 mg/3 mL solution for inhalation 90 μg/inhalation MDI	One vial by nebulizer up to 3–4 times/d over 5–15 min, or 2 inhalations q 4–6 h as needed; 2 inhalations 15 min before exercise for exercise-induced symptoms	
Alprazolam (Xanax)	0.25 mg, 0.5 mg, 1 mg, 2 mg tabs	Initial: 0.25–0.5 mg TID; may increase at 3–4 d intervals to max 4 mg/d	See Chapter 23. Benzodiazepines may be habit-forming. Monitor blood counts and hepatic function. Pregnancy category D.
Aluminum chloride hexahydrate (Drysol)	20% solution (35 mL)	Apply once daily at bedtime, wash next morning Maintenance: apply once–twice weekly	High toxicity in overdose. Monitor levels, EKG, liver enzymes. Monitor closely for suicidality.
Amitriptyline (Elavil)	10 mg, 25 mg, 50 mg, 75 mg, 100 mg, 150 mg tabs	Initial: 25–50 mg once daily at bedtime; may increase gradually to max 150 mg/d Migraine prophylaxis: 10–25 mg once daily at bedtime; may increase q 2–4 wk to 100 mg daily if needed	
Amlodipine (Norvasc)	2.5 mg, 5 mg, 10 mg tabs	2.5–5 mg daily	
Amoxicillin (several)	250 mg, 500 mg caps 500 mg, 875 mg tabs	Mild–moderate ENT, skin, GU: 500 mg q 12 h or 250 mg q 8 h Lower respiratory, severe ENT, skin, GU: 875 mg q 12 h or 500 mg q 8 h Uncomplicated gonorrhea: 3 g once	Not recommended first line for gonococcal infections; may be used in pregnancy. Dosing and duration of therapy varies depending on condition being treated.
Amoxicillin + clavulanate (Augmentin)	250 mg/125 mg tabs 500 mg/125 mg tabs 875 mg/125 mg tabs	Usually: 500 mg/125 mg q 12 h or 250 mg/125 mg q 8 h Respiratory or more severe infections: 875 mg/125 mg q 12 h or 500 mg/125 mg q 8 h	Take with meals. Additional formulations available. Dosing and duration of therapy varies depending on condition being treated.

Drug	Formulation	Dosing	Comments
Amphetamine/ Dextroamphetamine mixed salts (Adderall, Adderall XR)	5 mg, 7.5 mg, 10 mg, 12.5 mg, 15 mg, 20 mg, 30 mg tabs 5 mg, 10 mg, 15 mg, 20 mg, 25 mg, 30 mg extended-release (XR) tabs	5–60 mg/d ÷ BID–TID; XR: 20 mg once daily; may increase weekly in 5 mg/d increments to max 40 mg/d	See Chapter 19. High abuse potential.
Ampicillin (Principen)	250 mg, 500 mg caps	250–500 mg QID Uncomplicated gonorrhea: 3.5 g with 1 g probenecid once	Dosing and duration of therapy varies depending on condition being treated. Monitor blood, renal, hepatic function in long-term use.
Atomoxetine (Strattera)	10 mg, 18 mg, 25 mg, 40 mg, 60 mg caps	Initial: 40 mg/d; may increase after at least 3 d to 80 mg/d, then after 2–4 wk may increase to max 100 mg/d as a single dose or divided BID	See Chapter 19. Monitor for hepatic dysfunction.
Azelaic acid (Azelex)	20% cream (30 g, 50 g)	Apply small amount to clean, dry skin BID.	See Chapter 8. Reduce dosing frequency if irritation develops.
Azithromycin (Zithromax)	250 mg, 500 mg, 600 mg tabs 1 g packet (for resuspension)	500 mg once daily × 1 d, then 250 mg once daily × 4 d Uncomplicated chlamydia or nongonococcal urethritis: 1 g once Uncomplicated gonorrhea: 2 g once	Dosing and duration of therapy varies depending on condition being treated. Use 1 g packet for single dose therapy only.
Beclomethasone dipropionate (Qvar)	40 µg/inhalation, 80 µg/ oral inhalation MDI	Initial: 40–80 µg BID Rinse mouth after use. Max. 320 µg BID	See Chapter 7.
Benzoyl peroxide (several)	5%, 10% gel (60 g) 2.5%, 5%, 10% aqueous-base gel (60 g); others	Apply small amount to clean, dry skin BID	See Chapter 8. Reduce dosing frequency if irritation develops. May bleach hair or fabrics.
Budesonide—inhaled (Pulmicort Turbohaler)	200 µg/inhalation powder for inhalation with MDI	1–2 inhalations BID Max 4 inhalations BID	See Chapter 7. Rinse mouth after use.
Budesonide—nasal (Rhinocort aqua)	32 µg/spray (8.6 g = 120 sprays)	1–4 sprays to each nostril once daily	Direct spray laterally, away from nasal septum. Use regularly for maximal effect. Consider initiating use 1 wk prior to exposure to known allergen or 2–4 wk prior to anticipated start of pollen season.

(continued)

Product	How supplied	Dosing	Comments
Bupropion HCl (Wellbutrin SR, Wellbutrin XL, Zyban)	100 mg, 150 mg, 200 mg sustained release (SR) tabs 150 mg, 300 mg extended-release (XL) tabs	SR: Initial: 150 mg once daily in AM for 3 d; if tolerated increase to 150 mg BID XL: Initial: 150 mg once daily in AM for 3 d; if tolerated increase to 300 mg once daily Smoking cessation: See Chapter 21	See Chapter 23. Monitor closely for suicidality.
Buspirone HCl (BuSpar)	5 mg, 10 mg, 15 mg, 30 mg tabs	Initial: 7.5 mg BID; may increase every 2–3 d by 5 mg/d up to 30 mg BID	See Chapter 23.
Captopril (Capoten)	12.5 mg, 25 mg, 50 mg, 100 mg tabs	Initial: 12.5 mg BID; may titrate up to 50 mg TID after 1–2 wk to max 450 mg/d	Take 1 h before meals; may add diuretic before increasing to max dose; pregnancy category D (2nd/3rd trimesters).
Carbamazepine (Tegretol, Carbatrol)	200 mg, 300 mg extended-release caps; others	Initial: 200 mg BID; increase weekly as needed to max 1.2 g/d Migraine prophylaxis: 10 mg/kg/d ÷ BID, may titrate up to 30 mg/kg/d	Monitor levels, hepatic, ophthalmic, renal function; may reduce effectiveness of hormonal contraceptives via increased metabolism of estrogen. Pregnancy category D.
Cefdinir (Omnicef)	300 mg caps	300 mg q 12 h or 600 mg q 24 h	Dosing and duration of therapy varies depending on condition being treated.
Cefoxitin Sodium (Mefoxin)	1 g/50 mL, 2 g/50 mL, 1 g/vial, 2 g/vial for injection	Pelvic inflammatory disease: Inpatient: 2 g IV q 6 h [with doxycycline 100 mg BID × 14 d] Outpatient: 2 g IM once [with probenecid 1 g orally and doxycycline 100 mg orally BID × 14 d]	PID: See Chapter 27. Dosing and duration of therapy varies depending on condition being treated.
Cefpodoxime proxetil (Vantin)	100 mg, 200 mg tabs	100–400 mg q 12 h Uncomplicated gonorrhea: 200 mg once	Dosing and duration of therapy varies depending on condition being treated. Take with food.
Cefprozil (Cefzil)	250 mg, 500 mg tabs	250–500 mg q 12 h or 500 mg once daily	Dosing and duration of therapy varies depending on condition being treated.
Ceftibuten HCl (Cedax)	400 mg caps	400 mg once daily	Dosing and duration of therapy varies depending on condition being treated.

Drug	Forms/Strengths	Dosing	Comments
Ceftriaxone Sodium (Rocephin)	250 mg, 500 mg, 1 g, 2 g powder for reconstitution and injection	Uncomplicated gonorrhea: 125 mg IM once Pelvic inflammatory disease (outpatient treatment): 250 mg IM once [with doxycycline 100 mg BID × 14 d].	PID: See Chapter 27. Dosing and duration of therapy varies depending on condition being treated.
Cefuroxime (Ceftin)	250 mg, 500 mg tabs	Usual: 250–500 mg BID Uncomplicated gonorrhea: 1 g once	Dosing and duration of therapy varies depending on condition being treated. Not recommended first line for gonococcal infections; may be used in pregnancy.
Cephalexin (Keflex)	250 mg, 500 mg caps	250 mg q 6 h or 500 mg q 12 h	Dosing and duration of therapy varies depending on condition being treated.
Cetirizine HCl (Zyrtec)	5 mg, 10 mg tabs	5–10 mg q d	
Cetirizine HCl + pseudoephedrine HCl (Zyrtec-D 12 hour)	Cetirizine HCl 5 mg, pseudoephedrine HCl 120 mg tabs	1 tab twice daily	
Chlorpheniramine maleate (Chlor-trimeton)	4 mg tabs	4 mg q 4–6 h	Not recommended for use during pregnancy.
Ciclopirox (Loprox)	0.77% cream, gel	Apply BID up to 4 wk	
Cimetidine (Tagamet)	300 mg, 400 mg, 800 mg tabs	GERD: 200–400 mg BID for max 12 wk	
Ciprofloxacin (Cipro)	100 mg, 250 mg, 500 mg, 750 mg tabs	500–750 mg q 12 h Uncomplicated cystitis (E. coli or S. saprophyticus): 250 mg q 12 h × 3 d Other UTI: 250–500 mg q 12 h × 7–14 d Uncomplicated gonorrhea: 500 mg once	Not generally recommended for persons <18 yr of age; see literature for recommendations on use in this age group. Quinolones should not be used to treat gonococcal infections acquired in the Pacific Islands, Hawaii, or California.
Ciprofloxacin + hydrocortisone (Cipro HC Otic)	Ciprofloxacin 0.2%, hydrocortisone 1%, otic suspension (10 mL)	3 drops in affected ear BID × 7 d	Do not use with perforated tympanic membrane.
Citalopram (Celexa)	10 mg, 20 mg, 40 mg tabs	Initial: 20 mg once daily; after 1 wk may increase to 40 mg daily; max 60 mg daily	See Chapter 23. Monitor closely for suicidality.
Clarithromycin (Biaxin, Biaxin XL)	250 mg, 500 mg tabs; 500 mg extended-release tabs (XL)	250–500 mg BID XL: 1 g once daily	Dosing and duration of therapy varies depending on condition being treated.

(continued)

Product	How supplied	Dosing	Comments
Clindamycin (Cleocin)	75 mg, 150 mg, 300 mg caps	150–450 mg q 6 h	Dosing and duration of therapy varies depending on condition being treated. Take with full glass of water.
	1% solution (30 mL, 60 mL), pledgets (no. 60), lotion (60 mL), gel (30 g, 60 g) 1% gel (42 g, 77 g) 1% solution (30 mL, 60 mL) 1%, with benzoyl peroxide 5% gel (45 g) 1%, with benzoyl peroxide 5% gel (25 g, 50 g)	Acne: Apply small amount to clean, dry skin once–twice daily.	Reduce dosing frequency if irritation develops. Benzoyl peroxide products may bleach hair or fabric. Generic solution significantly less expensive.
	2% vaginal cream	Bacterial vaginosis: 1 applicator-full intravaginally at bedtime × 3–7 d	
Clonazepam (Klonopin, Klonopin wafers)	0.5 mg, 1 mg, 2 mg tabs 0.125 mg, 0.25 mg, 0.5 mg, 1 mg, 2 mg orally-disintegrating tabs	Initial: 0.25 mg BID; may increase to 0.5 mg BID after 3 d, then by 0.125–0.25 mg BID every 3 d as needed to max dose of 4 mg/d.	Benzodiazepines may be habit-forming; monitor blood counts and hepatic function. Pregnancy category D.
Clotrimazole (Lotrimin AF, Gyne-Lotrimin)	1% cream, solution, lotion 100 mg, 500 mg vaginal tablet 1%, 2% vaginal cream	Apply BID up to 4 wk Vulvovaginal candidiasis: See Chapter 27.	
Cromolyn sodium—inhaled (Intal)	0.8 mg/inhalation MDI	Two inhalations QID Two inhalations 10–60 min before exercise	
Cromolyn sodium—nasal (Nasalcrom)	5.2 mg/spray (13 mL, 26 mL)	1 spray to each nostril q 4–6 h	Direct spray laterally, away from nasal septum. Use regularly for maximal effect. Consider initiating use 1 wk prior to exposure to known allergen or 2–4 wk prior to anticipated start of pollen season.
Cyclobenzaprine HCl (Flexeril)	5 mg, 10 mg tabs	5 mg TID; may increase to 10 mg TID, max 2–3 wk	Sedating.
Cyproheptadine (Periactin)	4 mg tabs	Migraine prophylaxis: 4 mg nightly-TID; may titrate up to max 32 mg/d ÷ TID	Stimulates appetite.

Drug	Preparations	Dosing	Notes
Desloratadine (Clarinex)	5 mg tabs; 5 mg orally-disintegrating tablet	5 mg once daily	
Desmopressin acetate (DDAVP)	0.1 mg, 0.2 mg tabs; 10 μg/spray, nasal spray (5 mL = 50 sprays)	Primary nocturnal enuresis: Initial: 0.2 mg oral (or 10–40 μg intranasal) once daily at bedtime; max 0.6 mg oral	When using nasal spray, give half of total dose in each nostril.
Dexmethylphenidate (Focalin)	2.5 mg, 5 mg, 10 mg tabs	Initial: 2.5 mg BID; may increase at 1 wk intervals to max 20 mg/d	See Chapter 19. When switching from racemic methylphenidate, use half of the dose.
Dextroamphetamine sulfate (Dexedrine, Dexedrine spansules)	5 mg, 10 mg tabs; 5 mg, 10 mg, 15 mg sustained release capsules (spansules)	Initial: 5 mg once–twice daily; may increase weekly by 5 mg/d to max 40 mg/d; spansules are given once daily	See Chapter 19. High abuse potential.
Diazepam (Valium)	2 mg, 5 mg, 10 mg tabs	2–10 mg BID–QID as needed	Sedating. Potentially addictive. Avoid abrupt cessation. Prolonged use not recommended. Not recommended for use in pregnancy.
Dicyclomine HCl (Bentyl)	10 mg caps, 20 mg tabs	Initial: 20 mg QID; increase to 40 mg QID if tolerated	Anticholinergic. Discontinue if not effective in 2 wk or not tolerated. Antacids may inhibit absorption.
Dihydroergotamine mesylate (with caffeine) (Migranal)	4 mg/mL intranasal preparation; 0.5 mg/spray	One spray to each nostril; may repeat in 15 min (max 3 mg/24 h)	Pregnancy category X. Avoid macrolides. Not for use in persons <18 yr old.
Diphenhydramine (Benadryl)	25 mg tabs	25–50 mg q 4–6 h; max 300 mg/d	
Divalproex sodium (Depakote, Depakote ER)	125 mg, 250mg, 500 mg tabs; 250 mg, 500 mg extended release tabs	Initial: 500–750 mg daily ÷ BID–TID; max 60 mg/kg/d Migraine prophylaxis: 250 mg BID–TID ER: 500 mg q d	Monitor levels, hepatic function, platelets. Pregnancy category D.
Docosanol (Abreva)	10% cream (2g)	Apply 5 times daily until healed	Begin treatment at earliest sign or symptom of outbreak. Avoid eyes and mucous membranes.
Docusate sodium (Colace)	50 mg, 100 mg	50–300 mg daily	
Doxycycline (several)	50 mg, 75 mg, 100 mg caps; 100 mg tabs	100–200 mg daily or ÷ BID	Dosing and duration of therapy varies depending on condition being treated. For Acne: See Chapter 8. Take with fluids. Avoid sun/UV light. Monitor blood, renal, and hepatic function with long-term use. Pregnancy category D.

(continued)

Product	How supplied	Dosing	Comments
Econazole nitrate (Spectazole)	1% cream (15 g, 30 g, 85 g)	Tinea pedis, t. cruris, t. versicolor, t. corporis: apply once daily × 2 wk Cutaneous candidiasis: apply bid × 2 wk	May treat t. pedis × 4 wk. Avoid in 1st trimester pregnancy.
Eflornithine HCl (Vaniqua)	13.9% cream (30 g)	Apply bid at least 8 h apart; do not wash area for at least 4 h	
Enalapril (Vasotec)	2.5 mg, 5 mg, 10 mg, 20 mg tabs	Initial: 2.5–5 mg daily; may titrate up to 10–40 mg/d in one or two divided doses	Pregnancy category D (2nd/3rd trimesters).
Epinastine HCl (Elestat)	0.05% solution (5 mL)	1 drop to each eye bid	Remove contact lenses; may reinsert in 10 min if eye is not red.
Erythromycin base (several)	250 mg, 333 mg, 500 mg tabs	250 mg q 6 h, 333 mg q 8 h, or 500 mg q 12 h Max 4g/d; max 1g/d for twice daily dosing	Dosing and duration of therapy varies depending on condition being treated.
Erythromycin ethylsuccinate (EES)	400 mg tabs	1.6 g/d divided bid–qid; max 4 g/d; max 1 g/d for twice daily dosing	Dosing and duration of therapy varies depending on condition being treated.
Erythromycin (topical)	2% saturated swab (no. 60) 2% solution (60 mL) 2% gel (30 g, 60 g) 3%, with benzoyl peroxide 5% gel (46.6 g)	Apply small amount to clean, dry skin twice daily	Generic solution significantly less expensive. Reduce dosing frequency if irritation develops. Benzoyl peroxide products may bleach hair or fabrics.
Escitalopram (Lexapro)	5 mg, 10 mg, 20 mg tabs	Initial: 10 mg daily; may increase to 20 mg daily after 1 wk	See Chapter 23. Monitor closely for suicidality.
Esomeprazole (Nexium)	20 mg, 40 mg caps	GERD: 20 mg once daily for 4 wk; may continue 4 more weeks	Take 1 h before food.
Famciclovir (Famvir)	125 mg, 250 mg, 500 mg tabs	See Chapter 27 for dosing in genital herpes infections	Not recommended for persons <18 yr old.
Famotidine (Pepcid)	20 mg, 40 mg tabs	GERD: 20 mg BID up to 6 wk	
Fexofenadine HCl (Allegra)	30 mg, 60 mg, 180 mg tabs	60 mg BID or 180 mg q d	
Fexofenadine HCl + pseudoephedrine HCl (Allegra-D)	Fexofenadine HCl 60 mg, pseudoephedrine HCl 120 mg tabs	1 tab twice daily	Do not take with food.
Fluconazole (Diflucan)	50 mg, 100 mg, 150 mg, 200 mg tabs	Vulvovaginal candidiasis: 150 mg once	Dosing and duration of therapy varies depending on condition being treated.

Drug	Formulation	Dosing	Comments
Flunisolide (AeroBid)	250 µg/inhalation MDI	Two inhalations BID	See Chapter 7. Rinse mouth after use.
Fluoxetine (Prozac)	10 mg, 20 mg, 40 mg caps	Initial: 10 mg daily; may increase to 20 mg daily after 2 wk; max 60 mg/d	See Chapter 23. Monitor closely for suicidality.
Fluticasone propionate—inhaled (Flovent)	44 µg/inhalation, 110 µg/inhalation, 220 µg/inhalation MDI	Two inhalations BID Initial use: 88 µg BID	See Chapter 7. Rinse mouth after use.
Fluticasone propionate—nasal (Flonase)	50 µg/spray (16 g = 120 sprays)	Initial: 2 sprays to each nostril once daily or 1 spray to each nostril twice daily. Maintenance: may reduce to 1 spray to each nostril once daily	Direct spray laterally, away from nasal septum. Use regularly for maximal effect. Consider initiating use 1 wk prior to exposure to known allergen or 2–4 wk prior to anticipated start of pollen season.
Fluticasone propionate + salmeterol–inhaled (Advair Diskus)	100 µg/50 µg per inhalation 250 µg/50 µg per inhalation 500 µg/50 µg per inhalation	One inhalation bid Begin with lowest dose; increase as needed every 2 wk	Do not initiate in significantly worsening or acutely deteriorating asthma.
Formoterol fumarate (Foradil)	12 µg/inhalation dry powder in capsules for inhalation, with inhaler device	One inhalation q 12 h One inhalation at least 15 min before exercise	Do not initiate in significantly worsening or acutely deteriorating asthma.
Gabapentin (Neurontin)	100 mg, 300 mg, 400 mg caps 600 mg, 800 mg tabs	300 mg TID; may increase to max 1800 mg/d ÷ TID Migraine prophylaxis: 300 mg TID, may titrate up to 800 mg TID	
Hydrochlorothiazide (Hydrodiuril, Microzide)	12.5 mg, 25 mg, 50 mg tabs	Initial: 25 mg once daily; may titrate up to max 50 mg/d in single or divided doses	
Hydrocodone + acetaminophen (Vicodin)	5 mg + 500 mg tabs	1–2 tabs q 4–6 h as needed Max 8 tabs/24 h	Sedating. High abuse potential. Avoid with acute or severe asthma.
Hydrocodone bitartrate + homatropine methylbromide (Hycodan)	5 mg + 1.5 mg tabs 5 mg + 1.5 mg per 5 mL syrup	1 tab (or 5 mL) q 4–6 h as needed	Sedating. Risk of abuse.
Hydromorphone (Dilaudid)	2 mg, 4 mg, 8 mg tabs	2–4 mg q 4–6 h as needed	Sedating. High abuse potential. Avoid with acute or severe asthma.
Hydroxyzine HCl (Atarax)	10 mg, 25 mg, 50 mg, 100 mg tabs	25 mg TID–QID	Do not use during early pregnancy.
Ibuprofen	200 mg, 400 mg, 600 mg tabs	400–800 mg q 6–8 h	
Imiquimod (Aldara)	5% cream (12 single-use packets)	Apply and rub in before bed q Monday, Wednesday, Friday; wash off 6–10 h later; use up to 16 wk	See Chapter 27.

(continued)

Product	How supplied	Dosing	Comments
Ipratropium bromide (Atrovent)	18 µg/inhalation MDI	Two inhalations qid	See Chapter 7.
Iron (Feosol)	65 mg (as sulfate 200 mg) tabs 50 mg (as carbonyl) caplets	One tab or caplet daily	Take with orange juice (vitamin C) to enhance absorption.
Iron (polysaccharide-iron complex) (Niferex)	50 mg tabs 150 mg caps	1–2 tabs BID 1–2 caps daily	Take with orange juice (Vitamin C) to enhance absorption.
Iron gluconate (Fergon)	27 mg (as gluconate 240 mg) tabs	One tab daily	Take with orange juice (vitamin C) to enhance absorption.
Isometheptene + dichloralphenazone + acetaminophen (Midrin)	65 mg/100 mg/325 mg caps	2 caps, followed by 1 cap q 1 h until relief (max 5/24 h)	Frequent use may lead to analgesic withdrawal headache. Dichloralphenazone may be sedating and addictive.
Isoniazid (INH)	300 mg tabs	Tuberculosis prophylaxis: 300 mg once daily	
Itraconazole (Sporanox)	100 mg caps	Onychomycosis: Toenail: 200 mg once daily for 12 wk. Fingernail: 200 mg BID for 1 wk, then 3 wk off, then 200 mg BID for 1 more wk	Dosing and duration of therapy varies depending on condition being treated. Monitor hepatic function.
Ketoconazole (Nizoral)	2% cream (15 g, 30 g, 60 g)	Tinea cruris, t. versicolor, t. corporis: apply daily for at least 2 wk Tinea pedis: treat 6 wk	Dosing and duration of therapy varies depending on condition being treated. Monitor hepatic function before and during prolonged therapy
	200 mg tabs	Initial: 200 mg daily Max. 400 mg daily	
Ketorolac tromethamine (Toradol)	10 mg tabs	20 mg, followed by 10 mg q 6 h (max 40 mg/24 h)	Maximum use 5 d.
Labetalol (Trandate)	100 mg, 200 mg, 300 mg tabs	Initial: 100 mg BID; may increase at 2–3 d intervals in increments of 100 mg twice daily	
Lactulose (Kristalose)	10 g, 20 g packets, crystals for reconstitution (no. 30)	10–20 g dissolved in 4 oz water daily	May be antagonized by nonabsorbable antacids.
Lamotrigine (Lamictal)	25 mg, 100 mg, 150 mg, 200 mg	Migraine prophylaxis: 50 mg q d, may titrate up to 50 mg BID	Stevens-Johnson syndrome, blood dyscrasias.
Lansoprazole (Prevacid)	15 mg, 30 mg caps	GERD: 15 mg once daily up to 8 wk	Take before eating. May give with antacids.

Drug	Forms	Dosing	Notes
Lansoprazole + amoxicillin + clarithromycin (Prevpac)	Lansoprazole 30 mg (2 caps), amoxicillin 500 mg (4 caps), clarithromycin 500 mg (2 tabs)	Lansoprazole 30 mg + amoxicillin 1 g + clarithromycin 500 mg, all BID × 10–14 d	For eradication of *H. pylori*.
Levofloxacin (Levaquin)	250 mg, 500 mg, 750 mg tabs	500–750 mg once daily Uncomplicated UTI: 250 mg q d × 3 d Uncomplicated gonorrhea: 250 mg once Pelvic inflammatory disease: 500 mg once daily × 14 d	Take with full glass of water. Not generally recommended for persons <18 yr of age; see literature for recommendations on use in this age group. Quinolones should not be used to treat gonococcal infections acquired in the Pacific Islands, Hawaii, or California. Avoid sun/UV light.
Levothyroxine sodium (Levoxyl, Synthroid)	25 µg, 50 µg, 75 µg, 88 µg, 100 µg, 112 µg, 125 µg, 137 µg, 150 µg, 150 µg, 175 µg, 200 µg, 300 µg tabs	1.7 µg/kg once daily; titrate as needed in increments of 12.5–25 µg/d every 4–6 wk	Take in AM on an empty stomach.
Loperamide HCl (Imodium)	2 mg caps	Initial: 4 mg, then 2 mg after each loose stool; max 16 mg/d	Stop after 48 h if ineffective.
Loratadine (Alavert, Claritin)	10 mg tabs; 10 mg orally-disintegrating tablet	10 mg q d	
Loratadine + pseudoephedrine sulfate (Claritin-D 24 h)	Loratadine 10 mg, pseudoephedrine sulfate 240 mg tabs	1 tab daily	
Loratadine + pseudoephedrine sulfate (Alavert D-12, Claritin-D 12 hour)	Loratadine 5 mg, pseudoephedrine sulfate 120 mg tabs	1 tab q 12 h	
Lorazepam (Ativan)	0.5 mg, 1 mg, 2 mg tabs	Initial: 2–3 mg daily ÷ BID–TID; may titrate to 1–10 mg daily	Consider 0.5 mg test dose to evaluate for behavioral activation. Pregnancy category D.
Losartan (Cozaar)	25 mg, 50 mg, 100 mg tabs	Initial: 0.7 mg/kg (max 50 mg) once daily; may titrate up to max 100 mg/d	Pregnancy category D (2nd/3rd trimesters).
Mebendazole (Vermox)	100 mg chew tabs	Enterobiasis (pinworm): 100 mg once	Dosing and duration of therapy varies depending on condition being treated.
Meclizine HCl (Antivert)	12.5 mg, 25 mg, 50 mg tabs	Motion sickness: 12.5–50 mg 1 h prior to departure, repeat q 24 h as needed Vertigo: 25–100 mg/d in divided doses	

(continued)

Product	How supplied	Dosing	Comments
Mefenamic acid (Ponstel)	250 mg tabs	500 mg once, then 250 mg q 6 hr	Primarily used for dysmenorrhea, up to 3 d.
Meperidine (Demerol)	50 mg, 100 mg tabs	50–100 mg q 4 h as needed	Sedating. High abuse potential.
Metformin HCl (Glucophage)	500 mg, 850 mg, 1 g tabs	Initial: 500 mg BID; may increase by 500 mg/d at 1-wk intervals Max 2 g/d	
Methocarbamol (Robaxin)	500 mg, 750 mg tabs	Initial: 750 mg–1.5 g QID × 2–3 d, then decrease to max of 4 g daily ÷ TID − QID	Sedating. Not recommended for persons <16 yr old.
Methylphenidate (Concerta, Metadate CD, Metadate ER, Ritalin, Ritalin LA, Ritalin SR)	18 mg, 27 mg, 36 mg, 54 mg extended-release tabs (Concerta); 10 mg, 20 mg, 30 mg (Metadate CD) 10 mg, 20 mg (Metadate ER) 5 mg, 10 mg, 20 mg (Ritalin) 10 mg, 20 mg, 30 mg, 40 mg extended-release caps (Ritalin LA) 20 mg sustained-release tab (Ritalin SR)	Initial: 18 mg once daily; may increase weekly to max 54 mg/d Initial: 20 mg daily; may increase weekly to max 60 mg/d as a single dose (CD) or divided (ER) Initial: 10 mg daily; may increase weekly to max 60 mg/d as a single dose (LA) or divided (regular or SR)	See Chapter 19. Monitor growth, blood pressure. High abuse potential for some formulations (especially immediate release).
Methylprednisolone (Medrol)	2 mg, 4 mg, 8 mg, 16 mg, 32 mg tabs	Initial: 4–48 mg daily, depending on condition being treated Asthma: See Chapter 7	Medrol Dosepak contains 21 4-mg tablets administered with a tapered regimen.
Metronidazole (Flagyl, MetroGel-Vaginal)	250 mg, 500 mg tabs 375 mg caps 0.75% vaginal gel	Bacterial vaginosis: 500 mg orally BID × 7 d or 1 applicator intravaginally q d × 5 d Trichomoniasis: 2 g orally once or 500 mg orally BID × 7 d	Dosing and duration of therapy varies depending on condition being treated.
Miconazole nitrate (Lotrimin AF, Monistat)	2% spray powder, spray liquid 2% powder 100 mg, 200 mg, 1200 mg vaginal suppository 2% vaginal cream	Apply BID × 2–4 wk Vulvovaginal candidiasis: see Chapter 27	

Medication	How Supplied	Dose	Notes
Minocycline (Minocin)	50 mg, 100 mg caps	200 mg once then 100 mg q 12 h	Dosing and duration of therapy varies depending on condition being treated. For Acne: See Chapter 8. Swallow whole; take on empty stomach with fluids. Monitor blood, renal, hepatic function in long-term use. Pregnancy category D. Avoid sunlight and/or use sunscreen.
Mometasone furoate (Nasonex)	50 µg/spray (17 g = 120 sprays)	2 sprays to each nostril once daily	Direct spray laterally, away from nasal septum. Use regularly for maximal effect. Consider initiating use 1 wk prior to exposure to known allergen or 2–4 wk prior to anticipated start of pollen season.
Montelukast (Singulair)	10 mg tabs	10 mg once daily in the PM	See Chapter 7.
Naphazoline HCl + pheniramine maleate (Naphcon A)	Naphazoline HCl 0.025%, pheniramine maleate 0.3% solution (15 mL)	1–2 drops to affected eye(s) up to QID daily	Remove contact lenses.
Naproxen (Naprosyn)	250 mg, 375 mg, 500 mg tabs	250–500 mg q 8–12 h	
Naproxen sodium (Aleve, Anaprox, Anaprox DS)	220 mg, 275 mg, 550 mg tabs	220–550 mg q 8–12 h	
Naratriptan (Amerge)	1 mg, 2.5 mg tabs	1–2.5 mg; may repeat once in 4 h (max 5 mg/24 h)	
Nedocromil sodium (Alocril)	2% solution (5 mL)	1–2 drops to each eye bid	Remove contact lenses during therapy.
Nicotine replacement (Nicoderm CQ, Nicorette, Nicotrol)	7 mg/24 h, 14 mg/24 h, 21 mg/24 h transdermal patch 5 mg/16 h, 10 mg/16 h, 15 mg/16 h transdermal patch 2 mg, 4 mg chewing gum 0.5 mg/spray nasal spray 10 mg (4 mg delivered) inhalation device	See Chapter 21 for recommended use	Concurrent smoking or use of other nicotine products is prohibited. Pregnancy category D.
Nifedipine (Adalat CC, Procardia XL)	30 mg, 60 mg, 90 mg extended release tabs	Initial: 30 mg once daily; may titrate up to max 120 mg/d over 7–14 d	

(continued)

Product	How supplied	Dosing	Comments
Nitrofurantoin (Macrobid, Macrodantin)	25 mg, 50 mg, 100 mg caps 100 mg macrocrystal caps	50–100 mg q 6 h macrocrystal: 100 mg BID	Dosing and duration of therapy varies depending on condition being treated. Take with food.
Nizatidine (Axid)	150 mg, 300 mg caps	GERD: 150 mg BID up to 12 wk	
Norethindrone acetate (Aygestin)	5 mg tabs	2.5–10 mg daily for 5–10 d during 2nd half of theoretical menstrual cycle after estrogens if needed	Pregnancy category X.
Ofloxacin (Floxin, Floxin Otic)	200 mg, 300 mg, 400 mg tabs	Respiratory: 400 mg q 12 h Uncomplicated gonorrhea: 400 mg once Pelvic inflammatory disease: 400 mg q 12 h × 14 d Uncomplicated cystitis (E. coli, K. pneumoniae): 200 mg q 12 h × 3 d Other uncomplicated UTI: 200 mg q 12 h × 7 d	Take on empty stomach with full glass of water. Not generally recommended for persons <18 yr of age; see literature for recommendations on use in this age group. Quinolones should not be used to treat gonococcal infections acquired in the Pacific Islands, Hawaii, or California. Avoid sun/UV light.
	0.3% otic solution (5 mL, 10 mL; singles 0.25 mL [5 drops] - no. 20)	Otitis externa: 10 drops in affected ear once daily × 7 d Chronic suppurative otitis media: 10 drops BID × 14 d	May use with perforated tympanic membrane and/or tympanostomy tubes.
Olopatadine HCl (Patanol)	0.1% solution (5 mL)	1 drop to affected eye(s) bid	Remove contact lenses; may reinsert in 10 min if eye is not red.
Omeprazole (Prilosec)	10 mg, 20 mg, 40 mg caps	GERD: 20 mg once daily up to 4 wk	Take before eating. May give with antacids.
Oxycodone (Oxycontin)	10 mg, 20 mg, 40 mg, 80 mg controlled-release tabs	10 mg q 12 h as needed	Sedating. High abuse potential. Not recommended for persons <18 yr old. Avoid with acute or severe asthma.
Oxycodone HCl + acetaminophen (Percocet)	2.5 mg + 325 mg 5 mg + 325 mg 7.5 mg + 325 mg 7.5 mg + 500 mg 10 mg + 325 mg 10 mg + 650 mg tabs	1 tab q 6 h as needed; Max 4 g acetaminophen/d	Sedating. High abuse potential. Avoid with acute or severe asthma.
Paroxetine (Paxil)	10 mg, 20 mg, 30 mg, 40 mg tabs	Initial: 10–20 mg daily; may increase by 10 mg/d weekly to max dose of 60 mg/d	See Chapter 23. Monitor closely for suicidality.

Drug (Brand)	Formulation	Dosing	Notes
Penciclovir (Denavir)	1% cream (2 g)	Apply q 2 h while awake × 4 d	Begin treatment at earliest sign or symptom of outbreak. Avoid eyes and mucous membranes.
Penicillin V (Veetids)	250 mg, 500 mg tabs	125–500 mg q 6–8 h	Dosing and duration of therapy varies depending on condition being treated. Take on empty stomach.
Permethrin (Acticin, Elimite, Nix)	5% cream (60 g) 1% cream rinse (2 oz, with comb)	Scabies (5%): apply and massage in from head to soles of feet; wash off 8–14 h later. Lice (1%): apply to washed, towel-dried hair × 10 min, rinse; remove nits with provided comb	Clean bedding, clothing appropriately. Retreat if living mites are visible after 7–14 d.
Phenazopyridine HCl (Pyridium)	100 mg, 200 mg tabs	200 mg TID after meals; max 2 d therapy when used with antibacterials	
Pimecrolimus (Elidel)	1% cream (15 g, 30 g, 100 g)	Apply BID	Avoid sun/UV light. May increase cancer risk.
Pirbuterol (Maxair)	200 µg/inhalation breath actuated MDI (Autohaler) 200 µg/inhalation MDI (Inhaler)	1–2 inhalations q 4–6 h as needed; Max 12 inhalations/d	
Podofilox (Condylox)	0.5% topical solution, gel	Apply q 12 h × 3 d, then discontinue × 4 d; repeat up to 4 treatment cycles	See Chapter 27. Avoid mucous membranes.
Polyethylene glycol (PEG) (Glycolax, Miralax)	PEG 3350 powder for reconstitution (255 g, 527 g with dosing cup; single-dose packets [17 g] - no. 12)	17 g dissolved in 8 oz water once daily, up to 2 wk	
Polymyxin B + neomycin + hydrocortisone (Cortisporin Otic)	Polymyxin B sulfate 10,000 units, neomycin sulfate 3.5 mg, hydro-cortisone 10 mg per mL solution, suspension (10 mL)	3–4 drops in affected ear TID–QID up to 10 d	Do not use with perforated tympanic membrane.
Prednisone (Deltasone)	2.5 mg, 5 mg, 10 mg, 20 mg, 50 mg tabs	Initial: 5–60 mg daily, depending on condition being treated Asthma: See Chapter 7	Avoid if bowel obstruction is a possibility.
Prochlorperazine (Compazine)	5 mg, 10 mg tabs	5–10 mg BID–QID as needed	
Promethazine HCl (Phenergan)	12.5 mg, 25 mg, 50 mg tabs	Motion sickness: 25 mg 30–60 min before travel; may repeat in 8–12 h; maintenance 25 mg BID	

(continued)

Product	How supplied	Dosing	Comments
Propranolol (Inderal, Inderal LA)	10 mg, 20 mg, 40 mg, 60 mg, 80 mg tabs 60 mg, 80 mg, 120 mg, 160 mg sustained-release caps	Initial: 1 mg/kg/d (max 80 mg/d) ÷ BID; may titrate up to max 16 mg/kg/d or 640 mg/d Migraine prophylaxis: 40 mg BID, may increase weekly. Typical effective dose 160–240 mg/d	Contraindicated in persons with asthma.
Ranitidine (Zantac)	75 mg, 150 mg, 300 mg tabs	75–150 mg once–twice daily	May give with antacids.
Rifampin (Rifadin)	150 mg, 300 mg caps	600 mg daily For eradication of meningococci from nasopharynx in asymptomatic carriers: 600 mg BID × 4 doses	Dosing and duration of therapy varies depending on condition being treated. Give one hour before or two hours after meals. Reduces efficacy of oral contraceptive pills.
Rimantadine (Flumadine)	100 mg tabs	100 mg BID	Dosing and duration of therapy varies depending on condition being treated. Begin treatment within 24–48 h of onset of symptoms.
Rizatriptan (Maxalt, Maxalt ODT)	5 mg, 10mg tabs 5 mg, 10 mg orally-disintegrating tabs	5–10 mg; may repeat q 2 h (max 30 mg/24 h)	Interacts with propranolol.
Salmeterol (Serevent)	50 μg/inhalation dry powder for inhalation	1 inhalation q 12 h; 1 inhalation at least 30 min before exercise	See Chapter 7. Do not initiate in significantly worsening or acutely deteriorating asthma.
Selenium sulfide (Selsun)	2.5% lotion (4 oz)	Tinea versicolor: apply once daily, lather with small amount of water, wait 10 min, rinse, repeat × 7 d	May treat weekly for additional 1–2 mo.
Senna (Senokot)	8.6 mg tabs 15 mg/teaspoon granules (2 oz, 6 oz, 12 oz)	Tabs: 2 tabs at bedtime; max 4 tabs twice daily Granules: 1 tsp swallowed or mixed into food at bedtime; max 2 tsp twice daily	Avoid with acute abdomen, severe abdominal pain, nausea, vomiting.
Sertraline (Zoloft)	25 mg, 50 mg, 100 mg tabs	Initial: 25 mg daily; increase to 50 mg daily after 1 wk; may thereafter increase at 1-wk intervals to max 200 mg/d	See Chapter 23. Monitor closely for suicidality.

Spironolactone (Aldactone)	25 mg, 50 mg, 100 mg tabs	50–100 mg/d in single or divided doses; titrate at 2-wk intervals	May be used for hirsutism as well.
Suloconazole nitrate (Exelderm)	1% cream (15 g, 30 g, 60 g)	Tinea pedis: apply BID × 4 wk Tinea cruris, t. versicolor, t. corporis: apply once–twice daily × 3 wk	
Sumatriptan (Imitrex)	25 mg, 50 mg, 100 mg tabs 5 mg, 20 mg nasal spray 6 mg SQ injection	25–100 mg by mouth 5–20 mg intranasal 6 mg subcutaneous May repeat once in 2 h (max 2 doses/24 h)	
Tacrolimus (Protopic)	0.03%, 0.1% ointment (30 g, 60 g)	Apply BID	Avoid sun/UV light.
Tazarotene (Tazorac)	0.1% gel (30 g, 100 g), cream (15 g, 30 g, 60 g)	Apply small amount to clean, dry skin once daily at bedtime	For Acne: See Chapter 8. Pregnancy category X. Reduce dosing frequency or strength if irritation develops. Avoid sunlight and/or use sunscreen.
Terbinafine (Lamisil, Lamisil AT)	250 mg tabs	Onychomycosis: 250 g once daily × 6 wk (fingernail) or 12 wk (toenail)	Dosing and duration of therapy varies depending on condition being treated. Not recommended for persons <18 years old. Do baseline liver function tests.
Terconazole (Terazol)	0.4%, 0.8% vaginal cream	Apply BID × 1–2 wk Vulvovaginal candidiasis: see Chapter 27	Improvement may continue for several weeks after treatment.
Tetracycline (Sumycin)	250 mg, 500 mg tabs	250–500 mg QID	Dosing and duration of therapy varies depending on condition being treated. For Acne: See Chapter 8. Take on empty stomach, with non-dairy fluids. Avoid sun/UV light. May reduce efficacy of oral contraceptives.
Tinidazole (Tindamax)	250 mg, 500 mg tabs	Trichomoniasis: 2 g once	Take with food.
Tolnaftate (Tinactin)	1% cream, powder, solution, aerosol powder or liquid	Apply BID up to 4 wk	

(continued)

Product	How supplied	Dosing	Comments
Topiramate (Topamax)	15 mg, 25 mg caps 25 mg, 100 mg, 200 mg tabs	Initial: 25–50 mg once daily; may increase weekly to target dose of 400 mg/d ÷ BID Migraine prophylaxis: 50 mg once daily at bedtime, may titrate to 100–200 mg nightly	May reduce effectiveness of hormonal contraceptives via increased metabolism of estrogen.
Tramadol (Ultram)	50 mg tabs	50–100 mg q 4–6 h (max 400 mg/d)	Do not give to opioid-dependent patients.
Trazodone HCl (Desyrel)	50 mg, 100 mg, 150 mg, 300 mg tabs	Initial: 150 mg daily ÷ BID–TID; may increase by 50 mg/d as needed at 3–4 d intervals to max 400 mg/d	See Chapter 23. Very sedating; often used for insomnia related to depression and/or SSRI use. Take with food. Monitor closely for suicidality.
Tretinoin (Avita, Retin-A, Retin-A Micro)	0.025% cream, gel (20 g, 45 g) 0.025%, 0.05%, 0.1% cream (20 g, 45 g) 0.01%, 0.025% gel (15 g, 45 g) 0.05% liquid (28 mL) 0.04%, 0.1% microspheres, aqueous gel (20 g, 45 g) 0.025%, 0.05%, 0.1% cream (20 g, 45 g)	Apply small amount to clean, dry skin once daily at bedtime	For Acne: See Chapter 8. Reduce dosing frequency or strength if irritation develops. Avoid sunlight and/or use sunscreen.
Triamcinolone acetonide (Azmacort)	100 µg/inhalation MDI	Two inhalations TID–QID, or 4 inhalations BID Max. 12 inhalations/d	See Chapter 7. Rinse mouth after use.
Triamcinolone acetonide (Nasacort AQ)	55 µg/spray (16.5 g = 120 sprays)	2 sprays to each nostril once daily; may reduce dose as condition improves	Direct spray laterally, away from nasal septum. Use regularly for maximal effect. Consider initiating use 1 wk prior to exposure to known allergen or 2–4 wk prior to anticipated start of pollen season.
Trimethoprim + sulfamethoxazole (Bactrim, Bactrim DS, Septra)	80 mg/400 mg tabs 160 mg/800 mg tabs	TMP 160 mg/SMX 800 mg q 12 h	Dosing and duration of therapy varies depending on condition being treated. Avoid during 3rd trimester pregnancy.

Drug	Preparations	Dosage	Comments
Valacyclovir (Valtrex)	500 mg, 1 g caplets	See Chapter 27 for dosing in genital herpes infections	
Venlafaxine (Effexor XR)	37.5 mg, 75 mg, 150 mg caps	Initial: 37.5–75 mg daily; may increase by increments of 37.5–75 mg/d at intervals of at least 4 d; max 225 mg/d	See Chapter 23. Take with food. Monitor closely for suicidality.
Verapamil (Calan, Calan SR)	40 mg, 80 mg, 120 mg tabs 120 mg sustained-release caplet	Migraine prophylaxis: 80 mg TID, may titrate up to 720 mg/d ÷ TID	
Zanamivir (Relenza)	5 mg/blister dry powder for oral inhalation (Diskhaler)	2 inhalations BID (at least 2 h apart) on 1st d, then 2 inhalations q 12 h for next 4 d	Begin treatment within 48 h of onset of symptoms.
Zolmitriptan (Zomig, Zomig ZMT)	2.5 mg, 5 mg tabs 2.5 mg, 5 mg orally-disintegrating tabs	2.5–5 mg; may repeat once in 2 h (max 10 mg/24 h)	
Zolpidem tartrate (Ambien)	5 mg, 10 mg tabs	10 mg at bedtime	Safety not demonstrated for more than 1 mo of use.

Index